1998
YEAR BOOK OF
ANESTHESIOLOGY AND PAIN MANAGEMENT®

Statement of Purpose

The YEAR BOOK Service

The YEAR BOOK series was devised in 1901 by practicing health professionals who observed that the literature of medicine and related disciplines had become so voluminous that no one individual could read and place in perspective every potential advance in a major specialty. In the final decade of the 20th century, this recognition is more acutely true than it was in 1901.

More than merely a series of books, YEAR BOOK volumes are the tangible results of a unique service designed to accomplish the following:

- to *survey* a wide range of journals of proven value
- to *select* from those journals papers representing significant advances and statements of important clinical principles
- to provide *abstracts* of those articles that are readable, convenient summaries of their key points
- to provide *commentary* about those articles to place them in perspective

These publications grow out of a unique process that calls on the talents of outstanding authorities in clinical and fundamental disciplines, trained literature specialists, and professional writers, all supported by the resources of Mosby, the world's preeminent publisher for the health professions.

The Literature Base

Mosby and its editors survey more than 1,000 journals published worldwide, covering the full range of the health professions. On an annual basis, the publisher examines usage patterns and polls its expert authorities to add new journals to the literature base and to delete journals that are no longer useful as potential YEAR BOOK sources.

The Literature Survey

The publisher's team of literature specialists, all of whom are trained and experienced health professionals, examines every original, peer-reviewed article in each journal issue. More than 250,000 articles per year are scanned systematically, including title, text, illustrations, tables, and references. Each scan is compared, article by article, to the search strategies that the publisher has developed in consultation with the 270 outside experts who form the pool of YEAR BOOK editors. A given article may be reviewed by any number of editors, from one to a dozen or more, regardless of the discipline for which the paper was originally published. In turn, each editor who receives the article reviews it to determine whether the article should be included in the YEAR BOOK. This decision is based on the article's inherent quality, its probable usefulness to readers of that YEAR BOOK, and the editor's goal to represent a balanced picture of a given field in each volume of the YEAR BOOK. In addition, the editor indicates when to include figures and tables from the article to help the YEAR BOOK reader better understand the information.

Of the quarter million articles scanned each year, only 5% are selected for detailed analysis within the YEAR BOOK series, thereby assuring readers of the high value of every selection.

The Abstract

The publisher's abstracting staff is headed by a seasoned medical professional and includes individuals with training in the life sciences, medicine, and other areas, plus extensive experience in writing for the health professions and related industries. Each selected article is assigned to a specific writer on this abstracting staff. The abstracter, guided in many cases by notations supplied by the expert editor, writes a structured, condensed summary designed so that the reader can rapidly acquire the essential information contained in the article.

The Commentary

The YEAR BOOK editorial boards, sometimes assisted by guest commentators, write comments that place each article in perspective for the reader. This provides the reader with the equivalent of a personal consultation with a leading international authority—an opportunity to better understand the value of the article and to benefit from the authority's thought processes in assessing the article.

Additional Editorial Features

The editorial boards of each YEAR BOOK organize the abstracts and comments to provide a logical and satisfying sequence of information. To enhance the organization, editors also provide introductions to sections or individual chapters, comments linking a number of abstracts, citations to additional literature, and other features.

The published YEAR BOOK contains enhanced bibliographic citations for each selected article, including extended listings of multiple authors and identification of author affiliations. Each YEAR BOOK contains a Table of Contents specific to that year's volume. From year to year, the Table of Contents for a given YEAR BOOK will vary depending on developments within the field.

Every YEAR BOOK contains a list of the journals from which papers have been selected. This list represents a subset of the more than 1,000 journals surveyed by the publisher and occasionally reflects a particularly pertinent article from a journal that is not surveyed on a routine basis.

Finally, each volume contains a comprehensive subject index and an index to authors of each selected paper.

The 1998 Year Book Series

Year Book of Allergy, Asthma, and Clinical Immunology: Drs. Rosenwasser, Borish, Boguniewicz, Nelson, Routes, and Spahn

Year Book of Anesthesiology and Pain Management®: Drs. Tinker, Abram, Chestnut, Roizen, Rothenberg, and Wood

Year Book of Cardiology®: Drs. Schlant, Collins, Gersh, Graham, Kaplan, and Waldo

Year Book of Chiropractic®: Dr. Lawrence

Year Book of Critical Care Medicine®: Drs. Parrillo, Balk, Calvin, Franklin, and Shapiro

Year Book of Dentistry®: Drs. Meskin, Berry, Jeffcoat, Leinfelder, Roser, Summitt, and Zakariasen

Year Book of Dermatologic Surgery®: Drs. Greenway, Barrett, Papadopoulos, and Whitaker

Year Book of Dermatology®: Dr. Thiers

Year Book of Diagnostic Radiology®: Drs. Osborn, Groskin, Dalinka, Maynard, Pentecost, Rebner, Ros, Smirniotopoulos, and Young

Year Book of Drug Therapy®: Drs. Lasagna and Weintraub

Year Book of Emergency Medicine®: Drs. Wagner, Dronen, Davidson, King, Niemann, and Roberts

Year Book of Endocrinology®: Drs. Bagdade, Braverman, Horton, Kannan, Landsberg, Molitch, Morley, Nathan, Odell, Poehlman, Rogol, and Ryan

Year Book of Family Practice®: Drs. Berg, Bowman, Davidson, Dexter, and Scherger

Year Book of Gastroenterology®: Drs. Aliperti and Fleshman

Year Book of Geriatrics and Gerontology®: Drs. Burton, Beck, Ostwald, Rabins, Reuben, Roth, Shapiro, and Whitehouse

Year Book of Hand Surgery®: Drs. Amadio and Hentz

Year Book of Hematology®: Drs. Spivak, Bell, Ness, Quesenberry, Wiernik, and Horowitz

Year Book of Infectious Diseases: Drs. Keusch, Barza, Bennish, Poutsiaka, Skolnik, and Snydman

Year Book of Medicine®: Drs. Cline, Frishman, Jett, Klahr, Malawista, Mandell, McCallum, and Utiger

Year Book of Neonatal and Perinatal Medicine®: Drs. Fanaroff, Maisels, and Stevenson

Year Book of Nephrology, Hypertension, and Mineral Metabolism: Drs. Schwab, Bennett, Emmett, Hostetter, Kumar, and Toto

Year Book of Neurology and Neurosurgery®: Drs. Bradley and Gibbs

Year Book of Nuclear Medicine®: Drs. Gottschalk, Blaufox, Neumann, Strauss, and Zubal

Year Book of Obstetrics, Gynecology, and Women's Health: Drs. Mishell, Herbst, and Kirschbaum

Year Book of Occupational and Environmental Medicine®: Drs. Emmett, Frank, Gochfeld, and Hessl

Year Book of Oncology®: Drs. Ozols, Eisenberg, Glatstein, Loehrer, and Tallman

Year Book of Ophthalmology®: Drs. Wilson, Augsburger, Cohen, Eagle, Grossman, Laibson, Maguire, Nelson, Penne, Rapuano, Sergott, Spaeth, Tipperman, Ms. Gosfield, and Ms. Salmon

Year Book of Orthopedics®: Drs. Morrey, Beauchamp, Currier, Tolo, Trigg, and Swiontkowski

Year Book of Otolaryngology–Head and Neck Surgery®: Drs. Paparella and Holt

Year Book of Pathology and Laboratory Medicine®: Drs. Raab, Cohen, Olson, Sirgi, and Stanley

Year Book of Pediatrics®: Dr. Stockman

Year Book of Plastic, Reconstructive, and Aesthetic Surgery®: Drs. Miller, Bartlett, Garner, McKinney, Ruberg, Salisbury, and Smith

Year Book of Psychiatry and Applied Mental Health®: Drs. Talbott, Ballenger, Frances, Lydiard, Meltzer, Schowalter, and Tasman

Year Book of Pulmonary Disease®: Drs. Jett, Maurer, Ryu, Strollo, and Wenzel

Year Book of Rheumatology®: Drs. Panush, Hadler, LeRoy, Liang, Reichlin, Simon, and Weinblatt

Year Book of Sports Medicine®: Drs. Shephard, Drinkwater, Eichner, Torg, Alexander, and Mr. George

Year Book of Surgery®: Drs. Copeland, Bland, Deitch, Eberlein, Howard, Luce, Seeger, Souba, and Sugarbaker

Year Book of Thoracic and Cardiovascular Surgery®: Drs. Ginsberg, Wechsler, and Williams

Year Book of Urology®: Drs. Andriole and Coplen

Year Book of Vascular Surgery®: Dr. Porter

1998

The Year Book of ANESTHESIOLOGY AND PAIN MANAGEMENT®

Editor-in-Chief
John H. Tinker, M.D.

Editors
Stephen E. Abram, M.D.
David H. Chestnut, M.D.
Michael F. Roizen, M.D.
David M. Rothenberg, M.D.
Margaret Wood, M.D.

Contributing Editors
Richard S. Finn, M.D.
Carolyn P. Greenberg, M.D.
Mark J.S. Heath, M.D.
Eric J. Heyer, M.D., Ph.D.

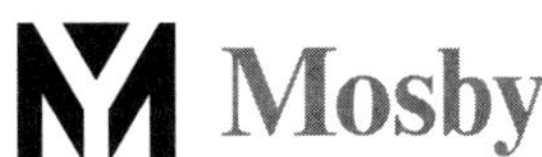

St. Louis Baltimore Boston Carlsbad Naples New York Philadelphia Portland London
Madrid Mexico City Singapore Sydney Tokyo Toronto Wiesbaden

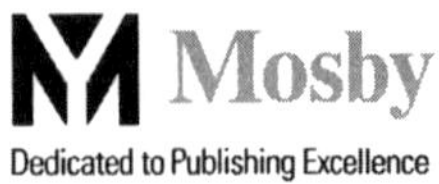

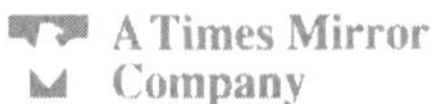

Associate Publisher: Gretchen C. Murphy
Developmental Editor: Jaime Chatman
Manager, Periodical Editing: Kirk Swearingen
Manuscript Editor: Stephanie M. Geels
Project Supervisor, Production: Joy Moore
Production Assistant: Laura Bayless
Manager, Literature Services: Idelle L. Winer
Illustrations and Permissions Coordinator: Phyllis K. Thompson

1998 EDITION

Printed in the United States of America
Composition by Reed Technology and Information Services, Inc.
Printing/binding by Maple-Vail

Editorial Office:
Mosby, Inc.
11830 Westline Industrial Drive
St. Louis, MO 63146
Customer Service: customer.support@mosby.com
www.mosby.com/Mosby/CustomerSupport/index.html

International Standard Serial Number: 1073-5437
International Standard Book Number: 0-8151-8781-5

Editorial Board

Table of Contents

Journals Represented

Mosby and its editors survey more than 1,000 journals for its abstract and commentary publications. From these journals, the editors select the articles to be abstracted. Journals represented in this YEAR BOOK are listed below.

ASAIO Journal
Acta Anaesthesiologica Scandinavica
American Journal of Medical Quality
American Journal of Medicine
American Journal of Nephrology
American Journal of Obstetrics and Gynecology
American Journal of Pathology
American Journal of Surgery
American Surgeon
Anaesthesia
Anaesthesia and Intensive Care
Anesthesia and Analgesia
Anesthesiology
Annals of Internal Medicine
Annals of Thoracic Surgery
Archives of Internal Medicine
Archives of Physical Medicine and Rehabilitation
Artifical Organs
British Journal of Anaesthesia
British Journal of Surgery
British Medical Journal
Canadian Journal of Anaesthesia
Chest
Circulation
Clinical Drug Investigation
Clinical Pediatrics
Clinical Pharmacology and Therapeutics
Critical Care Medicine
European Journal of Surgery
Infection Control and Hospital Epidemiology
Intensive Care Medicine
International Journal of Obstetric Anesthesia
Journal of Applied Physiology: Respiratory, Environmental and Exercise Physiology
Journal of Bone and Joint Surgery (American Volume)
Journal of Cardiac Surgery
Journal of Cardiovascular Surgery
Journal of Clinical Anesthesia
Journal of Pain and Symptom Management
Journal of Pediatric Orthopedics
Journal of Pediatric Surgery
Journal of Pharmacology and Experimental Therapeutics
Journal of Reproductive Medicine
Journal of Thoracic and Cardiovascular Surgery
Journal of Urology
Journal of Vascular Surgery
Journal of the American College of Surgeons

Journal of the American Medical Association
Lancet
Mayo Clinic Proceedings
Nature
Neurology
New England Journal of Medicine
Obstetrics and Gynecology
Ophthalmology
Pain
Pediatrics
Plastic and Reconstructive Surgery
Proceedings of the National Academy of Sciences
Regional Anesthesia
Scandinavian Audiology
Spine
Stroke
Surgical Neurology

Standard Abbreviations

The following terms are abbreviated in this edition: acquired immunodeficiency syndrome (AIDS), cardiopulmonary resuscitation (CPR), central nervous system (CNS), cerebrospinal fluid (CSF), computed tomography (CT), deoxyribonucleic acid (DNA), electrocardiography (ECG), health maintenance organization (HMO), human immunodeficiency virus (HIV), intensive care unit (ICU), intramuscular (IM), intravenous (IV), magnetic resonance (MR) imaging (MRI), and ribonucleic acid (RNA).

Note

The Year Book of Anesthesiology and Pain Management® is a literature survey service providing abstracts of articles published in the professional literature. Every effort is made to ensure the accuracy of the information presented in these pages. Neither the editors nor the publisher of the Year Book of Anesthesiology and Pain Management® can be responsible for errors in the original materials. The editors' comments are their own opinions. Mention of specific products within this publication does not constitute endorsement.

To facilitate the use of the Year Book of Anesthesiology and Pain Management® as a reference tool, all illustrations and tables included in this publication are now identified as they appear in the original article. This change is meant to help the reader recognize that any illustration or table appearing in the Year Book of Anesthesiology and Pain Management®may be only one of many in the original article. For this reason, figure and table numbers will often appear to be out of sequence within the Year Book of Anesthesiology and Pain Management®.

Introduction

It is again a privilege to report that this YEAR BOOK contains a wide variety of solid and interesting reports. As always, I have asked our editorial board to favor studies and reports likely to be of interest and use to practicing clinicians. As in the past, clinical anesthesiology, critical care topics, and acute and chronic pain management issues are widely represented. This year there is a new section containing reports of studies in the medicolegal/ethical arenas. For example, in Chapter 10 there are several reports regarding physician-assisted suicide (Abstracts 10–1 through 10–4) and an interesting paper from the American Society of Anesthesiologists' Closed Claims Study which examines the "variability" of "expert" opinion and testimony (Abstract 10–6). I trust you can read between the lines!

The toxicity issues of last year with respect to sevoflurane seem to have diminished, possibly related to the large accumulating patient experience and absence of clear toxicity, either renal or hepatic. The "low flow" issue with this agent seems to be poised to disappear (Abstracts 4–1 through 4–10).

Interest in obstetric anesthesia topics (Abstracts 3–1 through 3–38), regional anesthesia complications (Chapter 6), and acute and chronic pain management (Chapter 8) remains high. New drug testing seems largely in these fields.

The "bispectral" EEG analysis (using a proprietary "black box" that does whatever it does to a four-lead EEG and generates a number which, perhaps, indicates "depth" of anesthesia) is the subject of a number of studies in this YEAR BOOK (Abstracts 5–1, 5–2, and 5–3). The notion that money can be saved by titrating to "lighter" anesthetic levels, while assuring obliteration of awareness, is perhaps fanciful, but perhaps allowing us to "feel" more secure during "lighter" anesthesia might actually result in lower doses of agent. This, in turn, might be an improvement. Several papers on this hot topic in the YEAR BOOK will allow the reader to judge and contemplate the issue. Rumors that the "black box" is actually multiplying the power spectrum by the inventor's social security number are probably untrue, but it would be nice if we could be told how it works.

We may be nearer to practical general anesthesia with Xenon. Two studies of this "noble" anesthetic are included (Abstracts 4–26 and 4–27). Studies of old friends including malignant hyperthermia (Abstract 6–22), atypical pseudocholinesterase (Abstract 6–25), train-of-four monitoring (Abstract 5–34), and many others, will reassure our readers that we're still doing, studying, improving and arguing about our familiar specialty topics. The academicians do not seem to be heading too far off in some wild and crazy direction that will force clinicians to acquire whole new fields of expertise. I predict testing of an integrated automated anesthesia delivery system in the not-too-distant future, but not this year. (That'll shake us up some!) Many of our "gurus" enjoy the sound of their voices as they jump on the bandwagon about something they call "perioperative medicine," something we old-timers thought we were doing all along. This year's YEAR BOOK will, I think, convince you that our core knowledge and expertise still revolves around provision of safe and cost-effective care before, during, and after performance of needed operations, and that our traditional spirit of solid inquiry is alive and well.

John H. Tinker, M.D.

1 Studies of Outcomes, Risks, and Costs

General Outcome/Risk/Cost Studies

Report of the Anaesthetic Mortality Committee of Western Australia 1990–1995
Eagle CCP, Davis NJ (Health Dept of Western Australia, Perth)
Anaesth Intensive Care 25:51–59, 1997 1–1

Introduction.—The Anaesthetic Mortality Committee (AMC) of Western Australia is responsible for investigating deaths possibly related to anesthesia. All deaths occurring within 48 hours of anesthesia or in which the anesthetic is believed to have played a role must be reported. Five hundred such deaths investigated by the AMC during a 5-year period are reported.

Findings.—On investigation, the anesthetic was found to be a cause or contributing cause of death in 26 cases. In 5 of these, there was no anesthetic error even though the anesthetic was the precipitating cause of death. For the remaining 21 cases, a total of 34 anesthesia-related causes were identified. The principal causes of death were, in order of frequency, inappropriate anesthetic dosage, 7 cases; inappropriate anesthetic technique, 6 cases; inadequate preoperative assessment, 2 cases; and 1 case each of inappropriate anesthetic drug selection, adverse drug reaction, inadequate crisis management, inappropriate postoperative management, inadequate postoperative supervision, and inadequate resuscitation. In 7 of the patients the ASA status was grade 1 or 2.

Conclusions.—Data on recent anesthesia-related deaths in Western Australia are reported. The analysis suggests that 1 in 40,000 operations performed in Western Australia led to death from anesthetic factors. These events led to death in 1 or 2 otherwise healthy people each year. There are many contributing causes to these deaths, but the major causes are inappropriate drug dosage and inappropriate technique.

► Starting with the work of Ross Holland more than 30 years ago in New South Wales (eastern Australia), that country has been the source of some of our very best anesthetic risk data and analysis. This new article is another example of that kind of quality, not to mention "guts." What do I mean by "guts"? The American-organized anesthesiology has chosen to try to convince the public that the risk of anesthesia death is extraordinarily low, using incidence figures between 1:100,000 and 1:220,000. Those numbers are so small that they are easy to say but difficult to confirm. On the basis of anecdotal reports from various academic centers in the United States, I have long doubted that our anesthetic-related death rate is anywhere near that low (good). This figure—1 anesthetic death per 40,000 anesthetics—is "good data" from a country that is home to many superb anesthesiologists. I'll bet, though I can't prove it, that our anesthetic death rate in the United States is similar to this. If a major medical center in the United States reported this kind of death rate, would it be chastised by its administration for such "negative publicity"? Would the publication of such a death rate cause a number of other institutions to scurry around and obtain figures somehow or other to show "better" death rates in competition?

Data from such an impeccable source, with its long history of excellence in understanding how to perform these kinds of studies relatively free from outside interference, may be today's best estimate of genuine anesthesia death rates.

J.H. Tinker, M.D.

What Happens After Discharge? Return Hospital Visits After Ambulatory Surgery

Twersky R, Fishman D, Homel P (State Univ of New York, Brooklyn; Long Island College, New York;)

Anesth Analg 84:319–324, 1997 1–2

Objective.—One of the outcome measures of ambulatory surgery that is rarely reported to the ambulatory surgery unit is the frequency of return hospital visits. The frequency of return hospital visits after ambulatory surgery was examined retrospectively to identify predictor variables and to formulate interventions to reduce these return visits.

Methods.—Demographic data, including surgical service, procedure, anesthesia type, American Society of Anesthesiologists physical status class, interval between discharge and return visit, length of stay of readmission, insurance status, and provider profiles were obtained from hospital medical records for a 12-month period and used in a matched case control design to identify factors associated with an increased likelihood of a return hospital visit. Predictors of return were determined using univariate and multiple regression analysis.

Results.—Of 6,243 ambulatory surgery unit (ASU) visits, 187 returned to the hospital within 30 days, 54% to the emergency room and 46% as inpatients. Of those who returned to the emergency room, 29% sought treatment related to the ASU procedure. Urology had a significantly higher return rate (5.8%) than did general surgery, otolaryngology, and gynecology. Urology also had a significantly higher return rate for complications than did other specialties (2.7% versus 1.3%). Multivariate regression analysis established that ambulatory urology surgery was an independent predictor of return (OR 27.87), and showed that patients receiving monitored anesthesia care were almost 5 times more likely to return. Most patients who returned did so because of bleeding (41.5%), fever and infection (13%), and pain (9.8%). Patients undergoing hydrocelectomy/varicocelectomy were 8.3 times more likely to return because of complications, and patients undergoing dilation and curettage were 3.2 times more likely to return.

Conclusion.—Although the return visit rate is relatively low, the high return rate to the ER for bleeding needs to be addressed.

▶ Most interesting here is the finding that monitored anesthesia care was associated with a greater return to the emergency room, and to the hospital for problems—bleeding, pain, urinary retention, and wound dehiscence. The authors think that these issues might be related to the type of surgery for which monitored anesthesia care (MAC) is used, and that surgery predicts who returns. Another hypothesis might be that MAC did not allow enough relaxation for appropriate surgical intervention and that maybe these cases would be better served by using a general anesthetic. That is, of course, a hypothesis untested in this article.

The authors indicate that none of the cases that returned were due to anesthesia, but since a fair number related to postoperative pain, over 9% of the readmissions, one wonders whether the authors (and we as a specialty) believe that surgeons own the postoperative pain treatment arena.

One further group of data in this article deserves attention—that the vast majority of patients returned to and were treated in the ER for what can be called "nuisance" problems, that is, small amounts of bleeding, pain, urinary retention, or wound dehiscence. That is, more than 75% of the patients that went to the ER were treated in the ER and did not have to be admitted to the hospital. The authors then wonder if better preoperative education about what constitutes a serious problem or whether the patients could wait to go to a regular physician's office some time later in the day or the following day. That needs to be studied. The authors do point out one important limitation of the study in that it reported patients returning only to their healthcare facility; therefore, there may be an underreporting of the actual return rate, the authors go on to say. They further add that, because they had follow-up on more than 90% of patients, the underreporting would be, if anything, very small.

Thus, like all good studies, this one brings up more questions than it answers.

M.F. Roizen, M.D.

Discrepancies Between Meta-analyses and Subsequent Large Randomized, Controlled Trials

LeLorier J, Grégoire G, Benhaddad A, et al (Hôtel-Dieu de Montréal Hosp; Univ of Montreal)

N Engl J Med 337:536–542, 1997 1–3

Background.—Although large, randomized, controlled clinical trials are considered definitive treatment efficacy evaluations, they are not always available. In the absence of such trials, clinicians are increasingly relying on meta-analysis to interpret data available from multiple small trials available from the literature. To understand the accuracy of meta-analysis projections, the results of a series of large, randomized, controlled trials were compared to those of previously published relevant meta-analyses.

Study Design.—The *New England Journal of Medicine*, the *Lancet*, the *Annals of Internal Medicine*, and the *Journal of the American Medical Association* were searched for large, randomized, controlled trials published from 1991 through 1994. Prior meta-analyses on these same topics were sought. The results of each trial were compared to those of the corresponding meta-analyses. Both principal and secondary outcomes were evaluated.

Findings.—The literature search identified 12 large, randomized, controlled trials with 19 corresponding meta-analyses. Of the 40 primary and secondary outcomes analyzed, agreement between these 2 methods was only fair. The positive predictive value of the meta-analyses was 68% and the negative predictive value was 67%. In each case where findings disagreed, a significant treatment effect was determined by one method and no significant effect was found by the other method.

Conclusions.—The results of meta-analyses were not predictive of the results of large, randomized, controlled clinical trials in about one third of cases. This implies that on the basis of meta-analysis alone, an ineffective treatment would have been advocated one third of the time.

► Meta-analysis has been used to summarize a number of different but related studies so that the findings in essence are pooled. Often, only a small number of patients are studied for each report, resulting in a small sample size so that statistical analysis is not possible. However, reports are more often submitted for publication when they produce positive results and, thus, negative reports are less likely to be available for meta-analysis—a negative publication bias. Thus, there are problems with observational studies, and meta-analysis should be used to indicate the need for further confirmatory studies.

M. Wood, M.D.

Occupational Hazards of Operating: Opportunities for Improvement
Davis MS (DeKalb Med Ctr, Decatur, Ga)
Infect Control Hosp Epidemiol 17:691–693, 1996 1–4

Background.—The greatest threat to operating room personnel may be not HIV, but hepatitis C virus (HCV). Each year, more than 2,000 health care workers acquire HCV infection, the long-term lethal potential of which is greater than that of hepatitis B virus. The emergence of this and other bloodborne pathogens places a new light on the need for health care workers to protect themselves. Some possible steps to reduce the occupational hazards for operating room personnel are discussed.

Reducing the Hazards.—The best approach to protecting one's self against bloodborne pathogens in the operating room is to prevent exposure. Most exposures can be prevented through the use of current technology and knowledge. Many different safety-engineered devices have been designed to counteract the risk of bloodborne pathogens. These devices must be evaluated thoroughly before they are put into general use. Through education, communication, and access to safety technology, surgeons can be motivated to adopt safer practices. Some specific steps include creating a database of occupational exposures; holding monthly meetings to report exposures and discuss potential interventions; seeking appropriate help from vendors of safety-oriented technology; critically evaluating all new safety-engineered equipment, preferably by a multidisciplinary committee; and creating the position of "Safety Champion" to coordinate projects and act as a liaison to surgical staff.

Summary.—The health threat posed by HCV should lead to a new emphasis on reducing the occupational hazards for operating room personnel. Some key steps toward improvement in this regard are presented. Given information and the right tools, operating room personnel can be self-motivated to enact change.

► The author makes a good case for self-motivation to reduce the risk and improve protection for surgeons from infectious hazards in the operating room. The data in the literature do not indicate that self-motivation makes a difference, unless there is a quantitative tool and feedback or unless there is rigorous regulation mandating it.

M.F. Roizen, M.D.

National Symposium on Outcomes and Quality Assessment: State of the Art and Future Directions
McGee JL, Sessa EJ, Sirio CA (Pennsylvania Health Care Cost Containment Council, Harrisburg; Univ of Pittsburgh, Pa)
Am J Med Qual 11:S1–S3, 1996 1–5

Objective.—A National Symposium on Outcomes and Quality Assessment was sponsored by the Pennsylvania Health Care Cost Containment

Council to showcase the results of the council's efforts to make available to the public information about the cost and quality of health care, to survey severity of illness and outcomes assessment methodologies available in both commercial and academic arenas for patients requiring services other than those provided by general acute care hospitals, and to introduce to the participants some of the possibilities and challenges offered by emerging information technologies and trends toward health system integration. The goal of the symposium was to bring together providers and purchasers to talk about common interests.

Results.—A debate on outcomes data focused on whether such data are to be used in a quality improvement process or with the intent of punishing poor providers. Quality assessment and outcomes reporting have changed over the years, mainly as a result of the implementation of cost-saving guidelines for effective clinical practice. Essential to improving the process of care is the ability to measure outcomes, an understanding and acceptance by providers of measurement methodology, leadership and support of payors to change practice patterns, and increased availability of improved risk adjustment methodologies.

Conclusion.—The public availability of outcomes data has encouraged collaboration between purchasers and providers, has promoted greater understanding between purchasers and providers, and has encouraged increasing collaboration to solve challenges that remain.

▶ This is a report of the outcome by McGee, on the findings from Pennsylvania Health Care Cost Containment Council. Interestingly, this report from the Pennsylvania Health Care Cost Containment Council is to booster its own position. No one in this symposium, or in the report of their progress to date, takes account of the fact that the major driver in morbidity perioperatively appears to be morbidity preoperatively and not the individual skill of the providers. The success in dealing with the perioperative morbidity, that is, whether it results in a permanent disability or lack thereof, is related to the quality of the providers as reported in prior studies. Yet, these facts seem to bypass those more interested in boosting there own efforts by reporting numbers. It is interesting to read this article because it gives the position and the thought processes of one of the regulators and how their efforts to blend provider and purchaser community are intended to strengthen their own position and not intended to find truth, justice, or what is best for patients. These administrators may not understand the science of the issue and the science of risk adjustment well enough.

M.F. Roizen, M.D.

Risk/Outcome Studies in Obstetric Anesthesia

Anesthesia-related Deaths During Obstetric Delivery in the United States, 1979–1990

Hawkins JL, Koonin LM, Palmer SK, et al (Univ of Colorado, Denver; Natl Ctr for Chronic Disease Prevention and Health Promotion, Atlanta, Ga)

Anesthesiology 86:277–284, 1997 1–6

Background.—Complications of anesthesia are the sixth most frequent cause of pregnancy-related death in the United States. Although the total number of anesthesia-related obstetric deaths in the United States is known, the national data have never been analyzed in detail. The characteristics of anesthesia-related obstetric deaths in the United States from 1979 to 1990 were studied, including the causes of death, the types of anesthetics and obstetric procedures implicated, and the associated maternal conditions.

Methods.—The analysis included deaths occurring within 1 year of delivery, as reported to the Pregnancy Mortality Surveillance program of the Centers for Disease Control and Prevention. Maternal death certificates from 1979 to 1990 were matched with birth or fetal death certificates from the same years. From these records were identified deaths caused by anesthesia, as well as the cause of death, the delivery procedure, and the type of anesthesia. Maternal mortality was calculated per million live

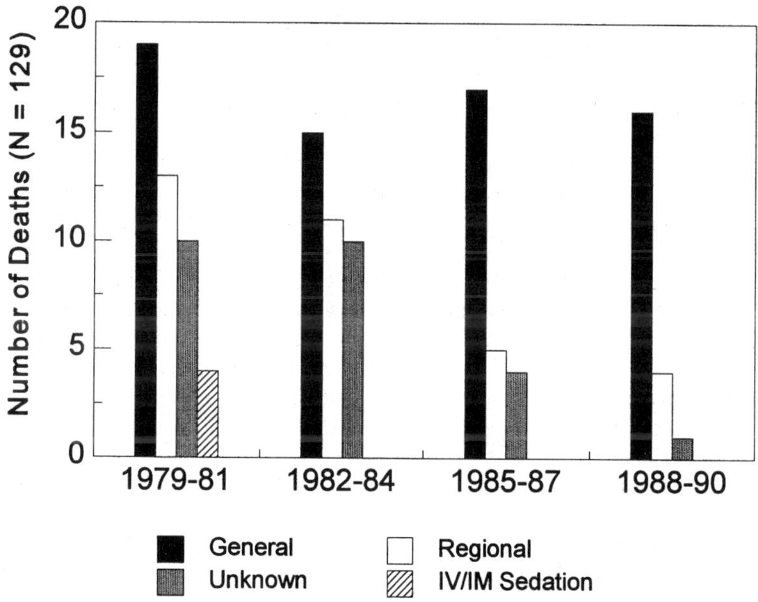

FIGURE 1.—Anesthesia-related maternal deaths by types of anesthesia, United States, 1979–1990. (Courtesy of Hawkins JL, Koonin LM, Palmer SK, et al: Anesthesia-related deaths during obstetric delivery in the United States, 1979–1990. *Anesthesiology* 86:277–284, 1997. Copyright American Society of Anesthesiologists, Inc. Used with permission of Lippincott-Raven Publishers.)

TABLE 4.—Anesthesia-related Maternal Mortality Rates for the United States and England and Wales by Triennium: 1979–1990

Triennium	United States MMR*	England and Wales MMR†
1979–1981	4.3	8.7
1982–1984	3.3	7.2
1985–1987	2.3	1.9
1988–1990	1.7	1.7

*Per million live births.
†Estimated rate per million maternities.
Abbreviation: MMR, maternal mortality rates.
(Courtesy of Hawkins JL, Koonin LM, Palmer SK, et al: Anesthesia-related deaths during obstetric delivery in the United States, 1979–1990. *Anesthesiology* 86:277–284, 1997. Copyright American Society of Anesthesiologists, Inc. Used with permission of Lippincott-Raven Publishers.)

births. For women undergoing cesarean section, the role of general vs. regional anesthesia was assessed.

Results.—Of 129 deaths, 82% were in women undergoing cesarean delivery. A significant drop in the rate of anesthesia-related maternal deaths occurred during the study period: from 4.3 per million live births in 1979–1981 to 1.7 per million in 1988–1990. The decline reflected a reduction in the rate of deaths related to regional anesthesia since 1984, with no change in the number of deaths related to general anesthesia (Fig 1). From 1979 to 1985, the case-fatality risk ratio for general anesthesia was 2.3 times higher than that of regional anesthesia; after 1985, the case-fatality risk ratio for general anesthesia rose to 16.7. Most of the general anesthesia-related deaths were caused by problems with aspiration and intubation, whereas the regional anesthesia-related deaths more often resulted from local anesthetic toxicity. The declining pattern of anesthesia-related maternal mortality rates was similar to that demonstrated in data covering the same period in the United Kingdom (Table 4).

Conclusions.—The majority of anesthesia-related maternal deaths occur in women receiving general anesthesia for cesarean section. Death is also possible with regional anesthesia, however, related to the toxicity of local anesthetics and excessively high regional blocks. Maternal deaths related to regional anesthesia are declining, whereas the number of deaths related to general anesthesia has remained stable. The reduction in maternal mortality attributable to regional anesthesia is ascribed to better awareness of the toxic effects of local anesthetics and improvements in anesthetic techniques.

► The authors have presented results of the first national study of anesthesia-related maternal mortality in the United States. They observed an overall decline in the anesthesia-related maternal mortality rate during the 12 years of the study. The absolute number of regional anesthesia-related maternal deaths decreased during the 12 years of the study, despite the increased utilization of regional anesthesia for labor and cesarean section. Unfortunately, the number of general anesthesia-related deaths did not decrease, despite an apparent decrease in the use of general anesthesia for cesarean section, and despite the widespread use of better monitoring techniques (i.e., pulse oximetry, end-tidal carbon dioxide monitoring) during the latter half of the study. Further, the estimated rate of maternal death from complications of general anesthesia actually increased during the second half of the study. This study provides support for the argument that general anesthesia entails greater maternal risk than regional anesthesia for most patients undergoing cesarean section.

D.H. Chestnut, M.D.

Quality and Retrieval of Obstetrical Anaesthesia Randomized Controlled Trials

Bender JS, Halpern SH, Thangaroopan M, et al (Women's College Hosp, Toronto; McMaster Univ, Hamilton, Ont)

Can J Anaesth 44:14–18, 1997 1–7

Background.—High-quality, easily retrieved randomized, controlled trials (RCTs) are needed for meta-analyses and systematic reviews. The quality of RCTs in obstetric anesthesia in a sample of available journals indexed in MEDLINE was determined.

Methods.—Both MEDLINE and hand searches were conducted of RCTs published from 1985 through 1994. Seven anesthetic and 3 obstetric

Instrument for Measuring Quality of RCTs

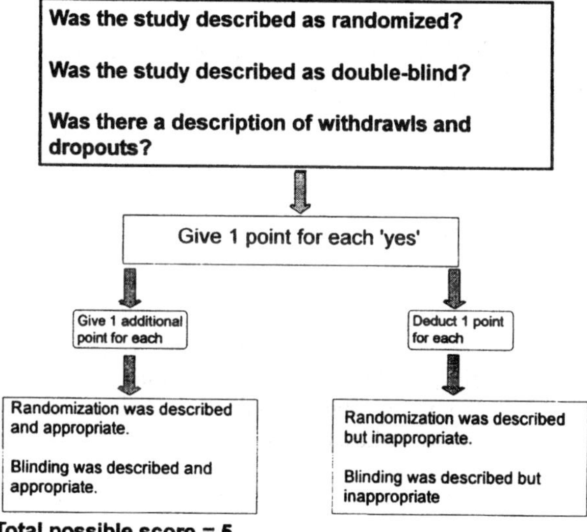

FIGURE 1.—Instrument for measuring quality scores. (Courtesy of Bender JS, Halpern SH, Thangaroopan M, et al: Quality and retrieval of obstetrical anaesthesia randomized controlled trials. *Can J Anaesth* 44:14–18, 1997.)

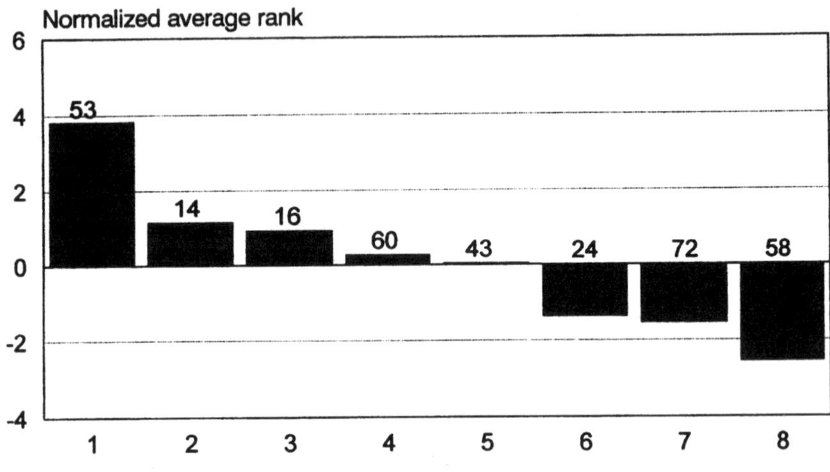

FIGURE 3.—Normalized average quality scores are shown by journal. The journals ranking greater than 1.96 or less than −1.96 are statistically different from the mean. The number of papers in each journal is shown above each *bar*. (Courtesy of Bender JS, Halpern SH, Thangaroopan M, et al: Quality and retrieval of obstetrical anaesthesia randomized controlled trials. *Can J Anaesth* 44:14–18, 1997.)

journals were included. A blinded rater assigned a quality score to each RCT using a reliable, validated scale.

Findings.—The searches identified 340 RCTs. Sixty-five percent of these studies were identified by the MEDLINE search alone. Ninety-eight percent were found by the hand search. The median quality score was 3 on a 5-point scale. The median score did not change over time. The highest and lowest median scores were assigned to *Anesthesiology* and *Anaesthesia*, respectively. Studies of poor quality were likely to be biased in favor of a new treatment (Figs 1 and 3).

Conclusions.—Care is needed when reviewing the obstetric anesthesia research. Because more than one third of the RCTs found in the current study were missed using a MEDLINE search alone, additional strategies are needed to identify such studies. Sensitivity analyses based on quality are needed to increase the validity of meta-analyses and reviews.

▶ Perhaps the most important finding in this study is that the quality of RCTS differs among journals. In this study, *Anesthesiology* had the highest median quality score. The authors correctly noted that "care must be exercised when including studies of low quality in meta-analyses...."

D.H. Chestnut, M.D.

Infection Risk Studies

Acute Non-A–E Hepatitis in the United States and the Role of Hepatitis G Virus Infection

Alter MJ, for the Sentinel Counties Viral Hepatitis Study Team (Ctrs for Disease Control and Prevention, Atlanta, Ga; et al)

N Engl J Med 336:741–746, 1997 1–8

Introduction.—Non-A–E hepatitis is said to be present in patients who have parenterally transmitted non-A, non-B hepatitis but no evidence of hepatitis C virus (HCV). The recently discovered hepatitis G virus (HGV) is related to HCV. Surveillance data were used to study the possible role of HGV in acute non-A–E hepatitis.

Methods.—The study included patients with acute viral hepatitis reported to the Sentinel Counties surveillance system during 2 periods: 1985–1986 and 1991–1995. Of more than 10,500 patients reported to this system from 1982–1995, 48% had hepatitis A, 34% had hepatitis B, 15% had hepatitis C, and 3% had non-A–E hepatitis. In the study groups, polymerase chain reaction was used to test serum samples for HGV RNA. Clinical outcome data were evaluated as well.

Findings.—The study included sera from 100 patients each with hepatitis A and B, 45 patients with non-A–E hepatitis, and 116 patients with hepatitis C. Hepatitis G virus RNA was found in 25% of patients with hepatitis A, 32% of those with hepatitis B, 23% of those with hepatitis C, and 9% of patients with non-A–E hepatitis. Hepatitis G virus was significantly more prevalent among patients with hepatitis B than among those with hepatitis C or non-A–E hepatitis. There were 4 patients infected with HGV only—none had evidence of chronic hepatitis during a follow-up period of 1–9 years.

Conclusions.—Although HGV RNA can be detected in the sera of many patients with acute viral hepatitis, it does not appear to be a causative agent of non-A, non-B hepatitis. Rather than being a hepatotropic agent, HGV may lead to hepatitis only when certain other circumstances are present, as observed with other viruses such as cytomegalovirus and yellow fever virus. Although HGV is clearly a unique virus that can be transmitted by blood, its link with disease remains uncertain.

The Incidence of Transfusion-associated Hepatitis G Virus Infection and Its Relation to Liver Disease

Alter HJ, Nakatsuji Y, Melpolder J, et al (NIH, Bethesda, Md; Genelabs Technologies, Redwood City, Calif)

N Engl J Med 336:747–754, 1997 1–9

Background.—Hepatitis C virus (HCV) is not involved in perhaps 20% of cases of community-acquired hepatitis and 10% of cases of transfusion-acquired hepatitis. Molecular amplification and cloning studies have led to the discovery of the hepatitis G virus (HGV). The role of HGV in transfusion-related hepatitis was studied.

Methods.—Four groups of serum samples were studied: 357 from transfusion recipients, 157 from controls who had not received transfusions, 500 from randomly selected blood donors, and 230 from donors who gave blood to a patient with transfusion-associated HGV infection. Polymerase chain reaction assays were used to test these samples for HGV RNA. Also studied were pretransfusion and posttransfusion samples from 79 patients with transfusion-related non-A, non-B hepatitis.

Results.—Eighty percent of patients with transfusion-associated hepatitis had HCV infection, and another 4% had pre-existing HCV infection and no apparent cause of the acute hepatitis episode. This left 13 patients, 3 of whom had acute HGV infection and 10 of whom had an unidentified infecting agent. Ten percent of patients infected with HCV who were tested also had HGV infection. Hepatitis was mild for the 3 patients with HGV infection only—none had jaundice, and their mean peak alanine aminotransferase level was 198 U/L. The severity of hepatitis was not strongly related to the level of HGV RNA. Patients with combined HCV–HGV infection had no more severe hepatitis than those with HCV infection only.

Of the transfusion recipients studied, 10% had HGV infection, but less than 1% had HGV as their sole viral marker. Hepatitis G virus RNA was detected in 1.4% of random blood donors. There were 8 testable patients with acute HGV infection after transfusion—all had received blood from at least 1 donor with HGV-positive status.

Conclusions.—Hepatitis G virus is demonstrated in 1% of a random sample of blood donors. This virus can be transmitted by transfusion, although most such infections do not lead to hepatitis. When a patient infected with HCV is infected with HGV, a worsened severity of hepatitis does not occur. This study finds no evidence that the so-called HGV actually causes hepatitis.

Estimates of Infectious Disease Risk Factors in US Blood Donors

Williams AE, for the Retrovirus Epidemiology Donor Study (Am Red Cross Holland Laboratory, Rockville, Md; et al)

JAMA 277:967–972, 1997 1–10

Background.—Various methods have been employed to increase the safety of the blood supply in the United States. Protective strategies include a voluntary blood donor pool, intensive blood donor education and history-based screening procedures, and extensive laboratory testing. Studies of donors who test positive for HIV and other infectious diseases, however, suggest that a larger proportion of seronegative donors may have behavioral risks that are not detected at screening. Anonymous mail surveys were sent to recent donors in an attempt to estimate the current prevalence of undetected behavioral and other risks.

Methods.—Surveys were administered to individuals who had donated blood within the previous 2 months at 5 geographically and demographically diverse blood centers. These centers had all participated in the Retrovirus Epidemiology Donor Study (REDS) since 1989. Monthly probability samples were selected from the REDS donation database for the months of April through July and October through December 1993. The survey instrument contained 53 questions designed to collect demographic, medical, and behavioral information. Responses were used to estimate the prevalence rate for risk behaviors that would have been a basis for deferral if reported at the time of screening.

Results.—Completed questionnaires were received for 34,726 donors, 69.2% of the sample. Despite the sensitive nature of some questions, 98.1% of respondents answered all the risk questions. A total of 186 per 10,000 respondents (1.9%) reported at least 1 risk that should have resulted in deferral; 39 per 10,000 (0.4%) reported such behavior within the 3 months before blood donation. The most prevalent deferrable risk behaviors among men were history of injection drug use, sexual contact with a homosexually active man since 1977, and having paid women for sex within the past year. Among women, sexual contact with an injection drug user in the past year was the most prevalent reported risk behavior. Overall, reported risk activities were more likely to have occurred episodically or in the distant past than as ongoing or recent behaviors.

Conclusion.—Transfusion safety has reached a high degree in the United States, but a measurable percentage of active blood donors still fail to report risks for HIV and other infections at the time of screening. The current transfusion transmission of HIV, estimated at approximately 2 per 1 million units, is almost entirely the result of donations made in the HIV window period. Further improvements are needed, both in laboratory testing and in the donor screening process.

► The first 2 articles in this group (Abstracts 1–8 and 1–9) discuss a relatively new viral agent, hepatitis G, and its role in transfusion-associated hepatitis. Unlike hepatitis C virus, which is responsible for the majority of non-A, non-B hepatitis, hepatitis G appears to have a minimal role in post-transfusion hepatitis. From these 2 studies, it is difficult to predict whether this virus will prove to be clinically important. The third article (Abstract 1–10) is by far more worrisome because it estimates that 2% to 3% of blood donors fail to report the type of behavior that puts themselves, and therefore potential recipients, at risk for having HIV or other serious infections.

D.M. Rothenberg, M.D.

Magnitude and Duration of the Effect of Sepsis on Survival

Quartin AA, for the Department of Veterans Affairs Systemic Sepsis Cooperative Studies Group (Univ of Miami, Fla)

JAMA 277:1058–1063, 1997 1–11

Introduction.—Sepsis is viewed as a deadly acute disease, with most studies addressing outcomes of 30 days or less. In the long-term after an episode of sepsis, the risk of death appears to be higher than explained by comorbidity, suggesting that the sepsis has some prolonged effect beyond the episode itself. The magnitude and duration of the effect of an episode of sepsis on patient survival were analyzed.

Methods.—The study included 1,505 patients who had probable sepsis and were screened for inclusion in the Department of Veterans Affairs Cooperative Study of Corticosteroids in Systemic Sepsis during the 1980s. The controls were 91,830 nonpsychiatric patients who were free of infection and discharged from the same medical centers during the same approximate time span. The 2 groups were compared for mortality through the 8 years after the index hospitalization, based on a proportional hazards model constructed from the characteristics of the control group. The relative contributions of sepsis and underlying disease to mortality were assessed.

Results.—Throughout the 8-year follow-up period, risk of death was higher for the patients with sepsis than for the control group. One-year mortality from nonseptic causes among patients with sepsis, as predicted from the model, was 26%. This figure was similar for patients with uncomplicated or severe sepsis or septic shock. For the first 5 years after screening, the daily risk of death for patients with sepsis was greater than predicted by the model. Thereafter, risk was similar to that observed in patients with similar underlying disease but without sepsis. For the first year, the hazard rate associated with sepsis rose along with the severity of the septic episode. For patients in the septic group who survived for 30 days, mean life span was reduced from a predicted 8.03 years to 4.08 years. The septic group had 452 more deaths than predicted within the first 30 days after screening, 192 more deaths within the first year among 30-day survivors, and 51 more deaths within 5 years among 1-year survivors.

Conclusions.—Sepsis increases mortality risk, not only within the first 30 days but also for up to 5 years after the septic episode. This is so even with adjustment for comorbid conditions. The severity of sepsis influences the risk of death for the first year after the episode. Studies of treatment for sepsis should consider the possible late benefits, as some of these treatments may improve long-term survival without apparent immediate benefits.

▶ This is a tremendously disheartening study which suggests that unless early intervention in the setting of systemic inflammatory response syndrome is accomplished, mean life expectancy is dramatically reduced following the initial event. It is not surprising that the control population survival model predicted that patients with cancer or end-stage single organ disease were at increased risk of death over the study interval. It is clear that long-term follow-up studies such as these are necessary in determining the effects of supportive and "magic bullet" therapies.

D.M. Rothenberg, M.D.

Dialysis and Aggressive Critical Care

Outcomes and Cost-effectiveness of Initiating Dialysis and Continuing Aggressive Care in Seriously Ill Hospitalized Adults

Hamel MB, Phillips RS, Davis RB, et al (Beth Israel Deaconess Med Ctr, Boston; Univ of Tennessee, Chattanooga; Univ of Virginia, Charlottesville; et al)

Ann Intern Med 127:195–202, 1997 1–12

Introduction.—Patients who require dialysis for renal failure during the course of a serious illness have a poor prognosis. The question of whether to initiate dialysis and continue aggressive care is a difficult one for patients, their families, and physicians. The clinical outcome and cost-effectiveness of initiating dialysis and providing aggressive care for patients in whom renal failure developed during hospitalization for serious illness were examined prospectively.

Methods.—Study participants were drawn from 5 geographically diverse teaching hospitals and enrolled in the Study to Understand Prognoses and Preferences for Outcomes and Risks of Treatments (SUPPORT). All had renal failure after enrollment and were treated with hemodialysis or peritoneal dialysis. Data collected by chart abstraction and interview included diagnoses, comorbid conditions, resource utilization, patients' functional status 2 weeks before and 6 months after study entry, and quality of life. Estimates were obtained for hospital costs, outpatient costs of long-term dialysis, and life expectancy.

Results.—Of the 9,105 patients enrolled in SUPPORT, 490 had dialysis initiated during the study period. The median age of these patients was 61 years; 69% had acute respiratory failure or multiorgan system failure with sepsis. Median survival after the initiation of dialysis was 32 days, and only 27% of patients were alive 6 months later. Among survivors, 62% rated their quality of life as "good" or better. Survivors had a median of 1 dependency in activities of daily living. The SUPPORT patients had been assigned to 5 prognostic groups defined by survival estimates. Among those who received dialysis, actual survival closely approximated predicted survival. Overall estimated costs per quality-adjusted life-year saved with dialysis and aggressive care vs. withholding dialysis was $128,200; cost estimates ranged from $61,900 for the best prognostic category to $274,100 for the worst prognostic category.

Conclusions.—The few patients who survived after undergoing dialysis for renal failure that developed during the course of a serious illness had a fairly good quality of life and functional status. For the majority of patients, however, the cost of this decision far exceeded the commonly cited upper limit for cost-effective care ($50,000 per quality-adjusted life-year).

▶ The development of acute renal failure in critically ill patients continues to portend a high mortality. This study not only supports the 70% to 80% mortality rates in critically ill patients in whom acute renal failure develops, but also the tremendous economic impact dialysis has in attempting to treat patients with extremely poor prognoses. This SUPPORT study attempts to provide scientific basis for assigning risk and hence potentially limiting expensive and often futile therapy. This of course raises tremendous ethical concerns as they relate to the rationing of health care.

D.M. Rothenberg, M.D.

Renal Risk Estimation

Preoperative Renal Risk Stratification

Chertow GM, Lazarus JM, Christiansen CL, et al (Brigham and Women's Hosp, Boston; Harvard School of Public Health, Boston; Univ of Colorado, Denver)

Circulation 95:878–884, 1997 1–13

Background.—One percent to 5% of patients undergoing cardiac surgery experience acute renal failure (ARF), necessitating dialysis postoperatively. This complication is strongly related to perioperative morbidity and mortality. Previous research has attempted to identify predictors of ARF but has not had sufficient power to perform multivariate analysis or to develop risk stratification algorithms.

Methods.—Data were obtained prospectively from a cohort of 43,642 patients undergoing coronary artery bypass or valvular heart surgery in 43 veterans hospitals between April 1987 and March 1994. Logistic regression analyses were performed, and a risk stratification algorithm was derived from recursive partitioning and validated on an independent sample of 3,795 patients undergoing surgery between April and December 1994.

Findings.—Overall, the risk of ARF necessitating dialysis was 1.1%. Patients with ARF had a 30-day mortality rate of 63.7%, compared with 4.3% among patients without ARF. Independent risk factors for ARF requiring dialysis were valvular surgery, estimated creatinine clearance, intra-aortic balloon pump, previous heart surgery, New York Heart Association functional class IV, peripheral vascular disease, ejection fraction lower than 35%, pulmonary rales, chronic obstructive pulmonary disease, and systolic blood pressure. The risk stratification algorithm classified patients as at low risk, medium risk, or high risk, based on several of these factors and their interactions.

Conclusions.—The risk of ARF after cardiac surgery can be quantified accurately based on data readily available before surgery. Physicians and surgeons may use the findings reported here to provide improved risk estimates and to target patients at high risk for appropriate interventions.

▶ Acute renal failure after cardiac surgery is considered a major problem to these authors. Perhaps so, but I think acute renal failure after other kinds of major surgery is an even bigger one. I chastise these authors for spending so much time and effort studying (as usual) coronary bypass patients. I can't imagine why they didn't test their "risk stratification algorithm" on patients other than those who underwent cardiopulmonary bypass (e.g., patients who underwent aortic reconstruction, major vascular surgery, thoracic surgery, etc.) Nonetheless, renal risk predictors are important because we need to get cracking on trying to figure out how to prevent renal failure, an area that hasn't changed much in the last 20 years.

J.H. Tinker, M.D.

Risks Associated With Regional Anesthesia

Severe Complications Associated With Epidural and Spinal Anaesthesias in Finland 1987–1993: A Study Based on Patient Insurance Claims

Aromaa U, Lahdensuu M, Cozanitis DA (Helsinki Univ)

Acta Anaesthesiol Scand 41:445–452, 1997 1–14

Introduction.—Since 1987, Finland has had a "no-fault" compensation scheme for patients injured in the course of medical treatment. Under the Patient Injury Act, injured patients file a claim with the Patient Insurance Association, rather than suing the implicated professional. Of the 23,500 claims made from 1987 through 1993, 40% led to a compensation award. Claims related to complications of spinal and epidural anesthesias were analyzed.

Methods.—Of the 132 claims related to various regional anesthesia techniques, 86 involved complications of spinal and epidural anesthesia. Data from these claims were analyzed to estimate the incidence of severe complications of this type, as well as the associated morbidity. The total number of spinal and epidural anesthesias given was estimated by responses from a questionnaire sent to every Finnish hospital.

Results.—The questionnaire responses suggested that 550,000 spinal anesthesias and 170,000 epidural anesthesias were administered during the 6-year study period. The Patient Insurance Association cases included 25 serious complications of spinal anesthesia: 7 cases of neurologic deficit, 6 of peroneal nerve paresis, 5 of paraplegia, 4 of bacterial infection, 2 of cardiac arrest, and 1 of permanent cauda equina syndrome. There were 9 serious complications of epidural anesthesia: 2 cases of bacterial infection, 2 of acute toxic reaction to the anesthetic used, and 1 each of paraparesis, permanent cauda equina syndrome, peroneal nerve paralysis, neurologic deficit, and opioid overdose. The estimated incidence of serious complications was 0.45:10,000 with spinal anesthesia and a 0.52:10,000 with epidural anesthesia.

Conclusions.—Serious complications of spinal and epidural anesthesia appear to be rare. However, they have the potential to cause catastrophic injury, including permanent disability and even death. Steps to avoid serious complications of epidural and spinal anesthesia include atraumatic technique, careful patient selection, and early recognition and treatment of complications.

▶ Finland has its own "closed-claims" study now; 86 claims were associated with 720,000 regional anesthetics (550,000 spinals, the rest epidurals). The authors contend that this produces an incidence figure for these complications. In that, they are making an enormous assumption, namely that all such "injuries" did in fact result in a claim. They have made a case for believing this because of the "patient injury act" in Finland, which creates a sort of "no-fault" system.

On the other hand, in other countries including the United States, it is well known that such closed-claim studies of legal cases grossly underestimate the incidence of such injuries for various reasons. One such reason has to do with the fact that our U.S. adversarial malpractice system likely discriminates greatly against the elderly because of the contingency fee system. Elderly people often do not have enormous economic future horizons and, therefore, in the lexicon of today's legal system, their cases may not be "worth" pursuing on a contingency basis. I imagine that something like this is true in Finland, although the authors will be unlikely to admit it. If so, the true incidence of these complications is likely worse. This incidence, namely 1 per 10,000 cases, is considerably worse than is being touted in the United States (though without data). This incidence is also much higher (worse) than that generally reported for general anesthesia. (I just *had* to throw in that zinger!)

J.H. Tinker, M.D.

Studies of Nausea and Vomiting—Propofol vs. Nitrous Oxide

Meta-analytic Comparison of Prophylactic Antiemetic Efficacy for Postoperative Nausea and Vomiting: Propofol Anaesthesia *vs* Omitting Nitrous Oxide *vs* Total I.V. Anaesthesia With Propofol

Tramèr M, Moore A, McQuay H (Oxford Radcliffe Hosp, Headington, England)

Br J Anaesth 78:256–259, 1997 1–15

Introduction.—During the past 30 years, many pharmacologic interventions for preventing postoperative nausea and vomiting have been discussed, but the efficacy of these interventions has been documented poorly and a gold standard is lacking. To compare the antiemetic efficacy of 3 different anesthetic interventions, an appropriate range of control event rates for postoperative nausea and vomiting were defined: propofol maintenance, omitting nitrous oxide, and total IV anesthesia with propofol.

Methods.—To compare the antiemetic efficacy of 3 different anesthetic regimens, data from 2 published and 1 new meta-analysis were reviewed.

Odds ratio and number-needed-to-treat methods were used to estimate efficacy measured as prevention of postoperative nausea and vomiting when compared with a control.

Results.—For early efficacy or within 6 hours, the efficacy rate was 20% to 60% when compared with controls, and it was 48% to 80% for late efficacy or within 48 hours. Omitting nitrous oxide or propofol anesthesia had similar effects on vomiting, both early and late. The incidence of nausea was decreased with propofol when nitrous oxide was not omitted. There was poor documentation with total IV anesthesia, and it was impossible to compare this with other interventions.

Conclusions.—The same effect on early and late postoperative vomiting was found with a propofol maintenance anesthetic and with omitting nitrous oxide in general anesthesia. The present evidence shows that total IV anesthesia with propofol cannot be recommended. Nitrous oxide with propofol reduces the risk of intraoperative awareness and eventually decreases costs.

Propofol Anaesthesia and Postoperative Nausea and Vomiting: Quantitative Systematic Review of Randomized Controlled Studies

Tramèr M, Moore A, McQuay H (Oxford Radcliffe Hosp, Headington, England)

Br J Anaesth 78:247–255, 1997 1–16

Introduction.—To decrease the incidence of postoperative nausea and vomiting, propofol is thought to be antiemetic and useful; however, its mechanism is obscure. There is evidence that when propofol is used for induction or maintenance of anesthesia, it decreases the incidence of postoperative nausea and vomiting when compared with other anesthetic techniques. A meta-analysis was conducted to test this theory.

Methods.—An analysis was done of 84 studies with 6,069 patients. Recordings were taken of cumulative data on early (up to 6 hours) and late (up to 48 hours) postoperative nausea and vomiting as accurrence of nonoccurrence of nausea or vomiting. To determine whether propofol was an induction or a maintenance regimen, early or late outcomes and different emetic events (combined odds ratio and number needed to treat) were calculated.

Results.—The method of administration, time of measurement, and range of control event rates affected the efficacy of propofol on postoperative nausea and vomiting. When used for induction of anesthesia, the number needed to treat to prevent postoperative nausea and vomiting with propofol was more than 9. When used for maintenance, the number needed to treat was at best 6. Best results were achieved with propofol maintenance to prevent early postoperative nausea and vomiting within the 20% to 60% control event range. The number needed to treat to prevent early nausea within the 20% to 60% control event rate range was 4.7; for vomiting, the number was 4.9, and for any emetic event, the number was 4.9. Of 5 patients treated with propofol for maintenance of anesthesia within the 20% to 60% control event rate, 1 (who would otherwise have vomited or been nauseated) did not vomit or become nauseated in the immmediate postoperative period. This had clinical relevance. Statistical significance may have been reached in all other situations studying the difference between propofol and control, such as propofol for induction, late outcomes, or low control event rates, but the clinical relevance is doubtful.

Conclusions.—In the short term, propofol may have a clinically relevant effect on postoperative nausea and vomiting when given as a maintenance regimen and when the event rate without prophylaxis is more than 20%. To expect that propofol can act as an antiemetic in every clinical setting is overly optimistic, particularly if the event rate without prophylaxis is low. For meaningful estimates of efficacy and for comparison, treatment efficacy should be established within a defined range of control event rates.

► There have been an enormous number of studies on pharmacologic intervention for prevention of postoperative nausea and vomiting, and one wonders what more can be said on this issue. However, I selected these 2 articles (Abstracts 1–15 and 1–16) because there has been discussion on whether propofol itself is an antiemetic. A large sample size is required to study the incidence of postoperative nausea and vomiting; therefore, the authors used a meta-analysis (whereby an analysis of combined data from a number of studies is performed) to compare the effect of propofol on nausea and vomiting. The data, however, were inconclusive, and the jury has still not returned a verdict on this issue.

M. Wood, M.D.

Patient Satisfaction—The Iowa Scale

Development of a Measure of Patient Satisfaction With Monitored Anesthesia Care: The Iowa Satisfaction With Anesthesia Scale

Dexter F, Aker J, Wright WA (Univ of Iowa, Iowa City)

Anesthesiology 87:865–873, 1997 1–17

Background.—When determining the quality of monitored anesthesia care (MAC), the patient's opinion is at least as important as the anesthesiologist's. Continuous quality checks can indicate areas for improvement and document patient preferences over time. These authors developed the Iowa Satisfaction with Anesthesia Scale (ISAS) to measure patient satisfaction with MAC.

Methods.—The goal of the ISAS is to measure the patient's satisfaction with anesthesia, and not to investigate the perioperative experience. Each of the 11 items is a direct statement that addresses 1 idea (i.e., "I felt relaxed," "I felt safe"). Patients mark their responses on a 6-point scale (from −3, "disagree very much" to +3, "agree very much"). Scoring for "negative" items is reversed, so that a patient who "disagrees very much" with a statement like "I felt pain" actually gets a score of +3.

Responses are averaged for a total score, and the maximum score is +3. Investigators tested the 11 items with 80 patients admitted to a phase II postanesthesia care unit and 32 anesthesia care providers. Specific measures of validity include the fact that the instrument must be internally consistent (i.e., all questions must measure some aspect of patient satisfaction), it must have convergent validity (i.e., its results correlate well with those of other measurements), and it must be reliable (i.e., patient responses should not change drastically over time).

Findings.—The mean score was 2.1 ± 0.87, and 12 of 80 patients (15%) had the maximum score of 3. In particular, 77 of 80 patients (96%) agreed at least moderately with the item, "I was satisfied with my anesthetic care." The average time to complete the questionnaire was 4.6 ± 2.1 minutes. The internal consistency of the 11 items was high as assessed by a Cronbach's α of 0.80. Its convergent validity was also high in that answers from patients and their anesthesia care provider had a significant positive correlation ($r^2 = 0.23$). Furthermore, a patient's responses to the other 10 questions were significantly correlated (Kendall's $\tau = +0.41$) with his or her response to the question, "I was satisfied with my anesthetic care." Finally, reliability was also high in that scores on the first postoperative day and those by day 4.4 ± 1.7 days postoperatively were significantly and positively correlated ($r^2 = 0.76$).

Conclusion.—The ISAS scale is an internally consistent, valid, and reliable measure of patient satisfaction with MAC. It can be easily completed in less than 5 minutes, and its results will help anesthesia care providers deliver the most satisfying care possible.

▶ Interest in patient satisfaction measurement and quantification is high, partly because anesthesia is increasingly viewed as a commodity that can be "marketed" as competition for "covered lives" as managed health care grows. This paper contains elegant medical validations for a reliable and relatively simple scale of satisfaction with anesthesia. With this kind of validation as its foundation, this satisfaction scale should prove widely useful as we try to understand our "product" from the patient's point of view.

J.H. Tinker, M.D.

Cost/Efficacy Studies

Cost-effectiveness Analysis of Spinal Cord Stimulation in Treatment of Failed Back Surgery Syndrome

Bell GK, Kidd D, North RB (Charles River Assoc Inc, Boston; Johns Hopkins Univ, Baltimore, Md)

J Pain Symptom Manage 13:286–295, 1997 1–18

Background.—For selected patients with failed back surgery syndrome (FBSS), spinal cord stimulation (SCS) is an effective form of therapy. With advances in technology and refinements in patient selection, the overall efficacy of SCS has improved. The initial costs of permanent implantation are high; however, if successful, SCS has the potential to reduce direct

TABLE 6.—Five-Year Medical Costs of Spinal Cord Stimulation

	Actual Costs			Present Value of SCS Savings (Costs)*	
	Chronic maintenance	SCS Internal	SCS External	SCS Internal	SCS External
Base case					
Average charges	$82,630	$80,000	$74,060	$840	$6460
Medicare fees	$49,780	$49,680	$46,010	($1140)	$2500
SCS Payback					
Average charges		4.3 yr	3.2 yr	4.7 yr	3.4 yr
Medicare fees		5.0 yr	3.7 yr	5.5 yr	3.9 yr
Increase of 10% in clinical efficacy (from 46% to 56%					
Incremental savings		($4290)	($5060)	$3990	$4690
Charges					
Incremental savings-costs		($2510)	($3000)	$2300	$2760
SCS Payback (at 56% efficacy):					
Average charges		3.5 yr	2.5 yr	3.8 yr	2.6 yr
Medicare fees		4.1 yr	3.0 yr	4.5 yr	3.1 yr
SCS (at 100% efficacy)					
Average charges	$82,630	$50,540	$38,340	$27,970	$39,340
Medicare fees	$49,780	$32,950	$25,100	$14,230	$21,550
SCS payback (at 100% efficacy)					
Average charges		1.4 yr	1.0 yr	1.5 yr	1.0 yr
Medicare fees		2.1 yr	1.4 yr	2.1 yr	1.4 yr

*Present values are calculated assuming a 5% real discount rate.
Abbreviation: SCS, spinal cord stimulation.
(Reprinted by permission of Elsevier Science Inc. from Bell GK, Kidd D, North RB: Cost-effectiveness of spinal cord stimulation in treatment of failed back surgery syndrome. *J Pain Symptom Manage* 13:286–295. Copyright 1997 by the U.S. Cancer Pain Relief Committee.)

medical costs, disability costs, and other social costs. The cost effectiveness of SCS for the treatment of FBSS was analyzed.

Methods.—A cost model was constructed to compared the costs of SCS with those of traditional palliative treatment for FBSS. The study included separate analyses of externally powered and fully internalized SCS systems. A variety of sources were used to construct clinical management models of each of the treatment alternatives: the clinical literature, retrospective data sets, expert opinion, and published diagnostic and treatment protocols. Costs were calculated on the basis of average charges and Medicare fees. The model assumed that 83% of patients screened would go on to receive an implant and that 46% of these patients—38% overall—would have long-term clinical efficacy of SCS. The model put no economic value on pain relief by SCS, nor on the resulting improvements in quality of life.

Results.—Both external and internal SCS systems reduced total medical costs for the treatment of FBSS. For positive responders, the costs of SCS system implantation are counterbalanced by the avoidance of repeat back surgery. The costs of caring for SCS complications and providing maintenance care were significantly less than costs for nonsurgical chronic care. Based on current screening and efficacy rates, SCS would pay for itself within 5.5 years on average and within 2.1 years for patients in whom SCS is clinically efficacious. Sensitivity analyses suggested that still greater cost reductions could be achieved through improved efficacy of SCS, perhaps through better patient screening. For patients in whom SCS was clinically efficacious, 5-year savings were estimated at $28,000 for internal systems and $39,000 for external systems (Table 6).

Conclusion.—Spinal cord stimulation can significantly reduce the costs of care for patients with FBSS by reducing the demand for medical care. Even considering the high costs of initial system placement, the need for periodic replacement and revision, and the significant failure rate, both internally and externally powered SCS systems offer substantial cost reductions. The reported savings do not even consider the value of improvements in activities of daily living, neurologic function, and ability to work.

► The authors' approach of assessing only the savings in medical costs achieved through the use of SCS is to be commended, as other outcomes—such as return to work and quality of life—are ignored in the current health care reimbursement models, which appear to be concerned mainly with profits and returns for stockholders. Future studies should be done to compare the costs, efficacy, and complications of SCS with those of implanted intrathecal drug infusion systems, as both of these techniques are being used in patients with FBSS.

S.E. Abram, M.D.

Cost-effective Reduction of Neuromuscular-blocking Drug Expenditures

Freund PR, Bowdle TA, Posner KL, et al (Univ of Washington, Seattle)
Anesthesiology 87:1044–1049, 1997 1–19

Purpose.—Health care cost-control initiatives have targeted expenditures for anesthetic drugs. Various approaches—including educational initiatives, practice guidelines, and formulary restrictions—have been tried. However, few studies have looked at the cost-effectiveness of these efforts. The cost-effectiveness and clinical impact of a program to reduce spending on neuromuscular-blocking (NMB) agents were prospectively studied.

Methods.—The goal of the program was to persuade anesthesiologists to use inexpensive NMB agents (i.e., pancuronium or a metocurine-pancuronium combination) instead of a more expensive agent (i.e., vecuronium). The program used a variety of approaches to change anesthesiologists' behavior, including education, practice guidelines, and paperwork barriers. Neuromuscular-blocking drug use was studied in 3 periods: a 6-month historical control period, including 4,804 patients; and 2 consecutive 1-year intervention periods, including 9,761 and 10,695 patients, respectively. The patient data were used to compare expenditures for vecuronium and all NMB drugs during the 3 periods. Continuous quality improvement data were used to assess patient outcomes, including complications related to NMB agents. The study hypothesis was that vecuronium use, spending for vecuronium, and spending for all NMB drugs would be decreased during the intervention periods, with no increase in NMB-related complications.

Results.—After the intervention, vecuronium use decreased by 76%. Costs for NMB drugs were reduced by 31% during the first year and 47% during the second year. This translated into savings of $34,000 and $51,000, respectively. The rate of NMB-related complications remained stable: 0.081% during the historical period and 0.11% and 0.093% during the intervention periods. All reported problems involved prolonged neuromuscular blockade, sometimes leading to prolonged recovery room stay and short-term mechanical ventilation. Mean recovery room stay was similar for patients receiving vecuronium vs. pancuronium vs. metocurine-pancuronium.

Conclusions.—Substituting less expensive NMB agents for vecuronium leads to substantial reductions in spending. The savings are maintained over a 2-year period, and are achieved with no increase in complication rates. Achieved through a combination of approaches to changing clinician behavior, substitution of pancuronium or pancuronium-metocurine for vecuronium is truly cost effective.

▶ The use of vecuronium (intermediate-duration muscle relaxant) decreased, resulting in reduced cost. However, the authors did not really examine outcome in a statistically pure manner, but rather only by a quality assurance/improvement program. Contrast this article with the one by Berg et al. (Abstract 6–3).

M. Wood, M.D.

Risks of Complications

Body Mass Index as a Correlate of Postoperative Complications and Resource Utilization

Thomas EJ, Goldman L, Mangione CM, et al (Harvard Med School of Boston; Univ of California, San Francisco; Univ of California, Los Angeles)
Am J Med 103:277–283, 1997 1–20

Background.—Overweight individuals have a higher risk of coronary artery disease, hypertension, diabetes, and other diseases. It is unclear whether being overweight also increases the risk of postoperative complications. There is little information on the effect of body weight on use of postoperative resources.

Methods.—Prospective data were collected from 2,964 patients undergoing elective noncardiac surgery. All patients were aged 50 years or older and were expected to stay at least 2 days in the hospital. Cardiac and noncardiac complications were detected by ECG, creatine kinase level, the level of the isoenzyme of creatine kinase containing M and B subunits, and chart review. The length of stay and costs were also analyzed.

Results.—The complication rates were similar among the various body mass index groups. The wound infection rate was significantly higher in

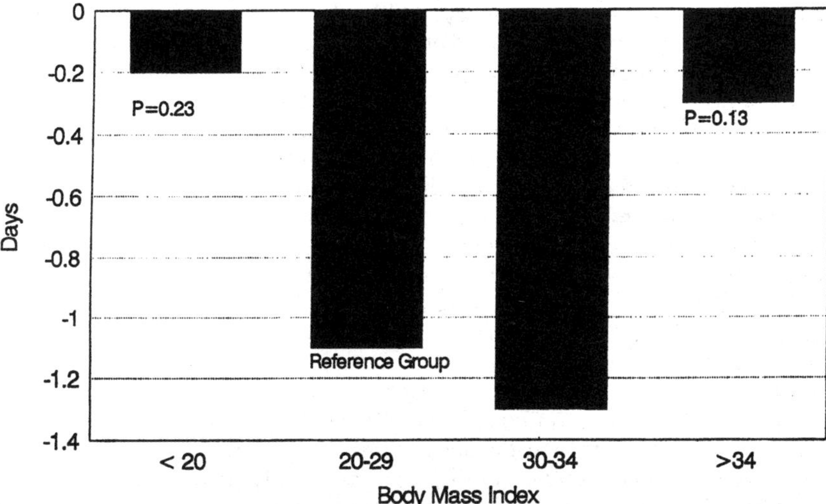

FIGURE 1.—Deviation from average diagnosis-related group length of stay (adjusted for age, race, sex, co-morbid diseases, insurance, and smoking history). The *P* value is for comparison of body mass index 20–29 to greater than 34 and 20–29 to less than 20. (Reprinted from Thomas EJ, Goldman L, Mangione CM, et al: Body mass index as a correlate of postoperative complications and resource utilization. *American Journal of Medicine* 103:277–283, Copyright 1997, with permission from Excerpta Medica, Inc.)

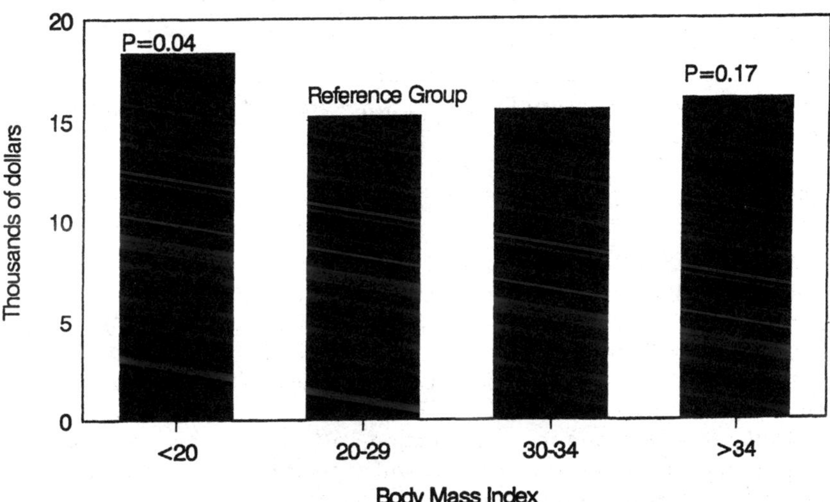

FIGURE 2.—Total costs (adjusted for procedure, age, race, sex, co-morbid diseases, insurance, and smoking history). The *P* value is for comparison of body mass index 20–29 to greater than 34 and 20–29 to less than 20. (Reprinted from Thomas EJ, Goldman L, Mangione CM, et al: Body mass index as a correlate of postoperative complications and resource utilization. *American Journal of Medicine* 103:277–283. Copyright 1997, with permission from Excerpta Medica, Inc.)

patients with a body mass index of 30–34 or greater than 34 who had abdominal or gynecologic operations than in patients of normal weight or underweight patients. After adjusting for age, race, sex, co-morbid diseases, smoking history, procedure type, and insurance, the trends toward higher use of resources by the most overweight patients were insignificant. These overweight patients stayed an average of 0.8 days longer (Fig 1) and had costs more than $800 higher than patients of normal weight. Underweight patients stayed an average of 0.9 days longer and had costs more than $3,150 higher than patients of normal weight (Fig 2). Quadratic models tested for a U-shaped relationship between body mass index and length of stay. There was no correlation found between body mass index and length of stay, but body mass index was significantly associated with total costs, even when patients with complications were excluded from analysis.

Discussion.—These findings show that higher body mass index is not significantly associated with a higher complication rate after major elective noncardiac surgery. These findings may not apply to patients with more co-morbid diseases, patients having nonelective surgery, or all surgical procedures. The analysis did not adjust for the severity of underlying illness or the overall health of the patients. Being overweight or underweight alone is not a sufficient reason to deny elective noncardiac surgery.

► This is a fascinating study from a well-established group of investigators in the area of the epidemiology of perioperative outcomes.

M. Wood, M.D.

Perioperative Respiratory Events in Smokers and Nonsmokers Undergoing General Anaesthesia

Schwilk B, Bothner U, Schraag S, et al (Univ of Ulm, Germany)

Acta Anaesthesiol Scand 41:348–355, 1997 1–21

Background.—Recent surveys of tobacco smoking and anesthesia report that smoking has negative effects on various organ systems, including the incidence of arrhythmia, formation of carboxyhemoglobin, closing capacity, altered mucus transport, and bronchial hyperreactivity. There is limited information on immediate perioperative problems during anesthesia and in the recovery unit.

Methods.—Demographic information, risk factors, and perioperative respiratory events were documented and analyzed in 26,961 patients given general anesthesia during a period of 30 months. There were 7,122 smokers and 19,839 nonsmokers.

Results.—The prevalence of chronic bronchitis in smokers was 23.3%. Overall, there were 1,573 perioperative respiratory events that occurred in 1,397 patients. Of these events, 459 were problems with intubation and technical airway management, and 1,114 were specific respiratory events such as re-intubation, laryngospasm, bronchospasm, aspiration, and hypoventilation/hypoxemia. The prevalence of specific respiratory events was 5.5% in smokers and 3.1% in nonsmokers. The relative risk of specific respiratory events was 1.8 in all smokers, 2.3 in young smokers, and 6.3 in young obese smokers. The relative risk of perioperative bronchospasm was 25.7 in young smokers with chronic bronchitis.

Discussion.—These results indicate that smoking is a serious risk factor in anesthesia. Results in young smokers and young nonsmokers were very different. It is unclear whether otherwise healthy smokers should be classified as American Society of Anesthesiologists physical status I. Perhaps elective smoking could be delayed by 2 months so that the patient can be weaned from tobacco and perhaps benefit from a lower risk of perioperative morbidity.

▶ When we take our "social" history, and we teach our medical students to do so, we ask about smoking and drinking but tend to ignore the facts that may (or may not) be revealed. We tend to ignore this particular aspect of the history for several reasons: (1) patients are not necessarily truthful about the extent to which they consume either cigarettes or alcohol; (2) they tend to minimize symptoms related to either of these "social" problems; (3) the prevalence of heavy smoking and heavy drinking is so great that there is an element of "familiarity breeding contempt." That is why this paper is so interesting. It clearly demonstrates, in no uncertain terms, the enormous impact on perioperative morbidity that smoking adds.

Mark Warner and I did a review several years ago of patients undergoing cardiac valve surgery. Unless smoking was stopped about 4 months before surgery, the major negative effect of smoking on perioperative respiratory morbidity were not reversed. In other words, telling the patient to stop smoking a few days before surgery is not much help. Somehow, this kind of information needs to be disseminated among our surgical colleagues.

J.H. Tinker, M.D.

End-tidal Carbon Dioxide and Outcome of Out-of-Hospital Cardiac Arrest

Levine RL, Wayne MA, Miller CC (Baylor College of Medicine, Houston; City of Bellingham Emergency Med Services, Wash)

N Engl J Med 337:301–306, 1997 1–22

Objective.—Fewer than 3% of individuals survive an out-of-hospital cardiac arrest unless advanced life support is immediately available. Even then, few survive long-term. End-tidal carbon dioxide level may be a reliable indicator of irreversible cardiac arrest. Whether quantitative end-tidal carbon dioxide measurements could be used to predict death in victims of cardiac arrest associated with electric activity but no pulse was studied prospectively.

Methods.—A prospective observational study was conducted between 1991 and 1995 in 150 consecutive individuals aged 18 years or older with

TABLE 1.—End-tidal Carbon Dioxide Values in Patients Who Survived to Hospital Admission and in Those Who Did Not

Variable	Nonsurvivors (N = 115)	Survivors (N = 35)	P Value*
	mean ± SD (range)		
Age (yr)	68.0 ± 13.8 (31–95)	71.5 ± 13.0 (27–90)	0.19
End-tidal carbon dioxide (mm Hg)†			
Initial	12.3 ± 6.9 (2–50)	12.2 ± 4.6 (5–22)	0.93
Final	4.4 ± 2.9 (0–10)	32.8 ± 7.4 (18–58)	<0.001

**P* values were calculated with the Wilcoxon rank-sum statistic.

†Initial end-tidal carbon dioxide levels were determined immediately upon intubation. Final end-tidal carbon dioxide levels were determined after 20 minutes of advanced cardiac life support.

(Reprinted by permission of *The New England Journal of Medicine,* from Levine RL, Wayne MA, Miller CC: End-tidal carbon dioxide and outcome of out-of-hospital cardiac arrest. *N Engl J Med* 337:301–306. Copyright 1997, Massachusetts Medical Society. All rights reserved.)

out-of-hospital cardiac arrest in Whatcom County, Washington, population 160,000, with advanced life support provisions. Patients with ventricular tachycardia or ventricular fibrillation without pulse and patients who remained in asystole despite therapy were not included. End-tidal carbon dioxide levels were measured by mainstream sampling from an endotracheal tube connected to a combined pulse oximetercapnograph. Resuscitation was continued for at least 20 minutes unless spontaneous circulation returned.

Results.—After 20 minutes, there was a significant difference in end-tidal carbon dioxide levels for survivors and nonsurvivors (Table 1). The sensitivity, specificity, and positive and negative predictive values of an end-tidal carbon dioxide level of 10 mm Hg or less were 100%. Of the 16 patients released from the hospital, 14 were alive 6 weeks later, and 8 were neurologically normal. Five had minor neurologic problems but could take care of themselves; 1 patient required skilled nursing care. Survivors were significantly younger than nonsurvivors (65.2 years vs. 76.8 years).

Conclusion.—End-tidal carbon dioxide level at 20 minutes after advanced life support is initiated is a reliable predictor of survival after an out-of-hospital cardiac arrest.

▶ Defining medical futility in out-of-hospital cardiac arrest situations is currently a medical, social, and ethical dilemma. Currently, most emergency medical services do not allow paramedical personnel to diagnose death in the field. In large rural areas, for example, excessive time spent during resuscitation, or in transporting patients with no hope of survival, severely impairs systems with otherwise limited resources. In addition, high speed ambulance rides impart great risk to both paramedical personnel and other innocent third parties. These data, coupled with the economic impact of futile resuscitation, have prompted the need to develop predictable parameters that would allow for futile resuscitation to be discontinued in the field. In this regard, this article provides the scientific basis for determining futile resuscitation in out-of-hospital cardiac arrest related to pulseless electric activity. Should corroborative data validate this study, end-tidal CO_2 monitoring might become the standard of care for both inhospital and out-of-hospital cardiac arrest.

D.M. Rothenberg, M.D.

Cost-efficient Carotid Surgery: A Comprehensive Evaluation
Ammar AD (Univ of Kansas, Wichita)
J Vasc Surg 24:1050–1056, 1996 1–23

Introduction.—Cost-reducing strategies for carotid endarterectomies (CEAs) typically address only 1 or 2 aspects of cost reduction. Comprehensive cost-cutting strategies were assessed to determine whether they would adversely affect outcome in 237 patients undergoing CEA.

Methods.—From December 1994 to December 1995, 237 consecutive patients who underwent 260 CEAs were prospectively evaluated. Costs were analyzed for the following:

- Carotid arteriography
- Preoperative laboratory tests
- Electrocardiograms and chest radiography
- Use of carotid shunts during operation
- Use of pathology department
- Intensive care
- Oxygen therapy
- Telemetry
- Hospital stay
- Complications of CEA

Results.—All variables evaluated were routinely ordered before the cost analysis. When cost-containment strategies were initiated for 237 patients who underwent 260 CEAs, the routine ordering of all tests was reduced to the following percentages: 22% arteriography, 62% preoperative complete blood cell count and SMA-7, 71% preoperative electrocardiograms, 73% preoperative chest radiographs, 32% carotid shunts, 11% intensive care unit, 13% oxygen therapy, and 7% telemetry. Hospital stay was reduced from an average of 2.6–1.3 days. The total savings for 237 patients, based on average hospital and physician charges, was $2.3 million. There were no deaths. Complications were 4 strokes and 1 myocardial infarction. No patients were readmitted, and there were no recurrent or new neurologic or cardiac findings at 1 and 4 weeks after surgery.

Conclusion.—In this series of 237 patients who underwent CEA, it was possible to significantly decrease cost without compromising patient outcome. Because physicians are ultimately responsible for most health care expenditures, they are in a position to assess the need for each charge incurred and educate medical students, residents, nurses and other health care providers, and patients about cost-containment efforts.

▶ The majority of the reduction in charges that they found were the result of a reduction of arteriograms. One hopes that there are not so many surprises from not doing arteriograms that patient outcome is hindered in a small percentage of cases. Nevertheless, it does seem that an arch and bilateral selective carotid arteriogram costing $8,100 on average can be eliminated in the vast majority of patients who have ultrasonograpy studies of their carotid. I would caution against reducing some of the other things such as routine oxygen therapy in patients whose carotid chemoreceptor function is indeed impaired. Some other things they do are also questionable, such as routinely using low–molecular weight dextran during the procedure when this has not been shown to be a benefit. Thus, the majority of the charge savings were for not doing radiography that they deemed unnecessary, and those reductions clearly can be continued. I think we need to be cautious before we recommend discontinuance of other things that might have a real benefit even if they are unstudied, or even if they have benefit in only 6% or 8% of patients and cannot be shown in a small study. The authors are to be commended for instituting this clinical pathway. I think it shows what one physician can do when he or she is devoted to reducing unnecessary cost of care.

M.F. Roizen, M.D.

2 Perioperative Cardiac and Vascular Evaluation, Risks, and Outcomes

Cardiac Risk of Noncardiac Surgery: Influence of Coronary Disease and Type of Surgery in 3368 Operations
Eagle KA, for the CASS Investigators and University of Michigan Heart Care Program (Univ of Michigan, Ann Arbor)
Circulation 96:1882–1887, 1997 2–1

Objective.—The most common cause of death after surgery is a cardiac complication. There is little information about surgery-specific risks of noncardiac procedures. The interaction between the extent of coronary disease and procedure-related stresses on the heart can be assessed by using the Coronary Artery Surgery Study (CASS) registry.

Methods.—Of the 24,959 patients enrolled at 15 clinical sites between 1974 and 1979, 3,368 patients had undergone at least 1 noncardiac surgery. Patients were stratified into those who had coronary artery disease (CAD), those who did not, and those who had undergone coronary bypass surgery (CABG) before noncardiac operations (abdominal 36%, urologic 21%, orthopedic 15%, vascular 9%, head and neck 7%, thoracic 5%, and breast 2%). The end point was operative mortality, myocardial infarction, or perioperative death. Univariate analysis was used to compare patients with and without myocardial infarction or perioperative death and risk factors.

Results.—Patients with known coronary disease, described as "high-risk" for noncardiac surgery, had a lower preoperative risk if they had undergone CABG (Figure). Multivariate predictors of 30-day death or myocardial infarction after noncardiac surgery, in addition to coronary disease not treated by CABG in patients with CAD, included congestive heart failure, advanced age, and hypertension. Multivariate predictors of 30-day death or myocardial infarction after higher-risk noncardiac surgery

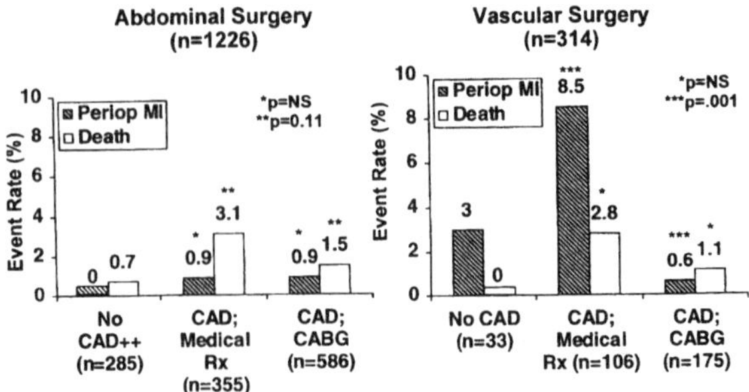

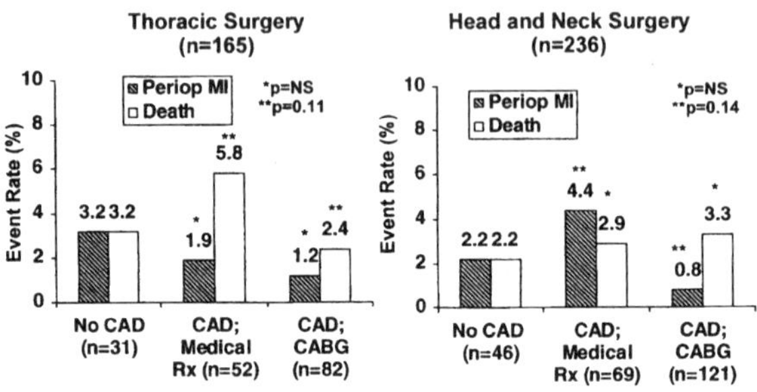

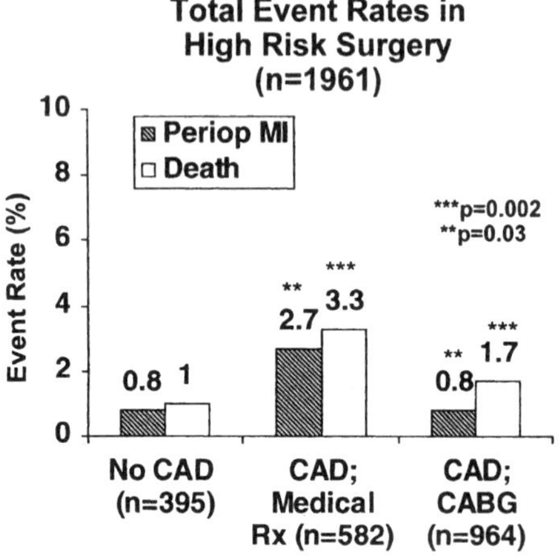

FIGURE.—Type of noncardiac surgery and postoperative myocardial infarction (MI) or death among higher-risk procedures (combined MI and death rate of 4% or higher in medically treated patients). Rates of MI or death among patients undergoing abdominal, vascular, thoracic, and head and neck surgeries are stratified by the presence or absence of coronary artery disease (CAD) and whether it was previously treated medically or with coronary artery bypass surgery (CABG). (Reproduced with permission from Eagle KA, for the CASS Investigators and University of Michigan Heart Care Program: Cardiac risk of noncardiac surgery: Influence of coronary disease and type of surgery in 3368 operations. *Circulation* 96[6]:1882–1887, 1997. Copyright 1997 American Heart Association.)

TABLE 7.—How Long Does Prior Coronary Artery Bypass Surgery Protect Against Perioperative Myocardial Infarction or Death After Noncardiac Surgery?

Years From CABG to Noncardiac Surgery	Perioperative Risk Death	MI
0–2	7/420 (1.7%)	3/420 (0.7%)
2–4	3/531 (0.6%)	6/531 (1.1%)
4–6	6/357 (1.7%)	2/357 (0.6%)
>6	5/324 (1.5%)	7/324 (2.2%)

Abbreviations: CABG, coronary artery bypass surgery; *MI,* myocardial infarction.

(Reprinted with permission from Eagle KA, for the CASS Investigators and University of Michigan Heart Care Program: Cardiac risk of noncardiac surgery: Influence of coronary disease and type of surgery in 3368 operations. *Circulation* 96[6]:1882–1887, 1997. Copyright 1997 American Heart Association.)

in patients with known CAD included coronary disease not treated by CABG, congestive heart failure, hypertension, and smoking. Patients having urologic, orthopedic, breast, and skin surgery were at no increased risk, regardless of whether pre-existing coronary disease was treated medically or surgically. Coronary bypass surgery protected noncardiac surgical patients for at least 6 years (Table 7).

Conclusion.—Patients undergoing low-risk surgical procedures such as urologic, orthopedic, breast, and skin operations, and patients who have undergone CABG will probably not benefit from extensive coronary evaluations. Mortality and myocardial infarction risks are reduced in patients with coronary disease having noncardiac surgery if they have undergone CABG.

► This is one of many articles from the CASS study, which has been ongoing for many years. It identifies over 3,300 operations in almost 25,000 participants in the CASS study who underwent one or more episodes of noncardiac surgery during the 10-year period *after* their initial coronary bypasses. As we and others have found several times in the past, performance of prior CABG is clearly associated with better coronary outcomes after noncardiac surgery in these patients. Whether CABG "protects" patients against a perioperative Myocardial infarction (MI) or other ischemic event after subsequent noncardiac surgery or, alternatively, whether the CABG simply constitutes a "survival test,"(i.e., if a perioperative MI was destined to happen) it may have happened surrounding the CABG and was thus not "available" to occur after subsequent noncardiac surgery. This "survivalist" view is mitigated against by the long follow-up in this study. As has been reported many times, noncardiac operations involving the thorax, abdomen, and major vasculature were associated with greater risk of perioperative MI. In this study, head and neck operations were also associated with greater risk, something which hasn't been reported, possibly because of the preponderance of carotid endarterectomies in that population.

I think the most important aspect of this study is that it does definitively show that coronary bypass is associated with decreased risk of anesthesia and surgery in patients undergoing subsequent noncardiac operations. Of interest also is the length of time since the CABG with respect to performance of subsequent noncardiac surgery. The authors have contributed here also, showing that the risk increases somewhat but not alarmingly. I find this article to be of considerable value in our continuing efforts to understand and quantitate the true value of CABG.

J.H. Tinker, M.D.

Risks of Cardiac Operations for Elderly Patients: Reduction of the Age Factor

Katz NM, Chase GA (Georgetown Univ, Washington, DC)

Ann Thorac Surg 63:1309–1314, 1997 2–2

Background.—Although hospitalization of elderly patients for cardiovascular surgery may be more costly than for a less invasive procedure, surgical intervention offers the possibility of more sustained clinical improvement and fewer total days of hospitalization in the long term. Thus, it is important to define the current risks and outcomes.

Methods.—A study was made of 285 consecutive patients 70 years of age and older and 568 patients younger than 70 years undergoing surgery from 1991 through 1995. Treatment consisted of antegrade and retrograde cold and warm cardioplegia, epicardial echocardiography, retrosternal dissection for repeat surgery, maintenance of normal arterial pressure, and measures to avoid renal dysfunction.

Findings.—The 30-day mortality rate for both age groups was 1.8%. The hospital mortality rate was 3.2% among the elderly patients and 2.5% in the younger group, a nonsignificant difference. The frequencies of complications also did not differ. During the 5-year study, length of stay declined from 12.5 to 8.9 days for more elderly patients and from 11.5 to 6.4 days for the younger patients. Hospital charges were 13% higher for the more elderly patients (Tables 4 and 6).

Conclusion.—With current management strategies, mortality rates among the more elderly patients undergoing cardiac surgery approached that for younger patients. These findings support the continued performance of cardiac procedures in selected elderly patients.

TABLE 4.—Mortality by Age Group in Elderly Patients

Age (y)	No. of Patients	30-Day Mortality*	
		No.	%
70–74	153	1	0.7
75–79	82	3	3.7
≥80	50	1	2
Overall	285	5	1.8

*There were no significant differences between age groups.

(Reprinted with permission from the Society of Thoracic Surgeons, courtesy of Katz NM, Chase GA: Risks of cardiac operations for elderly patients: Reduction of the age factor. *Ann Thorac Surg* 63:1309–1314, 1997.)

TABLE 6.—Major Complications

Complication	Age < 70 Years (n = 568) No.	%	Age ≥ 70 Years (n = 285) No.	%
Reoperation	33	5.8	19	6.7
MI	5	0.9	2	0.7
Sternal dehiscence	1	0.2	1	0.4
Sepsis	5	0.9	4	1.4
Reintubation	13	2.3	8	2.8
Tracheostomy	1	0.2	2	0.7
Dialysis	6	1.1	7	2.5
GI bleed	9	1.6	6	2.1
Stroke	4	0.7	4	1.4

Note: There were no significant differences between the 2 groups.
Abbreviations: GI, gastrointestinal; *MI,* myocardial infarction.
(Reprinted with permission from the Society of Thoracic Surgeons, courtesy of Katz NM, Chase GA: Risks of cardiac operations for elderly patients: Reduction of the age factor. *Ann Thorac Surg* 63:1309–1314, 1997.)

► We are continually being asked to treat older, sicker patients and, consequently, we are getting better and better at it!

M. Wood, M.D.

Rapid Recovery After Coronary Artery Bypass Grafting: Is the Elderly Patient Eligible?

Ott RA, Gutfinger DE, Miller MP, et al (Univ of California Irvine, Orange)
Ann Thorac Surg 63:634–639, 1997 2–3

Background.—Though rapid recovery protocols are successful in young patients with normal ventricular function after coronary artery bypass grafting, the success of such protocols in elderly patients has not been thoroughly validated. At some centers, there is still reluctance to discharge such elderly patients early. The success of an accelerated recovery program in a group of elderly patients requiring coronary artery bypass grafting was investigated.

Methods.—In this retrospective analysis, 152 consecutive patients younger than 70 years were compared with 167 patients aged 70 years or older undergoing isolated coronary artery bypass grafting using cardiopulmonary bypass. The rapid recovery program, applied to all patients, consisted of an anesthetic protocol for early extubation, decreased cardiopulmonary bypass time, and perioperative administration of corticosteroids and thyroid hormone. Early identification and management of postoperative atrial fibrillation, a proactive negative fluid balance, rapid return of bowel function, mobilization of the patient, and aggressive use of the intra-aortic balloon pump preoperatively were emphasized.

Findings.—The younger patient group had a 30-day mortality of 3.3%. The 30-day mortality of 4.2% in the older group was not significantly greater. Postoperative complications also did not differ significantly between groups. Nineteen percent of the older patients and 48% of the younger patients were discharged before postoperative day 5. The younger and older groups were discharged at a mean 5.7 and 8.0 days, respectively, after surgery.

Conclusions.—This rapid recovery protocol expedited recovery for all patients undergoing isolated coronary bypass grafting using cardiopulmonary bypass, regardless of age, acuity of illness, or related conditions. Though the postoperative duration of stay was significantly briefer for the younger patients, the older patients also proved to be suitable candidates for rapid recovery protocols.

▶ This paper is included in the YEAR BOOK to stimulate consideration of the current fad, namely, "fast-tracking" (i.e., earliest possible extubation and earliest possible exit from the intensive care unit and then from the hospital). This paper concludes that, even in the elderly, fast-tracking is doable. How ethical is it to shove old people out the door of the hospital days, even weeks, before they would have been discharged just a few years ago? Has the government's wonderful "DRG" system dramatically changed the humanitarian aspects of medicine or the rate of healing (certainly not *faster* in older patients)? The recent hue and cry over 1-day discharges after labor and delivery was stimulated by several cases of new mothers who were not properly trained to breast feed their infants and who unknowingly allowed their infants to become severely dehydrated, and at least in one case to die. Lay people and the profession of obstetrics and gynecology properly rose up against this insurance company–mandated practice, and in many instances got it changed! We in anesthesiology facilitate all kinds of practices with our competent modern performance of high-quality anesthesia. Early extubation and discharge after cardiac surgery is in major part facilitated by us. Therefore, perhaps we should have something to say about it. I have long believed that anesthesiologists facilitate all sorts of medical practices, ethical and otherwise. Because we usually don't actually initiate the practices ourselves, we tend to remain quiet on many ethics questions. Perhaps we shouldn't stay so quiet.

J.H. Tinker, M.D.

Perioperative Maintenance of Normothermia Reduces the Incidence of Morbid Cardiac Events: A Randomized Clinical Trial

Frank SM, Fleisher LA, Breslow MJ, et al (Johns Hopkins Med Insts, Baltimore, Md; Vanderbilt Univ, Nashville, Tenn)

JAMA 277:1127–1134, 1997 2–4

Introduction.—Administration of anesthesia, the use of IV fluids, and other factors contribute to development of hypothermia in most surgical patients. Even mild hypothermia (from 0.5°C to 1.2°C below normal core temperature) can trigger sympathetically mediated hypertension and place increased demands on the cardiovascular system. A randomized control trial designed to assess the relationship between body temperature and cardiac morbidity in the perioperative period compared groups of patients receiving routine thermal care and supplemental warming care.

Methods.—The study enrolled 300 patients during a 3-year period. Those eligible were older than 60 years; were scheduled for peripheral vascular, abdominal, or thoracic surgical procedures and for postoperative admission to the ICU; and had documented coronary artery disease (CAD) or were at high risk for CAD. Patients were also required to have a preoperative tympanic temperature between 36°C and 38°C. Routine thermal care included warming of IV fluids and blood and the use of paper surgical drapes and warmed cotton blankets. The normothermic group had routine care plus an upper- or lower-body forced-air warming cover with therapy continued through the first 2 hours of postoperative care. Eight body sites were monitored for temperature, and an investigator blinded to clinical information determined morbid cardiac events.

Results.—Hypothermic and normothermic groups were similar in preoperative demographic variables, anesthetic technique, level of invasive hemodynamic monitoring, and intraoperative blood and fluid requirements. Mean core temperature was significantly lower after surgery in the hypothermic group (35.4°C) than in the normothermic group (36.7°C), and remained lower during the early postoperative period. The incidence of perioperative morbid cardiac events was 6.3% in the hypothermic group vs. 1.4% in the normothermic group. Maintenance of normothermia was associated with a reduction in postoperative ventricular tachycardia. In multivariate analysis, hypothermia was an independent predictor of morbid cardiac events (relative risk, 2.2).

Conclusion.—Active warming designed to maintained normothermia during the intraoperative and postoperative periods was associated with a decreased incidence of early postoperative morbid cardiac events in patients with cardiac risk factors undergoing noncardiac surgery.

► The results of this outcome analysis emphasize the benefit of both active perioperative warming and preoperative beta-blockade therapy to minimize postoperative cardiac morbidity. This study, coupled with previous results showing the decreased incidence of infection after colon surgery when patients are kept warm,[1] should mandate more careful attention to intraoperative temperature control. No more "cold hands–warm heart" theories.

D.M. Rothenberg, M.D.

Reference

1. Kurz A, for the Study of Wound Infection and Temperature Group: Perioperative normothermia to reduce the incidence of the surgical-wound infection and shorten hospitalization. *N Engl J Med* 334:1209–1215, 1996. (1997 Year Book of Anesthesiology and Pain Management, pp 180–182.)

► This paper is a continuation of a series of studies of patients undergoing major abdominal, thoracic, or vascular surgery, comparing regional vs. general anesthesia and asking other important questions. One question asked was the effect of postoperative hypothermia on various complications, especially serious ones.

In the age-old battle over operating room temperature between ourselves, the surgeons, and the OR nursing personnel, this paper should probably be posted in OR lounges all over the country.

J.H. Tinker, M.D.

Temperature During Cardiopulmonary Bypass for Coronary Artery Operations Does Not Influence Postoperative Cognitive Function: A Prospective, Randomized Trial

Plourde G, Leduc AS, Morin JE, et al (Royal Victoria Hospital, Montreal; McGill Univ, Montreal)

J Thorac Cardiovasc Surg 114:123–128, 1997 2–5

Objective.—Cardiopulmonary bypass (CPB) can cause CNS damage. By reducing cerebral metabolism, hypothermia during CPB may reduce the risk or severity of CNS damage. Two studies of this issue have been performed: 1 found no difference in postoperative cognitive function in patients receiving warm vs. cold CPB, whereas the other found a higher incidence of abnormalities with warm CPB. This randomized trial examined the effects of warm vs. cold CPB on postoperative cognitive function.

Methods.—The study included 62 patients scheduled for elective coronary revascularization. They were randomized to receive either cold (28°C) or warm (36°C) CPB. Neuropsychological studies were administered before and 7 days after CPB by an observer who was unaware of the patients' group assignment. The assessments included tests of attention, concentration, and mental tracking; conceptual and visuomotor tracking and flexibility; complex psychomotor function; verbal memory and learning; and verbal memory.

Results.—The final analysis included 54 patients. The duration of CPB was 18 minutes longer in the cold group. On analysis of the neuropsychological test results, no significant effect of temperature and no significant interactions were found. Two thirds of patients in each group had deterioration of 1 or more standard deviations on at least 1 test. Both groups had significant deterioration in performance on tests of psychomotor coordination and verbal memory.

Conclusion.—Temperature during CPB does not influence postoperative cognitive function. The longer duration of CPB in the cold group had no apparent impact on neuropsychological outcome. The authors note that their study was small and included patients at low risk of complications.

► Dr. Plourde and his group in Canada are leaders in monitoring patient awareness under anesthesia and understanding the cognitive effects of CPB. It is perfectly legitimate to ask the question as to whether depth of hypothermia during CPB adversely affects cognitive function. Although the answer in this study was "no" (i.e., it was a negative study) the authors have performed one of the more elegant studies you will see this year.

J.H. Tinker, M.D.

Reduction in Requirements for Allogeneic Blood Products: Nonpharmacologic Methods

Hardy J-F, Bélisle S, Janvier G, et al (Univ of Montreal; Centre Hospitalier Universitaire de Bordeaux, France; Université Paris)

Ann Thorac Surg 62:1935–1943, 1996 2–6

Objective.—For patients undergoing cardiac surgery, a number of different approaches have been tried to reduce bleeding and the need for allogeneic transfusion during the operative and postoperative periods. Some of these techniques are relatively harmless, but others have risks that must be weighed against the risks of autologous blood transfusion. Nonpharmacologic techniques of reducing requirements for allogeneic blood products (ABPs) in cardiac surgical patients were reviewed.

Methods.—The available blood conservation methods were reviewed in chronologic order, based on their order of availability in the perioperative period. A critical analysis of the literature for and against each procedure was performed.

Findings.—Two key approaches to reducing requirements for ABPs were identified from the literature: avoiding preoperative anemia and following published guidelines for transfusion. Effective measures for reducing the need for ABPs during the operation included allowing low hemoglobin concentrations and using autologous blood, whether predonated or collected before bypass. Ongoing debate was noted regarding the value of plateletpheresis, retransfusion of shed mediastinal fluid, and directed donations. Blood substitutes may one day be helpful in decreasing the need for ABPs, but they are not yet clinically available. Evidence indicates that maintaining normothermia during and after surgery helps to improve hemostasis.

Discussion.—Evidence shows that there are several effective nonpharmacologic approaches to reducing the need for ABPs in patients undergoing cardiac operations. In combination, these approaches can sometimes even eliminate the need for allogeneic blood products in cardiac surgical patients. The keys to reaching this goal are a thorough understanding of the pathophysiology of anemia and coagulopathy and adherence to recognized transfusion guidelines.

▶ This article is like the old review articles of the 70s and 80s that used to appear in *Anaesthesia* and other publications. Meta-analysis has replaced this qualitative analysis, so that more evidence-based appraisal can be obtained. Nevertheless, this is an important article. It reviews the material well and discusses the pharmacology of the issue.

M.F. Roizen, M.D.

Open Heart Operations Without Transfusion Using a Multimodality Blood Conservation Strategy in 50 Jehovah's Witness Patients: Implications for a "Bloodless" Surgical Technique

Rosengart TK, Helm RE, DeBois WJ, et al (Cornell Univ, New York)
J Am Coll Surg 184:618–629, 1997 2–7

Objective.—Because of the risks imposed by homologous blood transfusions, a variety of blood conservation techniques have been developed to decrease risks, particularly in patient groups such as Jehovah's Witnesses, who refuse to accept blood transfusions of any kind. A "bloodless" surgical technique for open heart operations is described.

Methods.—A blood conservation program of high-dose erythropoietin (800 U/kg loading dose followed by 500 U/kg every other day until surgery), a full Hammersmith regimen of intraoperative aprotinin (a total of 6 million U), intraoperative autologous blood donation, intraoperative cell salvage, reinfusion of blood recovered during surgery, and limited blood drawing was developed for 50 adult Jehovah's Witnesses, average age 61 years, undergoing heart operations. Results from this group were compared with a group of 30 consecutive control patients who underwent first-time coronary bypass surgery using standard blood conservation measures.

Results.—Operations performed in the Jehovah's Witnesses group included 30 primary coronary bypass grafting, and 20 multiple valve and combined valve-coronary procedures. The discharge hematocrit in the Jehovah's Witnesses group was 32%, and the in-hospital mortality was 4%. No deaths were anemia-related. Adverse neurologic events included 1 transient posterior circulation stroke in a patient requiring repair of a chronic aortic dissection and 1 patient in whom a deep vein thrombosis developed after discharge. There was no risk advantage for transfusion between the 30 Jehovah's Witnesses undergoing first-time coronary surgery and the 30 control patients. Compared with the control group, chest tube output was significantly lower in the 30 Jehovah's Witnesses patients undergoing first-time coronary surgery (470 vs. 160 mL). Postoperative hematocrit levels were higher in the 30 Jehovah's Witnesses than in the control group, despite the fact that baseline hematocrit levels were lower in the Jehovah's Witnesses. Duration of hospital stays and costs were similar for the 30 Jehovah's Witnesses and the controls. The 30 Jehovah's Witnesses did not require transfusions, but 17 control patients did.

Conclusion.—Open heart surgery can be performed as a "bloodless" operation with current blood conservation techniques.

▶ I found this paper fascinating. The authors actually included a "control" group of 30 patients undergoing first-time coronary bypass, who were not Jehovah's Witnesses. In the Jehovah's Witness group, there was 40% less chest-tube output and, amazingly, postoperative hematocrit levels were *higher* than the "control" group, despite the fact that red cells were given to patients in group 2. They explain this by use of the "multi-modality" approach to blood conservation, including erythropoietin, aprotinin, etc. They admit that this costs an extra $4,500 per case. I doubt the dramatic differences between these two groups are quite so easily explainable. Perhaps when you start out "behind the eight-ball"(i.e., constrained against giving any blood at all), could it be that you "tighten up" your practices (i.e., possibly do a little more thorough job of hemostasis in the first place)? I certainly can't prove that based on their results. Total operative time was only slightly greater in the Jehovah's group. The obvious question here is that if we can do such a good job in avoidance of transfusion in Jehovah's Witnesses, why not do the same for everybody?

J.H. Tinker, M.D.

Perfluorocarbon Emulsion in the Cardiopulmonary Bypass Prime Reduces Neurologic Injury

Cochran RP, Kunzelman KS, Vocelka CR, et al (Univ of Washington, Seattle)

Ann Thorac Surg 63:1326–1332, 1997 2–8

Background.—Neurologic function can be a devastating complication of cardiopulmonary bypass. Several causes for this damage have been proposed, including emboli and blood flow changes. This study evaluated whether adding a perfluorocarbon (PFC) emulsion to the prime solution during cardiopulmonary bypass could affect postoperative cerebral infarction.

Methods.—Fourteen pigs were anesthetized and intubated. They underwent cardiopulmonary bypass with either a standard crystalloid prime solution or a PFC-emulsified solution. An air or saline (control) bolus was administered 10 minutes into the bypass procedure. Cerebral infarction was determined from stained brain cross sections. Colored microspheres were injected to assess regional cerebral blood flow. Blood pressure, blood gas concentrations, an electroencephalogram, and an electrocardiogram were monitored through the 6-hour protocol.

Findings.—Cerebral infarctions were less common and less severe in the 5 pigs that received the PFC prime solution and an air insult (PFC-air group; with no infarctions), than in the 5 pigs that received the crystalloid solution and an air insult (crystalloid-air group; 3 of 5 animals had infarcts). Cerebral blood flow was unchanged or increased in the PFC-air group, whereas it decreased significantly 5 minutes after the air bolus in the crystalloid-air group. Cerebral blood flow normalized within 1 hour in both groups. Electroencephalographic activity recovered to 48% of the stable level in the PFC-air group, but only to 18% in the crystalloid-air group.

Conclusions.—Adding a PFC emulsion to the prime solution attenuated the effects of a cerebral air embolism during cardiopulmonary bypass. No cerebral infarcts occurred, cerebral blood flow was unchanged or even increased, and electroencephalographic activity recovered better and faster in the PFC-air group.

▶ It is obvious to those who study this problem that neurologic dysfunction after cardiopulmonary bypass is a persistent problem which causes major morbidity, and which seems to still be pretty much unchecked. Also agreed now is the fact that air embolism, probably coupled with particulate embolism, is the proximate cause of most of these problems. Because of the enormous oxygen and other gas solubility in solutions of liquid perfluorocarbons, the latter constitutes a fascinating potential "scavenger" for emboli when used to prime the pump for cardiopulmonary bypass. The problem with the perfluorocarbons is the fact that, once given, they don't go away easily if at all. The reticuloendothelial system takes them up, but then doesn't seem to be able to do much with them (shades of the silicone breast implant problem). What will happen several years after the use of perfluorocarbons in patients who have these substances "stored" at some sort of uneasy truce with their immune systems, is unknown, and, frankly, a bit scary. Nonetheless, the finding in this paper that air embolus can be prevented by perfluorocarbon usage is exciting.

J.H. Tinker, M.D.

Retrospective Review of 100 Cases of Endoluminal Aortic Stent-Graft Surgery From an Anaesthetic Perspective

Baker AB, Lloyd G, Fraser TA, et al (Royal Prince Alfred Hosp, Sydney, Australia; Univ of Sydney, Australia)

Anaesth Intensive Care 25:378–384, 1997 2–9

Background.—Endoluminal aortic stent-graft surgery offers a minimally invasive approach to treatment of a fatal condition. Compared with open surgery, the endoluminal approach significantly reduces patient morbidity and health care costs. The authors' hospital has had extensive experience with this procedure since 1992. The results of this experience were reviewed from an anesthetic perspective.

Methods.—The 4-year experience included 100 patients undergoing endoluminal aortic stent surgery. Anesthetic data analyzed included the form of anesthesia used, use of a pulmonary artery catheter or central venous line, use of IV mannitol, lowest recorded hemoglobin level, length of the procedure, and need for open repair of the aneurysm. Mortality and major morbidity were analyzed.

Results.—Ninety-seven patients had abdominal aneurysms and 3 had thoracic aneurysms. Anesthesia consisted of general anesthesia alone for 41 patients, general anesthesia plus midthoracic epidural anesthetic for 41, and lumbar epidural anesthesia with sedation in 9 patients. Sixteen patients died; overall mortality was comparable to that for open surgery. Mortality was 100% for patients with multiple organ failure, 78% for those with acute renal failure, and 55% for those with a serum creatinine increase of greater than 100 μmol/L. Forty-six patients received mannitol—16% had a serum creatinine increase of greater than 100 μmol/L, compared with 4% for patients who did not receive mannitol. Mortality was 22% for patients with intraoperative or postoperative anemia, defined as a hemoglobin level of 80 g/L or less, vs. 5% for those without anemia. Mortality rose to 15% for patients whose operation took more than 4 hours, compared with 3% for those with shorter operations.

Conclusions.—The findings have important implications for anesthetic management of patients undergoing endoluminal aortic stent-graft surgery. Some of the special considerations to be observed with this procedure include the need for the patient to remain perfectly still for an extended period, the need for IV heparin, preparation for sudden massive blood loss, careful blood pressure management at the time of balloon occlusion of the aorta, the possibility of postoperative renal impairment, and the need to prevent heat loss. Ongoing technical advances should simplify the anesthetic requirements of this procedure. However, the medical condition of these patients can make anesthetic management difficult.

► This outstanding article highlights the anesthetic problems for endoluminal aortic stent-graft surgery. Although it is anticipated that eventually these will not require anesthesia, the requirements for patients to hold absolutely still for positioning and to lower blood pressure for perfect stent placement at this time means that anesthesia care and vasoactive management are involved. The high mortality rate of these procedures currently may reflect, as the authors believe, the seriously ill nature of the patients and not a hazard of the technique itself.

M.F. Roizen, M.D.

Anatomical Suitability of Abdominal Aortic Aneurysms for Endovascular Repair

Armon MP, Yusuf SW, Latief K, et al (Univ Hosp, Nottingham, England)

Br J Surg 84:178–180, 1997 2–10

Introduction.—Aneurysm anatomy is important in determining suitability for endovascular repair. The proportions of patients with aortic aneurysms suitable for endovascular repair with 3 different graft-stent systems were assessed.

Methods.—The anatomy of 154 abdominal aortic aneurysms was examined via spiral CT. Measurements were determined for aneurysm neck length and diameter, renal artery to aortic bifurcation length, common iliac artery diameter and length, and external artery diameter. Aneurysms were evaluated for anatomic suitability of 3 currently available devices: aortoaortic, aortobi-iliac, and aortouni-iliac.

Results.—Of 154 patients, 6 (4%) had a distal neck suitable for implantation of a straight aortic graft, 15 (10%) had arterial anatomy suitable for implantation of a bifurcated graft, and 85 (55%) were suitable for endovascular repair using an aortouni-iliac graft. The reasons for unsuitability were: 44 had proximal neck lengths less than 1.5 cm, 12 had proximal neck diameters greater than 3.0 cm, 3 had angulations of the proximal neck, 4 had bilateral common iliac artery aneurysms, 4 had tortuous iliac arteries, and 2 had narrow external iliac arteries.

Conclusion.—Of the currently available endovascular systems, the aortouni-iliac device has the most extensive applicability. For most patients, open repair is the only viable option.

▶ One wonders whether, with the perfection of the endovascular technique, the need for anesthesia for vascular repair will substantially diminish. This article implied that perhaps as much as 50% of the anesthesia used for abdominal aortic aneurysms may disappear if the endovascular repair can be done without anesthesia.

M.F. Roizen, M.D.

Endotoxin Related Early Neutrophil Activation Is Associated With Outcome After Thoracoabdominal Aortic Aneurysm Repair

Foulds S, Cheshire NJ, Schachter M, et al (Imperial College School of Medicine St Mary's, London)

Br J Surg 84:172–177, 1997 2–11

Introduction.—Patients undergoing surgical repair of thoracoabdominal aortic aneurysm (TAAA) have a high mortality, particularly if they experience problems with renal and pulmonary function postoperatively. These complications may involve a systemic inflammatory response syndrome mediated by activated polymorphonuclear neutrophils (PMNs). Previous studies have documented PMN activation during surgery for thoracoabdominal and infrarenal aneurysms, but have not shown any link with postoperative complications. Patients undergoing TAAA surgery were studied to assess the potential relationship between intraoperative PMN activation and postoperative outcomes.

Methods.—The study included 21 consecutive patients undergoing TAAA repair. Flow cytometry measurement of surface CD11b expression was determined as an indicator of perioperative PMN activation. Plasma endotoxin, endotoxin core antibody, tumor necrosis factor (TNF), and interleukin-1 were measured as well. The occurrence of postoperative renal and respiratory failure was assessed.

Results.—Pulmonary or respiratory failure occurred in 11 patients; 10 recovered without complications. The patients with complications had significantly higher intraoperative PMN CD11b expression than those who recovered uneventfully. Plasma endotoxin level increased and antibody level decreased—reflecting binding by absorbed endotoxin—before CD11b expression during visceral reperfusion. These alterations were significantly greater in the group that experienced complications. There was a significant correlation between plasma endotoxin level and CD11b expression. Intraoperative plasma TNF and IL-1 were not significantly different between the complication and uncomplicated groups, nor were aortic cross-clamp times and blood transfusion volumes.

Conclusions.—In patients undergoing TAAA repair, neutrophil activation during surgery is related to the occurrence of postoperative renal and respiratory failure. Intraoperative neutrophil activation is also related to endotoxin absorption. If the mechanisms of PMN activation and neutrophil-mediated organ damage can be identified, it may lead to treatments to reduce the morbidity and mortality of TAAA surgery.

▶ This study shows that patients who have neutrophil activation during their surgery have more complications postoperatively. Although this is logical, it is probably unanticipated that such early activation would be detectable and so predictive. Perhaps it is like the epinephrine story, "that people who are stressed," or have (in this case) neutrophil activation stress, "go on to have adverse outcomes after surgery."

M.F. Roizen, M.D.

The Effect of Digoxin on Mortality and Morbidity in Patients With Heart Failure

Garg R, and the Digitalis Investigation Group (Mount Sinai Med Ctr, New York)

N Engl J Med 336:525–533, 1997 2–12

Background.—Digoxin is a commonly used to treat heart failure, but its long-term safety and efficacy are unclear. Recent studies have shown that discontinuing digoxin in patients with heart failure can worsen functional status, exercise capacity, and left ventricular ejection fraction. The effects of digoxin on hospitalization and mortality rates in patients with heart failure were assessed in a randomized, double-blind, placebo-controlled trial.

Methods.—Patients with heart failure and a left ventricular ejection fraction of 0.45 or less were treated with digoxin or placebo, plus angiotensin-converting enzyme inhibitors and diuretics. The median dose of digoxin was 0.25 mg per day. The average follow-up time was 37 months. In a substudy of patients with a left ventricular ejection fraction of 0.45 or more, 492 patients were treated with digoxin, and 496 were given placebo.

Results.—In the main study, mortality was similar in both groups of patients (Fig 3). In patients treated with digoxin, there was a trend toward a lower risk of death from worsening heart failure. Also, for patients treated with digoxin, the hospitalization rate was 6% less than for patients given placebo, and fewer patients were admitted for worsening heart failure. In the substudy, the mortality and hospitalization rates from worsening heart failure were consistent with the rates in the main study.

Discussion.—In these patients, digoxin did not affect overall mortality in patients also receiving angiotensin-converting enzyme inhibitors and

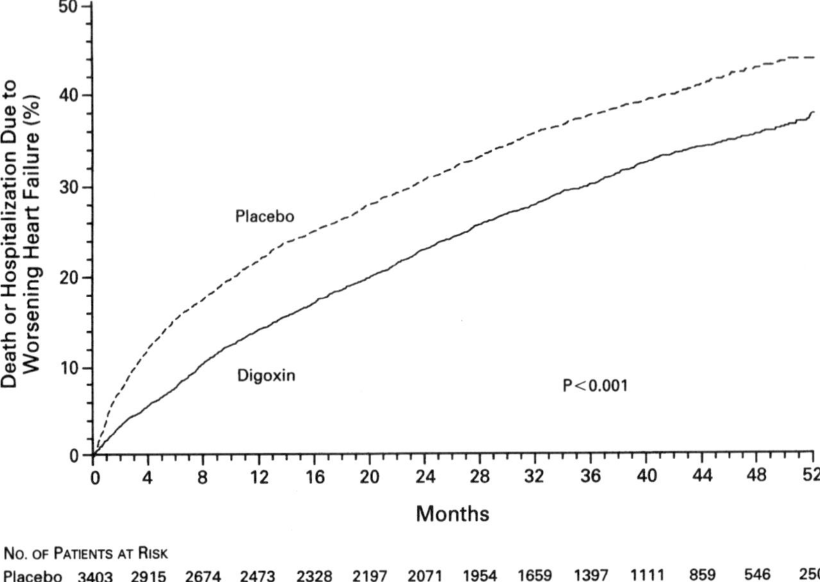

No. of Patients at Risk

Placebo	3403	2915	2674	2473	2328	2197	2071	1954	1659	1397	1111	859	546	250
Digoxin	3397	3120	2888	2696	2544	2392	2241	2115	1825	1521	1188	916	578	255

FIGURE 3.—Incidence of death or hospitalization due to worsening heart failure in the digoxin and placebo groups. The number of patients at risk at each 4-month interval is shown below the figure. (Reprinted by permission of *The New England Journal of Medicine*, from Garg R, and the Digitalis Investigation Group: The effect of digoxin on mortality and morbidity in patients with heart failure. *N Engl J Med* 336:525–533. Copyright 1997, Massachusetts Medical Society. All rights reserved.)

diuretics, but it did lower the death and hospitalization rates from worsening heart failure. In clinical practice, it is unlikely that digoxin would affect survival rates.

► It is hard to believe that a drug that has been in existence for over 200 years continues to be at the center of medical controversy. Unfortunately, this large multicenter study raises as many questions as it answers. Although it appears that digoxin decreases the risk of hospitalization and death from congestive heart failure (CHF), it may increase cardiac morbidity by predisposing patients to malignant arrhythmias and heart block, irrespective of serum digoxin levels. By showing that overall mortality is not altered by digoxin use, this study will be the basis for physicians who are concerned about digoxin toxicity to only prescribe this drug when other agents, such as angiotension-converting enzyme inhibitors or β-adrenergic antagonists, fail to improve CHF symptoms.

D.M. Rothenberg, M.D.

Laboratory Evaluation of Hemostasis Before Cardiac Operations
de Moerloose P (Universitaire de Genèva)
Ann Thorac Surg 62:1921–1925, 1996 2–13

Objective.—Preoperative coagulation tests are widely performed to determine patients' bleeding tendencies. However, research has shown that the clinical history is the best approach to screening for bleeding disorders. For patients undergoing cardiac operations with cardiopulmonary bypass, however, some routine coagulation tests may still be indicated. The literature was reviewed to make simple, clinically relevant recommendations for coagulation testing before cardiac operations.

Findings.—The literature of preoperative coagulation testing includes few carefully controlled, randomized trials. However, the available evidence suggests that it may be appropriate to perform a few, inexpensive tests of hemostasis in asymptomatic patients who are to undergo cardiac surgery. The main reason for these tests—including a platelet count, activated partial thromboplastin time, and prothrombin time—is to determine baseline values for patients who are about to experience a major hemostatic challenge. Other tests have been shown to be of little value in predicting bleeding during or after cardiac surgery in asymptomatic patients; these include fibrinogen testing, bleeding and thrombin times, and urea clot lysis.

More thorough coagulation testing may be indicated in patients who have a history of bleeding, physical signs of bleeding complications, or comorbid conditions affecting hemostasis. Tests to consider in this situation include bleeding time, fibrinogen testing, thrombin time, and sometimes even platelet aggregation tests, factor XIII dosage studies, and α_2-antiplasmin. Consultation with a specialist in hemostasis should be sought, since abnormal results of these tests could have important treatment implications.

Discussion.—The most important consideration in the detection of bleeding disorders before cardiac surgery is a careful medical history. For asymptomatic patients undergoing cardiac operations, only a limited coagulation profile is needed preoperatively. More extensive tests may be indicated for patients with a history of bleeding. The lack of randomized, controlled trials makes it difficult to make definitive recommendations about routine preoperative coagulation testing.

▶ This is an interesting article in that, after the authors reviewed the data, they find that nothing is useful but still recommend a platelet count, activated partial thromboplastin time, and prothrombin time before operation "as baseline." It is interesting that, as scientists, they could not find any reason to do anything, but as clinicians they still want something to hold in their hands, even though that something is more likely to lead to false-positive results than true-positive results.

M.F. Roizen, M.D.

Chlorhexidine Gluconate 0.12% Oral Rinse Reduces the Incidence of Total Nosocomial Respiratory Infection and Nonprophylactic Systemic Antibiotic Use in Patients Undergoing Heart Surgery

DeRiso AJ II, Ladowski JS, Dillon TA, et al (Lutheran Hosp of Indiana, Fort Wayne)

Chest 109:1556–1561, 1996 2–14

Background.—Selective decontamination of the digestive tract reduces aerobic bacterial colonization of the oropharyngeal and intestinal surfaces without changing anaerobic flora, thereby decreasing nosocomial infection rates. Most clinical trials of selective decontamination of the digestive tract have reported lower rates of nosocomial respiratory infection, but it has been difficult to evaluate the results of these trials because of differences in design, population, and definition of pneumonia. Most studies have also reported inconsistent effects on survival, and recent studies have documented the high cost of this treatment. There is also concern about the development of antibiotic-resistant bacteria from studies of aerosolized antibiotics.

Methods.—In a prospective, randomized, double blind, placebo-controlled trial, 353 consecutive patients received chlorhexidine gluconate, 0.12%, oral rinse, or placebo. Patients had undergone coronary artery bypass grafting, valve surgery, septal surgery, cardiac tumor excision, or combined coronary artery bypass grafting valve surgery.

Results.—Overall, the rate of nosocomial infection decreased by 65% in patients treated with chlorhexidine gluconate. The total number of respiratory tract infections was reduced by 69% in patients treated with chlorhexidine gluconate. Gram-negative organisms were involved in 59% fewer nosocomial infections and 67% fewer respiratory tract infections. There was no change in bacterial antibiotic resistance in either group. In patients treated with chlorhexidine gluconate, the use of nonprophylactic IV antibiotics was 43% less; mortality was also lower.

Discussion.—These findings show that treatment with chlorhexidine gluconate can reduce the rate of nosocomial infections and the use of nonprophylactic IV antibiotics after cardiac surgery. This treatment may improve mortality and can significantly reduce costs. Future research may be directed at assessing (1) the effect of chlorhexidine gluconate on mortality among groups of patients with similar mortality risks, (2) the value of chlorhexidine gluconate in patients with AIDS as protection against pneumocystis or other lung infection, and (3) its general value in patients in ICUs.

► Anesthesia gets blamed for many different types of adverse perioperative outcomes, including wound infections. Cardiac surgeons are among the most likely to blame us for external wound infections, despite the fact that they often stand there after bypass with the firestick, not just cooking the sternum, but actually charring it. They somehow have convinced themselves that that char is, in fact, not a full-thickness burn with extensive areas of tissue injury surrounding each blackened portion. Sometimes we do have the blood pressure a tad high, though.

This paper is one of several recent studies reporting that nosocomial infections have been reduced by simple measures such as oral and nasal application of antibiotics preoperatively. It is such a good idea, so simple, and without much expectation of side effects, that we probably should have been doing it routinely all along.

J.H. Tinker, M.D.

3 Perioperative Patient Care

Obstetric Anesthesia and Analgesia

Analgesia for Labor/Vaginal Delivery

Positional Effects on Maternal Cardiac Output During Labor With Epidural Analgesia
Danilenko-Dixon DR, Tefft L, Cohen RA, et al (Brown Univ, Providence, RI)
Am J Obstet Gynecol 175:867–872, 1996 3–1

Background.—To date, no one has quantified the effect of supine position on maternal cardiovascular response to epidural analgesia in labor. Supine gravid women were hypothesized to have greater decrements in cardiac output after epidural analgesia for labor than laterally positioned gravid women.

Methods.—By random assignment, 21 healthy women at term were placed in the left lateral or supine position in early labor. Cardiac output measures were obtained every 5 minutes, beginning before a 500-mL IV fluid bolus and ending 45 minutes after epidural injection.

Findings.—There were significant between-group differences at baseline in mean cardiac output, stroke volume, arterial pressure, and systemic vascular resistance. Heart rate was comparable in the 2 groups. In women placed supine, fluid bolus resulted in a significantly increased cardiac output and stroke volume and reduced mean arterial pressure and systemic vascular resistance. Heart rate was unchanged. Also, cardiac output and stroke volume declined significantly after epidural injection. Patients placed in the lateral position showed no hemodynamic changes after fluid bolus or epidural administration.

Conclusions.—The supine position is associated with a significant postepidural decrement in cardiac output that cannot be identified by a change in heart rate, probably reflecting an inability to maintain stable preload volume in the supine position. Placement in the lateral position does not produce such hemodynamic changes.

► The authors stated that the supine position "is commonly used in the immediate postepidural period, in an effort to optimize analgesic effect, and for vaginal examinations. . . ." Why? Posture has little or no effect on the onset and spread of epidural analgesia. Further, the obstetrician or nurse may perform an adequate examination of the cervix with the patient in the semilateral position. Similarly, the nurse may place a urethral catheter with the patient in the semilateral position.

This study illustrates the hazards of the supine position—with its attendant aortocaval compression—during administration of epidural analgesia in pregnant women. In this study, women in the supine-position group experienced a significant decrease in cardiac output after administration of epidural analgesia.

D.H. Chestnut, M.D.

Does Station of the Fetal Head at Epidural Placement Affect the Position of the Fetal Vertex at Delivery?

Robinson CA, Macones GA, Roth NW, et al (Univ of Pennsylvania, Philadelphia)

Am J Obstet Gynecol 175:991–994, 1996 3–2

Background.—Attempts to clarify the reason for the increased incidence of operative delivery associated with epidural analgesia have been inconclusive. Whether epidural placement before engagement of the fetal head results in an increased incidence of malposition at delivery was investigated.

Methods.—Three hundred twenty records of patients in spontaneous or induced labor who were receiving epidural analgesia were included in the retrospective review. Women with a contraindication to labor, antepartum fetal death, or twin gestations were excluded. Station was classified as high when the fetal vertex was above the level of the maternal ischial spines and low when the vertex was at or below the level of the ischial spines at the time of epidural placement.

Findings.—Placement of the epidural when the fetal station was high significantly increased the relative risk of occiput malposition. This risk persisted, even after controlling for age and birth weight. Cervical dilation was not correlated independently with occiput position at delivery.

Conclusions.—An increased incidence of malposition at delivery is associated with epidural placement before fetal head engagement. These data may help explain why operative delivery is variably increased among patients laboring with epidural anesthesia.

▶ This retrospective study suffers from the limitations that are common to other retrospective studies of epidural analgesia and obstetric outcome, namely, the authors were unable to eliminate the problem of selection bias. It is possible—perhaps even likely—that women with a pre-existing malposition of the fetal occiput are more likely to experience severe pain during early labor. Similarly, it is possible—perhaps even likely—that women with a pre-existing malposition of the fetal occiput are more likely to request epidural analgesia before engagement of the fetal head. Thus, this study calls attention to an association between station of the fetal head "at epidural placement and malposition of the fetal occiput at delivery." However, it does *not* establish a cause-and-effect relation.

D.H. Chestnut, M.D.

Safe Epidural Analgesia in Thirty Parturients With Platelet Counts Between 69,000 and 98,000 mm^{-3}

Beilin Y, Zahn J, Comerford M (Mount Sinai School of Medicine, New York)
Anesth Analg 85:385–388, 1997 3–3

Introduction.—A clinically significant coagulopathy is considered an absolute contraindication to the use of regional anesthetic during labor and delivery, and one author recommends withholding an epidural anesthetic if the patient's platelet count is less than 100,000 mm^{-3}. A retrospective chart review of patients who had such a platelet count during the peripartum period was conducted to determine whether they had neurologic complications related to regional anesthetic or to the labor process.

Methods.—Study participants had given birth during the period from March 1993 through February 1996. A complete blood count with platelets is routinely obtained from all parturients on admission to the labor floor. All epidural anesthetics were administered using the same kit. Charts were reviewed for the cause of thrombocytopenia, type of anesthesia, mode of delivery, and neurologic complications.

Results.—Of the 15,919 women admitted for labor and delivery during the study period, 80 (0.50%) had platelet counts of less than 100,000 mm^{-3}. Thirty (group 1) had an epidural anesthetic placed despite this platelet count, and 20 (group 2) had an epidural anesthetic placed when the platelet count was higher, but their count subsequently fell below 100,000 mm^{-3}. No regional anesthetic was given to 28 women (group 3); in 23 of these cases the anesthesiologist decided to withhold the anesthetic. Platelet counts ranged from 69,000 to 98,000 mm^{-3} in group 1, from 58,000 to 99,000 mm^{-3} in group 2, and from 28,000 to 94,000 mm^{-3} in group 3. No patient had any documented neurologic complication.

Discussion.—Although the minimum platelet count below which it is safe to place a regional anesthetic has not been determined, 30 women in this series safely received an epidural anesthetic when their platelet count was less than 100,000 mm^{-3}. None had a decreasing platelet count at the time of epidural placement and no evidence of bleeding. The decision to use a regional anesthetic should take into account the entire clinical presentation and should not be denied solely on the basis of platelet count.

► The authors correctly stated that "The size of the sample (n = 30) in this study is not large enough to support the claim that regional anesthesia in women with a platelet count of less than 100,000 mm^{-3} is safe." Hanley and Lippman-Hand[1] discussed the interpretation of zero numerators in their excellent article, "If nothing goes wrong, is everything all right?" Nonetheless, I agree with the authors of this study that a platelet count of less than 100,000 mm^{-3} does not represent an absolute contraindication to the administration of regional anesthesia in obstetric patients. I have administered spinal or epidural anesthesia to obstetric patients with a platelet count as low as 70,000 mm^{-3}, and I will continue to do so, provided there is no clinical evidence of abnormal bleeding or coagulopathy.

D.H. Chestnut, M.D.

Reference

1. Hanley JA, Lippman-Hand A: If nothing goes wrong, is everything all right? Interpreting zero numerators. *JAMA* 249:1743, 1983.

Low Dose Epidural Bupivacaine/Fentanyl Infusion Does Not Mask Uterine Rupture

Kelly MC, Hill DA, Wilson DB (Queen's Univ of Belfast, Northern Ireland)

Int J Obstet Anesth 6:52–54, 1997 3–4

Purpose.—In the past, epidural analgesia was not used in laboring women with a previous cesarean section for fear that the analgesia would mask the signs and symptoms of uterine rupture. Despite evidence against this belief, opioids are still frequently omitted in women with a previous cesarean section. A patient whose spinal-epidural analgesia did not mask symptoms and signs of uterine rupture was seen.

Case Report.—Woman, 25, was admitted at 39 weeks' gestation in spontaneous labor at 2-cm cervical dilation. She was para 1, the previous child having been delivered by lower uterine segment cesarean section because of fetal distress. After 4 hours, at the patient's request, she was given a combined spinal-epidural analgesia with epidural infusion of 0.1% bupivacine and 1.5 $\mu g/mL^{-1}$ fentanyl started at 12 mL hr^{-1}. This provided excellent analgesia. Two hours later, the membranes were artificially ruptured and oxytocin was started.

A while later, the patient had sudden, severe breakthrough pain with sweating and tachycardia. An additional 8 mL epidural bolus of 0.1% bupivacine and 1.5 $\mu g/mL^{-1}$ fentanyl did not relieve the patient's pain. Further questioning revealed shoulder pain that was distinct from the pain of uterine contractures. This raised suspicion of uterine rupture. The fundus was tender to palpation and the cervix was dilated 6–7 cm, with a small amount of vaginal bleeding. The patient was prepared for cesarean section, with 10 mL of 0.5% bupivacaine given epidurally. However, because of intense shoulder pain, the operation was performed using general anesthesia. When the parietal peritoneum was opened, a large amount of free amniotic fluid was discovered. Surgery showed a 2-cm dehiscence of the previous uterine scar. A live infant was delivered with 1 and 5 minute Apgar scores of 7 and 9, respectively. The patient lost an estimated 800 mL of blood.

Discussion.—In this patient, a low-dose epidural bupivacaine and fentanyl infusion did not mask the clinical signs and symptoms of uterine rupture. Prompt recognition of uterine rupture was possible, permitting immediate cesarean section. This case is consistent with the evidence that appropriate doses of local anesthetic and fentanyl do not eliminate pathologic pain in laboring women.

► This case report provides further evidence that epidural analgesia, using a dilute solution of local anesthetic and opioid, does not mask evidence of uterine rupture in patients who undergo a trial of labor after a previous low transverse cesarean section. However, not all patients who experience uterine scar dehiscence have pain, with or without epidural analgesia. Fetal heart rate abnormalities remain the most sensitive sign of uterine rupture.

D.H. Chestnut, M.D.

Anesthesia and the HIV-infected Parturient: A Retrospective Study

Gershon RY, Manning-Williams D (Emory Univ, Atlanta, Ga)

Int J Obstet Anesth 6:76–81, 1997 3–5

Background.—In healthy individuals, general anesthesia may be associated with a transient immunodepression. There is some concern that general anesthesia in HIV-infected parturients might lead to further immune function compromise and peripartum complications. However, there is no evidence to suggest that either general or regional anesthesia has any effect on HIV-related disease in parturients. Whether the mode of anesthesia in HIV-infected parturients had any effect on immunosuppression or acceleration of HIV-associated disease was investigated in a retrospective study.

Methods.—The study included 96 women with known HIV infection who delivered at 1 hospital over a 2-year period. Baseline health status, mode of delivery, mode of anesthesia, and peripartum or postpartum complications were reviewed for each patient.

Findings.—Although none of the patients had symptomatic disease at baseline, many had various types of predelivery morbidity, including venereal disease and IV drug abuse. Anesthesia included 36 regional anesthetics, 11 general anesthetics, and 22 local anesthetics with IV sedation. Twenty-seven patients received no anesthesia. Complication rates were no different among the various anesthetic groups, neither at 24–498 hours nor at 4–6 weeks post partum. In the 2 years after anesthesia, none of the women had neurologic sequelae. Data on CD4/CD8 T-cell lymphocyte counts from the second trimester and 24–48 hours post partum were available in 31 patients. These data showed no deterioration of immune status for women in the various anesthetic groups.

Conclusions.—For laboring women with asymptomatic HIV infection, regional and general anesthesia do not appear to be associated with immunodepression or acceleration of HIV-associated disease. Clinical outcomes and CD4/CD8 ratios are no different among women receiving various types of anesthesia or no anesthesia at all. The usual obstetric and clinical considerations apply in making anesthetic decisions with such patients.

► This study provides further evidence that asymptomatic HIV infection should not affect the choice of anesthesia in obstetric patients. Others have concluded that regional anesthesia is safe in obstetric patients who are infected with HIV. Likewise, autologous epidural blood patch appears to be safe in HIV-infected patients who experience postdural puncture headache.

D.H. Chestnut, M.D.

Addition of Epinephrine to Intrathecal Bupivacaine and Sufentanil for Ambulatory Labor Analgesia

Campbell DC, Banner R, Crone L-A, et al (Univ of Saskatchewan, Saskatoon)

Anesthesiology 86:525–531, 1997 3–6

Background.—The intrathecal combination of sufentanil and bupivacaine provides rapid, effective analgesia of a limited duration for women in labor. Many practitioners are concerned that the use of intrathecal local anesthetics precludes maternal ambulation. Whether adding epinephrine to the combination of sufentanil and bupivacaine would prolong intrathecal analgesia and affect ambulation among laboring women was studied.

Methods.—Thirty-nine patients were included in the prospective, randomized, double-blind study. The patients received either an intrathecal control dose of 10 μg sufentanil plus 2.5 mg bupivacaine plus 0.2 mL normal saline or 10 μg sufentanil plus 2.5 mg bupivacaine plus 0.2 mL of epinephrine.

Findings.—Three women in the control group and 4 in the epinephrine group delivered vaginally before requesting epidural analgesia, and 1 woman in each group needed cesarean delivery before epidural analgesia. In the remaining patients, epinephrine was found to prolong the duration of intrathecal labor analgesia significantly. All 19 women in the control group and 80% in the epinephrine group were able to ambulate (Fig 1).

Conclusions.—Adding epinephrine to the intrathecal combination of sufentanil and bupivacaine significantly prolongs labor analgesia without adversely affecting the mother or fetus. With or without epinephrine, this intrathecal combination provided rapid, profound labor analgesia in the patients studied, permitting most to ambulate.

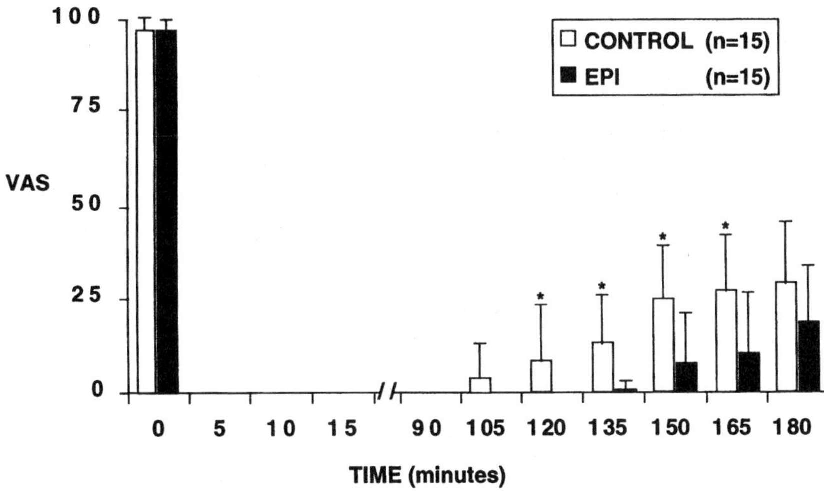

FIGURE 1.—Visual analog scale (VAS) pain scores are shown on the y axis and time (in minutes) after the intrathecal administration of the study solution on the x axis. Time 0 represents VAS scores reported immediately before the intrathecal administration of the study solution. Data are expressd as means ± SD. **P* < 0.05. (Courtesy of Campbell DC, Banner R, Crone L-A, et al: Addition of epinephrine to intrathecal bupivacaine and sufentanil for ambulatory labor analgesia. *Anesthesiology* 86:525–531, 1997. Copyright American Society of Anesthesiologists, Inc. Used with permission of Lippincott-Raven Publishers.)

▶ I have little experience with ambulatory spinal-epidural analgesia in laboring women. In our hospital, few parturients want to ambulate after receiving spinal-epidural analgesia during labor. I remain concerned about the potential for patient injury. The authors of this study correctly noted that "ambulation should only be attempted if there are no obstetrical contraindications; the patient is accompanied by a midwife, nurse, or physician; and there is no evidence of postural hypotension or motor blockade."

D.H. Chestnut, M.D.

Ambulatory Combined Spinal–Epidural Analgesia for Labor: Influence of Epinephrine on Bupivacaine–Sufentanil Combination

Gautier PE, Debry F, Fanard L, et al (Clinique Ste Anne-St Remi, Brussels, Begium)

Reg Anesth 22:143–149, 1997 3–7

Introduction.—The effects of subarachnoid sufentanil, 5 µg, in laboring women are variable. When bupivacaine, 1 mg, is added, the result is good labor analgesia lasting 100 minutes on average. The further effects of adding epinephrine, 25 µg, were investigated.

Methods.—The randomized, double-blind trial included 42 laboring women with cervical dilation of less than 5 cm. Through a combined spinal-epidural technique, all women received sufentanil 5 µg and bupivacaine, 1 mg. One group received epinephrine, 25 µg, as well. A visual analogue scale was used to evaluate analgesia. Also assessed were time until additional analgesia was required, blood pressure, heart rate, sensory levels, motor block, and side effects (pruritus, nausea, and sedation).

Results.—The mean duration of analgesia was 142 minutes in patients who received epinephrine vs. 104 minutes in those who did not. In addition, the median cephalad level of sensory block was T6 with epinephrine vs. T3 without epinephrine. There was no significant difference in the incidence of side effects or in motor performance. A 20% reduction in mean arterial blood pressure occurred in 9 patients in the epinephrine group vs. 5 patients in the control group, though the difference was nonsignificant.

Conclusions.—In laboring women, adding epinephrine to combined spinal-epidural analgesia significantly lengthens the duration of analgesia. Analgesia occurs with a low sensory block level and no motor block. Hypotension is a possible late side effect.

► The authors noted that administration of this regimen involves the mixing of 3 drugs—after prior dilution of 2 of the 3 drugs. The potential for human error is great, which dampens my enthusiasm for this regimen.

D.H. Chestnut, M.D.

Duration of Intrathecal Labor Analgesia: Early Versus Advanced Labor

Viscomi CM, Rathmell JP, Pace NL (Univ of Utah, Salt Lake City; Univ of Vermont, Burlington)

Anesth Analg 84:1108–1112, 1997 3–8

Objective.—The pain experienced during the early first stage of labor is mainly visceral in origin. In the late first stage and second stage, pain increases in intensity and shifts to somatic nociceptive input. Little is known about how the shift to nociceptive input affects the duration of intrathecal labor analgesia. This issue was studied in a prospective, observational study.

Methods.—The study included 41 laboring women receiving a combined spinal-epidural analgesia technique, consisting of 10 μg of intrathecal sufentanil and 2.5 mg of bupivacaine. Eighteen women received analgesia during early labor, at 3- to 5-cm dilation. The other 23 patients received analgesia during advanced labor, i.e., 7- to 10-cm dilation. The patients rated their pain on a verbal scale of 0–10 before and after injection of the intrathecal anesthetic. The women in early and advanced labor were compared for duration of analgesia, defined as the time to a pain score of greater than 5 or until a request for supplemental epidural analgesia.

Results.—The 2 groups were similar in their baseline characteristics, including baseline pain scores. The mean duration of spinal analgesia was 120 minutes for women injected in advanced labor vs. 163 minutes for those injected in early labor (Fig 1). Mean time from injection to delivery was 116 vs. 281 minutes, respectively. The outcomes of labor and neonatal Apgar scores were similar for the 2 groups.

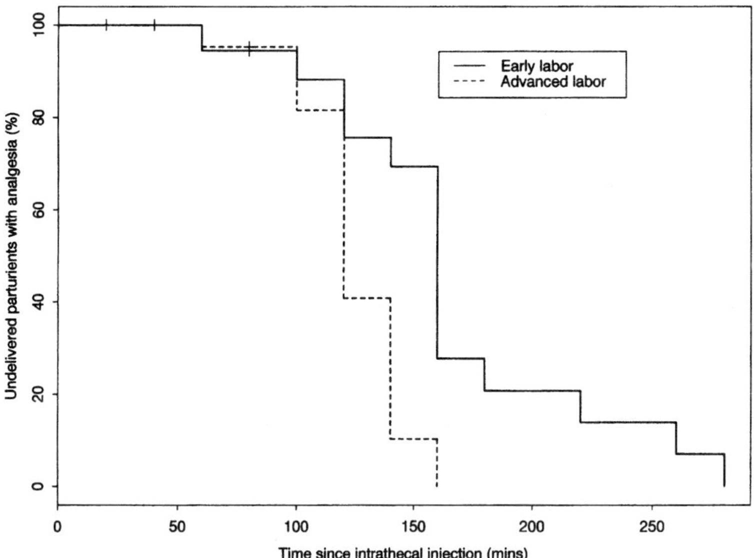

FIGURE 1.—Proportion of group E (early labor) and group A (advanced labor) patients with effective spinal analgesia vs. time after spinal injection. Patients delivering before the loss of spinal analgesia are included until the time of delivery. (Courtesy of Viscomi CM, Rathmell JP, Pace NL: Duration of intrathecal labor analgesia: Early versus advanced labor. *Anesth Analg* 84[5]:1108–1112, 1997).

Conclusions.—The duration of intrathecal sufentanil plus bupivacaine analgesia during labor is longer when the injection is made during early vs. advanced labor. Prompted by these results, the investigators now start epidural infusions about 45 minutes before loss of spinal analgesia is anticipated and give fewer single-shot spinal injections for analgesia during advanced labor. The difference in analgesia duration between early and advanced labor should be considered in future studies of labor analgesia techniques.

▶ These results are not surprising, given the fact that during advanced labor, uterine contractions typically have greater duration and intensity than during early labor. Further, during early labor, pain primarily results from cervical dilation. In contrast, during advanced labor, pain results from both cervical dilation and descent of the fetal head through the pelvis. Others have noted that intrathecal opioids relieve the visceral pain of cervical dilation more effectively than they relieve the somatic pain that occurs during advanced labor.

D.H. Chestnut, M.D.

A Comparison of Multiport and Uniport Epidural Catheters in Laboring Patients

D'Angelo R, Foss ML, Livesay CH (Wake Forest Univ, Winston-Salem, NC; Portsmouth Naval Hosp, Va)

Anesth Analg 84:1276–1279, 1997 3–9

Background.—It is commonly believed that the use of uniport catheters (those with a single distal port) and multiport catheters (those with 3 lateral ports) affects the incidence of insertion-related complications during epidural catheterization. However, there is debate concerning the risks and benefits of each type of catheter. The complication rates associated with multiport vs. uniport epidural catheters were compared in a randomized trial.

Methods.—The study included 500 women in active labor who requested epidural anesthesia. They were randomly assigned to epidural catheterization with a multiport or uniport catheter. Each catheter was inserted 6 cm into the epidural space. The results of catheterization, including complication rates, were compared for the 2 groups.

Results.—The final analysis included 487 patients. The 2 groups were comparable in their demographic characteristics, catheter insertion interspace, depth to the epidural space, and other characteristics. Patients in the multiport catheter group were less likely to have inadequate catheterization and to require catheter manipulation. There were no differences in the number of patients with no analgesia, IV cannulation, or epidural catheter dislodgment. There were no cases of multicompartment placement in the multiport catheter group.

Conclusions.—For women in labor receiving epidural analgesia, multiport catheters are associated with less inadequate analgesia and require manipulation less often than uniport catheters. There is no difference in the rate of other complications.

▶ This study confirms a long-standing bias of mine—namely, that multiport epidural catheters provide satisfactory analgesia more consistently than single-orifice catheters. Further, the multiport catheters require manipulation less often than single-orifice catheters. The authors observed no difference between multiport catheters and single-orifice catheters in the incidence of IV cannulation. Further, they observed no evidence of multicompartment placement of a multiport epidural catheter in the present study.

D.H. Chestnut, M.D.

Intrathecal Sufentanil for Labor Analgesia: Do Sensory Changes Predict Better Analgesia and Greater Hypotension?

Riley ET, Ratner EF, Cohen SE (Stanford Univ, Calif)

Anesth Analg 84:346–351, 1997 3–10

Introduction.—Intrathecal sufentanil (ITS), when given for pain relief during labor, can cause sensory changes and hypotension. Whether sensory changes predict hemodynamic changes or duration of pain relief was determined in a randomized study of women in active labor. Also examined was the effect of different concentrations of ITS on sensory and hemodynamic changes.

Methods.—Forty-five of 49 women enrolled in the study had complete data for analysis. All participants were ASA physical status I and II and were in the first stage of labor. Randomization was to 10 μg ITS in either 1, 2, or 3 mL or normal saline. Blocks were performed with the woman in the sitting position, using the L2-3 or L3-4 interspace. An observer blinded to treatment recorded verbal pain scores (VPS) on a scale of 0 (no pain) to 10 (worst imaginable pain), blood pressure, and sensory changes to light, touch, pinprick, and cold. Ten assessments were made during the 60 minutes after ITS injection.

Results.—All 3 groups experienced a marked decrease in mean VPS after ITS administration; pain relief was comparable in the 3 groups. Only 1 woman in each group failed to experience excellent anesthesia. Systolic blood pressure (SBP) also decreased to a similar degree in the 3 groups. Sensation to cold was lost by 66% of women and sensation to pinprick by 50%; sensation to light touch developed in 33%. Sensory changes affected equivalent numbers of women in the 3 groups and were relatively short-lived compared with the duration of analgesia. Data from the 3 groups were then pooled and the women divided into 2 groups: those who did and those who did not have blocks to cold and pinprick. Both groups had shown rapid decreases in VPS and SBP, and the presence of sensory changes was not related to the duration or quality of analgesia. The anesthesiologist gave ephedrine to 6 women whose SBP was less than 100 mm Hg and at least 30% less than baseline SBP. Maternal and neonatal outcomes were excellent in all groups.

Conclusion.—Sensory changes and decreased blood pressure were common in women given ITS during active labor, but the sensory changes were not predictive of duration or quality of analgesia or degree of hemodynamic change. Thus analgesia with ITS appears to be predominantly mediated via spinal cord opioid receptors rather than by a local anesthetic action.

► As in their earlier study,[1] the authors observed a high incidence of sensory changes and decreased blood pressure after intrathecal sufentanil administration. In the present study, the authors demonstrated "the separation of sensory changes and analgesia," which is inconsistent with a clinically important local anesthetic mechanism of intrathecal sufentanil analgesia.

Nonetheless, 6 patients required ephedrine for treatment of hypotension. This illustrates the importance of establishing IV access and monitoring maternal blood pressure in women who receive intrathecal opioid analgesia during labor.

D.H. Chestnut, M.D.

Reference

1. Cohen SE, Cherry CM, Holbrook RH, et al: Intrathecal sufentanil for labor analgesia: Sensory changes, side effects, and fetal heart rate changes. *Anesth Analg* 77:1155–1160, 1993.

Intrathecal Sufentanil for Labor Analgesia Does Not Cause a Sympathectomy

Riley ET, Walker D, Hamilton CL, et al (Stanford Univ, Calif)

Anesthesiology 87:874–878, 1997 3–11

Background.—Although intrathecal sufentanil (ITS), which is used to provide analgesia during labor, lowers blood pressure during labor, the mechanism of this effect is not known. These authors examined whether this decrease is caused by a sympathectomy or by pain relief in women during labor, by comparing patients given ITS with a control group of women receiving spinal anesthesia with bupivacaine (in whom sympathectomy was expected because of the anesthetic's blockade).

Methods.—The study group consisted of 10 parturients who received 10 µg of ITS. The control group consisted of 10 parturients undergoing elective cesarean section who received 12 mg hyperbaric bupivacaine, 200 µg morphine, and 10 µg fentanyl delivered as spinal anesthetics. No patient had diabetes or pregnancy-induced hypertension. Probes measured temperatures in the right great toe, the lateral midcalf, and the rectum or eardrum. Temperature changes between the toe and the calf were taken as a measure of vasodilation, because the toe temperature is very sensitive to vasodilation, whereas the calf temperature is relatively constant. Pain was assessed on a 10-item verbal pain scale.

Findings.—Both drugs achieved excellent pain control. In the group receiving ITS, none of the temperature measures changed significantly from a clinical point of view. In the control group, however, the toe temperature increased significantly, the change between the toe and the calf temperature decreased significantly, and tympanic or rectal temperatures decreased significantly, indicating vasodilation.

Conclusion.—The temperature changes in the control group were as expected and reflected the vasodilation and sympathetic blockade induced by the spinal anesthesia. However, no temperature changes occurred in the ITS group, indicating that no vasodilation occurred. Thus, the decrease in blood pressure after ITS is likely not caused by sympathectomy, but rather by pain relief. The authors speculate that this analgesic effect occurs via an opioid interaction in the afferent limb of the sympathetic nervous system.

► The authors used novel methods to confirm their hypothesis that the decrease in blood pressure often seen after intrathecal sufentanil administration during labor is not a result of a sympathectomy. Rather, the blood pressure decrease often observed after intrathecal sufentanil administration is, most likely, a result of pain relief.

D.H. Chestnut, M.D.

Maternal Posture Influences the Extent of Sensory Block Produced by Intrathecal Dextrose-free Bupivacaine With Fentanyl for Labor Analgesia

Richardson MG, Thakur R, Abramowicz JS, et al (Univ of Rochester, NY)
Anesth Analg 83:1229–1233, 1996 3–12

Background.—Intrathecal (IT) dextrose free local anesthetics and opioids produce a variable cephalad degree of sensory block. Most studies of the effects of IT analgesics have not controlled for patient posture. Because such agents are hypobaric relative to CSF, parturients who are sitting may have greater cephalad sensory block than those positioned laterally during IT injection.

Methods and Findings.—Twenty-four healthy women in labor were randomly assigned to a sitting or lateral position during IT administration of dextrose free bupivacaine 0.25% with fentanyl 0.005%. The extent of sensory block was assessed at different intervals. Free CSF flow was achieved in 20 participants. Women who were sitting during IT injection had a significantly greater maximal cephalad extent of block than those in a lateral position. The mean cephalad extent of block was greater in sitting parturients at 20 and 30 minutes. When sensory block was asymmetric, the extent of block was greater on the nondependent side.

Conclusions.—The position of the patient affects the extent of sensory block in laboring parturients after IT injection of a 0.25% bupivacaine and fentanyl mixture. Positioning did not influence other clinical variables in the series. Studies of the effects of non–dextrose-containing IT solutions need to specify patient posture at the time of and after IT injection.

► These results are not surprising. Posture affects the spread of *intrathecally* administered local anesthetics, opioids, or both. In contrast, posture has little—if any—effect on the spread of *epidurally* administered local anesthetics and opioids.

D.H. Chestnut, M.D.

Does Combined Spinal–Epidural Analgesia With Subarachnoid Sufentanil Increase the Incidence of Emergency Cesarean Delivery?

Albright GA, Forster RM (Bellevue Woman's Hosp, Niskayuna, NY)

Reg Anesth 22:400–405, 1997 3–13

Background.—It is suspected that the treatment of maternal pain with analgesics during labor causes an imbalance in plasma epinephrine and norepinephrine levels. This imbalance contributes to arterial spasm, which reduces uteroplacental blood flow and thus promotes fetal bradycardia. If so, might the speed of pain relief (and thus a more immediate epinephrine imbalance) be associated with a greater occurrence of fetal distress? The need for emergency cesarean section for fetal distress in women receiving combined spinal-epidural (CSE) analgesia with sufentanil (a quick-acting analgesic) was compared with that in women receiving systemic or no medications (S/NM) during labor.

Methods.—Over 14 months, 1,217 patients received CSE analgesia with subarachnoid sufentanil, 1,140 patients received S/NM, and 296 patients underwent an unplanned cesarean delivery. Cesarean sections were classified as emergencies (surgery needed immediately), urgent (first available operating time), semiurgent (when the surgery could be fit in without delaying the operating room schedule), and nonurgent (when convenient for the surgical team).

Findings.—The 168 cesarean deliveries (13.8%) in the CSE group included 16 emergency, 58 urgent, 70 semiurgent, and 24 nonurgent deliveries. The 128 cesarean deliveries (11.2%) in the S/NM group included 16 emergency, 43 urgent, and 69 semiurgent deliveries. There were 16 emergency cesarean deliveries in each group, for a rate of 1.3% in the CSE group and 1.4% in the S/NM group. Significantly more patients undergoing emergency cesarean delivery in the S/NM group required general anesthesia (8, or 50%) than those receiving CSE (1, or 6%). In all 5 of the cases in which fetal distress occurred less than 90 minutes after CSE, confounding obstetric factors were present, including rupture of the membranes, shoulder cord compression, oligohydramnios, and meconium fluid staining.

Conclusions.—Patients who received CSE analgesia with subarachnoid sufentanil were not at significantly higher risk of cesarean deliveries than patients receiving systemic or no analgesics. Rates of emergency surgeries were comparable between the groups, and in fact patients receiving CSE analgesia were significantly less likely to require general anesthesia. Fetal distress that developed within 90 minutes of CSE administration occurred only in cases with confounding obstetric factors. Although these results should be extrapolated with care to other types of patients, they do argue for further examination of the association between CSE analgesia and fetal distress during labor.

▶ Some anesthesiologists have expressed concern that intrathecal administration of a lipid-soluble opioid (e.g., sufentanil, fentanyl) might result in an increased incidence of fetal bradycardia and emergency cesarean section. In this retrospective review of outcome at a community women's hospital, women who received CSE analgesia with intrathecal sufentanil did not have a higher incidence of emergency cesarean section, when compared with women who received systemic opioids or no medication. The authors cautioned that these results are not necessarily applicable to "high-risk obstetric patients with a precarious uteroplacental blood flow."

D.H. Chestnut, M.D.

Epidural Analgesia Compared With Combined Spinal–Epidural Analgesia During Labor in Nulliparous Women

Nageotte MP, Larson D, Rumney PJ, et al (Long Beach Mem Med Ctr, Calif; Univ of California, San Diego)

N Engl J Med 337:1715–1719, 1997 3–14

Introduction.—For pain relief during labor, lumbar epidural analgesia is the most commonly used form of regional blockade. Substantial sensory and motor blockade commonly results with segmental analgesia, and women are unable to walk. The combination of spinal and epidural analgesia is an alternative but less commonly used form of intrapartum analgesia. The result is satisfactory analgesia without motor blockade. The use of conventional lumbar epidural analgesia for pain relief during labor has been associated with an increased rate of operative delivery. A study of the safety and benefits of spinal or epidural administration of a narcotic agent compared with conventional intrapartum epidural analgesia has not been conducted. In nulliparous women in spontaneous labor at term, continuous lumbar epidural analgesia was compared with the combination of spinal and epidural analgesia.

Methods.—A total of 761 nulliparous women in spontaneous labor at term requested epidural analgesia. They were randomly assigned to receive either a combination of spinal and epidural analgesia or continuous lumbar epidural analgesia. Some of the women who received combined spinal-epidural analgesia were discouraged from walking, whereas others were encouraged to walk. In the 2 groups, a comparison was made of maternal and neonatal outcomes, the incidence of dystocia necessitating cesarean section, and measures of patients' satisfaction.

Results.—Between the 2 groups, there were no significant differences in the overall rate of cesarean section, the frequency of maternal or fetal complications, the incidence of dystocia, the degree of overall satisfaction, or the patients' or nursing staff's assessment of the adequacy of analgesia. Pruritus occurred in significantly more women receiving combined spinal-epidural analgesia, and they requested additional epidural bolus doses of local anesthetic. When analgesia was administered with the fetal vertex at a negative station or at less than 4 cm of cervical dilatation, dystocia necessitating cesarean section was significantly more likely for all the women.

Conclusions.—An overall decrease in the incidence of cesarean delivery is not associated with the combination of spinal and epidural analgesia as compared with continuous lumbar epidural analgesia.

▶ Women have the right to receive safe, excellent analgesia during labor. Combined spinal and epidural analgesia is a new technique in which intrathecal administration of an opioid through a very fine spinal needle is combined with low-dose local anesthetic and opioid administration through a catheter. This is an important, well-performed prospective randomized study. However, as David Birnbach[1] states in an accompanying editorial, it does not answer the question—what is the effect of epidural analgesia on the risk of cesarean section? This question could not be answered because the authors did not include a control group of women who did not receive neuraxial analgesia.

M. Wood, M.D.

Reference

1. Birnbach DJ: Analgesia for labor (editorial). *N Engl J Med* 337:1764–1766, 1997.

The Effect of Instituting an Elective Labor Epidural Program on the Operative Delivery Rate

Lyon DS, Knuckles G, Whitaker E, et al (Univ of Florida, Jacksonville; United States Air Force Med Corps, Andrews Air Force Base, Md)

Obstet Gynecol 90:135–141, 1997 3–15

Introduction.—A policy change by the United States Department of Defense resulted in the immediate availability of elective labor epidural analgesia. Before October 1, 1993, the use of epidural analgesia for patients in labor was usually in response to urgent obstetrician requests. The labor outcome and maternal and neonatal morbidity before and after the initiation of elective labor epidural analgesia were assessed.

Methods.—Prelabor and labor characteristics and outcomes were examined for the year before policy change in 373 women (group 1) and 421 women in the year after policy change (group 2). All women evaluated were nulliparous and were delivering singleton, vertex fetuses at 36–42 weeks' gestation age. Forty-nine women who received labor epidurals before policy change were compared with the 247 women in the group who received epidurals after their ready availability.

Results.—Women in group 2 had a 10-minute prolongation of the second stage of labor and an increased incidence of diagnosed chorioamnionitis, compared to women in group 1. Women in each time frame were evaluated to determine epidural-related factors, compared to factors related to intrinsically more problematic labors. Findings related to epidural use were slight prolongation of the second stage of labor, increased use of oxytocin, and increased incidence of diagnosed chorioamnionitis.

Conclusion.—There was no increase in the rate of operative deliveries after a policy change that allowed elective labor epidural analgesia in a setting where it was previously available only upon urgent obstetrician requests. There was no increase in morbidity or mortality for mothers or fetuses after policy change. The epidural option may be offered without compromising safety for comfort.

▶ This is another study that demonstrates that an abrupt increase in the use of epidural analgesia during labor did not result in an increase in the cesarean section rate in nulliparous women at term.

D.H. Chestnut, M.D.

The Dermatomal Spread of Epidural Bupivacaine With and Without Prior Intrathecal Sufentanil

Leighton BL, Arkoosh VA, Huffnagle S, et al (Thomas Jefferson Univ, Philadelphia)

Anesth Analg 83:526–529, 1996 3–16

Background.—Combined intrathecal sufentanil and epidural bupivacaine often is used to provide labor analgesia. The influence of 27- or 24-gauge dural-puncture and intrathecal injection of sufentanil 10 μg on

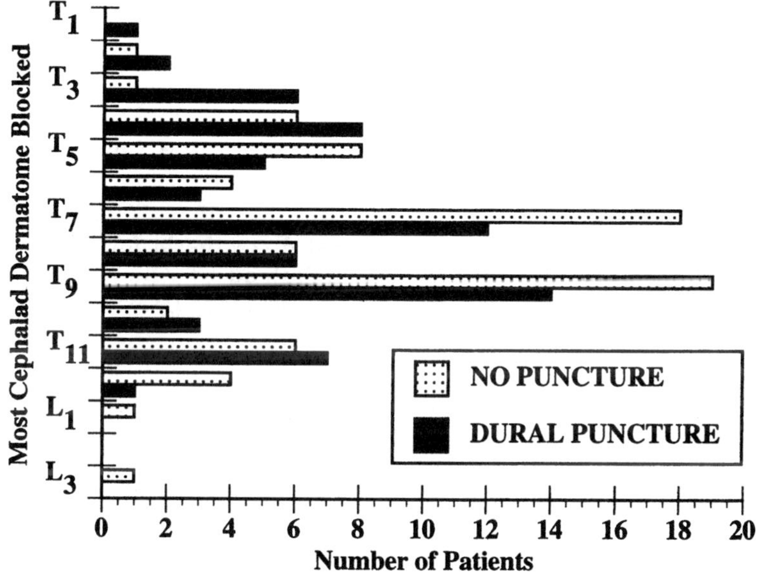

FIGURE 1.—Most cephalad dermatome blocked on either side in patients receiving 27- or 24-gauge dural puncture and intrathecal sufentanil 10 μg (dural-puncture group [*DPG*]) or no dural puncture (no-puncture group [*NPG*]) before epidural injection of 13 mL bupivacaine 0.25%. More patients in the DPG had sensory blockade T4 or higher (17 of 70 DPG patients vs. 8 of 77 NPG patients; $P < 0.05$). (Courtesy of Leighton BL, Arkoosh VA, Huffnagle S, et al: The dermatomal spread of epidural bupivacaine with and without prior intrathecal sufentanil. *Anesth Analg* 83[3]:526–529, 1996.)

the dermatomal spread of subsequent epidural bupivacaine in healthy women in labor was investigated prospectively.

Methods and Findings.—Seventy-seven healthy, laboring women received no dural puncture, 33 received dural puncture with a 27-gauge Whitacre needle, and 37 received a 24-gauge Sprotte needle and intrathecal sufantenil before epidural injection of 13 mL bupivacaine 0.25%. More dermatomes were anesthetized in the dural-puncture group than in the no-puncture group, mean numbers being 16.6 and 13.6. More patients in the former group had sensory blockade T4 or higher. None of the patients in either group had clinical evidence of respiratory compromise (Fig 1).

Conclusions.—Epidural bupivacaine anesthetized more dermatomes after intrathecal sufentanil than when given alone. The appropriate dose of epidural bupivacaine must be determined individually for each woman.

▶ The authors correctly noted that the higher sensory levels observed in the dural-puncture group may have resulted from 1 or both of 2 mechanisms. First, the dural puncture may have enhanced the physical spread of the bupivacaine. Second, the residual intrathecal sufentanil may have potentiated the epidural bupivacaine, even though the bupivacaine was administered 104 ± 42 minutes after intrathecal sufentanil administration.

The authors stopped short of recommending epidural administration of a smaller dose of bupivacaine in patients who have earlier received intrathecal sufentanil. In fact, they noted that the observed difference between the 2 groups (i.e., 2.8 dermatomes) is "unlikely to be important clinically given the large variation seen within each group." This is a curious comment, given that more patients in the dural-puncture group had sensory blockade of T4 or higher than in the no-puncture group.

D.H. Chestnut, M.D.

Anesthesia for Cesarean Section

Prevention of Hypotension During Spinal Anaesthesia for Caesarean Section: Ephedrine Infusion Versus Fluid Preload

Chan WS, Irwin MG, Tong WN, et al (Univ of Hong Kong, China)
Anaesthesia 52:896–913, 1997 3–17

Introduction.—Spinal anesthesia for cesarean section is associated with peripheral vasodilation and decreased systemic vascular resistance, which can cause rapid onset of maternal hypotension. The conventional technique of preloading with crystalloid solution (20 $mg \cdot kg^{-1}$) immediately before spinal anesthesia was compared with prophylactic IV infusion of ephedrine 0.25 $mg \cdot kg^{-1}$ over 3 minutes immediately after injection of intrathecal bupivacaine in 46 women undergoing elective cesarean section.

Methods.—Women were randomly assigned to either the fluid preloading or prophylactic ephedrine group. Both groups were evaluated for the extent of hypotension, uterine blood flow before delivery, neonatal Apgar score, umbilical blood gas data at delivery, and other adverse maternal effects. Moderate and severe hypotension were defined as a 20% or greater or 30% or greater decrease in systolic blood pressure.

Results.—The rate of moderate hypotension was similar for both groups. Compared to patients in the fluid group, patients in the ephedrine group had significantly lower incidence of severe hypotension (35% vs. 65%), higher mean umbilical venous pH (7.33 vs. 7.29), and more shivering (2 vs. 9 women). Baseline systolic pressure after spinal anesthesia was lower from the second to eighth minute in the ephedrine group and the first to the fourteenth minute in the fluid group. There were no significant between-group differences in pre- and postspinal uterine artery pulsatile indices.

Conclusion.—Prophylactic ephedrine infusion was at least as good as fluid preloading alone in preventing hypotension in women undergoing cesarean section. The incidence of severe hypotension and neonatal acidosis was significantly lower in the ephedrine group than the fluid group. These and earlier findings question the need for fluid preloading before spinal anesthesia for cesarean section.

▶ In this study, the incidence of hypotension was high in both groups. No regimen is completely effective in preventing hypotension during administration of spinal anesthesia for cesarean section. In my judgment, a combination of (1) fluid preloading, (2) prophylactic IV ephedrine, and (3) therapeutic ephedrine at the first sign of hypotension represents the most effective regimen for the prevention and treatment of hypotension during spinal anesthesia for cesarean section.

D.H. Chestnut, M.D.

Prevention of Maternal Hypotension by Epidural Administration of Ephedrine Sulfate During Lumbar Epidural Anesthesia for Cesarean Section

Fong J, Gurewitsch ED, Press RA, et al (New York Hosp–Cornell Med Ctr, New York)

Am J Obstet Gynecol 175:985–990, 1996 3–18

Objective.—Lumbar epidural anesthesia commonly results in arterial hypotension in women giving birth that can have deleterious effects on the fetus. Although ephedrine sulfate, a sympathomimetic agent, has been shown to be safe for mother and fetus when used to increase maternal blood pressure occurring after administration of lumbar epidural anesthesia, its prophylactic use has not been successful. The efficacy of epidurally administered ephedrine sulfate in preventing the onset of maternal hypotension when 2% lidocaine is buffered with bicarbonate was tested.

Methods.—In a double-blind, placebo-controlled trial, normal saline or ephedrine sulfate was administered coincidentally with lumbar epidural anesthesia to 50 normotensive pregnant women undergoing cesarean section. All patients were supine on a 15-degree, right-sided wedge when blood pressure was measured as baseline, immediately after induction, at 1-minute intervals for 10 minutes, and every 2.5 minutes after that. Hypotension was defined as a systolic blood pressure 90 mm Hg or less or 70% or less of baseline. Differences between groups were analyzed statistically.

Results.—The mean baseline blood pressures were similar between groups. The incidence of hypotension in the placebo group (24%) was similar to that for the treatment group (32%). There was no difference between groups in weight, prehydration status, attainment of a T4 level under or over 10 minutes, or demographic or operative characteristics.

Conclusion.—In this study, administration of ephedrine sulfate concurrently with lumbar epidural anesthesia did not reduce the incidence of hypotension in pregnant women undergoing cesarean section.

▶ The authors commented on the limitations of prophylactic ephedrine administered either IV or IM during administration of epidural anesthesia. They suggested that prophylactic *IV* ephedrine is ineffective because the circulatory effects occur before the onset of sympathetic blockade associated with epidural anesthesia. Similarly, they suggested that prophylactic *IM* ephedrine is ineffective because of delayed absorption, so that the peak circulatory effects occur after the onset of sympathetic blockade. They speculated that the circulatory effects of prophylactic *epidural* ephedrine might coincide with the circulatory effects of epidural lidocaine anesthesia. Interesting. But how many anesthesiologists give prophylactic ephedrine—by *any* route—during administration of epidural anesthesia for cesarean section? I do not. Further, I have some questions regarding the safety of epidural administration of 35 mg of ephedrine. Perhaps the question is moot, given that the authors of this study observed no benefit of epidural ephedrine.

D.H. Chestnut, M.D.

Maternal Experience During Epidural or Combined Spinal–Epidural Anesthesia for Cesarean Section: A Prospective, Randomized Trial

Davies SJ, Paech MJ, Welch H, et al (King Edward Mem Hosp for Women, Perth, Western Australia)

Anesth Analg 85:607–613, 1997 3–19

Background.—Epidural anesthesia (EA) and combined spinal–epidural anesthesia (CSEA) are common techniques for elective cesarean section. Maternal experience during these 2 techniques was compared in a randomized, blind study.

Methods.—One hundred twenty patients were enrolled in the study. Epidural anesthesia was established using alkalinized 2% lidocaine with epinephrine and fentanyl. Spinal anesthesia was done using 2.5 mL hyperbaric 0.5% bupivacaine and fentanyl through a single-space CSEA approach.

Findings.—Compared with EA, CSEA was associated with earlier onset times, a more intense motor block, and greater ephedrine use. Patients given CSEA had significantly less anxiety and higher satisfaction before the start of surgery. In addition, CSEA was associated with lower preoperative and intraoperative pain scores; the difference was significant during block placement and at delivery. The groups did not differ in the incidence or severity of hypotension and nausea or analgesic supplementation rate. There were also no differences in postoperative assessments of intraoperative pain, anxiety, satisfaction, or postpartum backaches or headaches.

Conclusions.—Both EA and CSEA were associated with low anesthetic failure rates, good operative conditions, and high maternal satisfaction. However, CSEA had several minor advantages over EA.

▶ These results are not surprising. The authors did not include a group of women who received spinal anesthesia alone. It is unclear whether CSEA offers advantages over spinal anesthesia alone for uncomplicated cesarean section. On the other hand, CSEA allows the anesthesiologist to maintain anesthesia during prolonged surgery, and it also allows the anesthesiologist to administer a continuous epidural infusion of a lipid-soluble opioid for postcesarean analgesia.

D.H. Chestnut, M.D.

Combined Spinal–Extradural Anaesthesia for Preterm and Term Caesarean Section: Is There a Difference in Local Anaesthetic Requirements?

James KS, McGrady E, Patrick A (Glasgow Royal Maternity Hosp, Scotland)

Br J Anaesth 78:498–501, 1997 3–20

Objective.—In the United Kingdom, the cesarean section rate is increasing, particularly for preterm births. Whereas some have suggested that preterm (32 weeks' gestation) women require the same amount of anesthesia as term (38 weeks' gestation) women to develop an adequate sensory block, clinical observations have suggested that preterm women need larger doses. Results of a nonblinded observational study testing the null hypothesis that there are no differences in anesthesia requirements between term and preterm women having a cesarean section are presented.

Methods.—A combined spinal-extradural anesthetic (2.25 mL of 0.5% hyperbaric bupivacaine) was administered in the sitting position to 25 term women, aged 29–36 years, and 25 preterm women, aged 25–33.5 years, prior to performing a cesarean section. A suitable sensory block was defined as T4. Block height after subarachnoid injection, supplementary extradural local anesthetic required, maximum block height, time to reach T4, and incidence of hypotension were recorded. The outcome was successful achievement of, or failure to achieve, a suitable block.

Results.—All term women achieved a suitable sensory block, but 21 of preterm women did not (Fig 1). The latter group required a median supplementary dose of 8 mL of 2% lignocaine with 1:200,000 adrenaline.

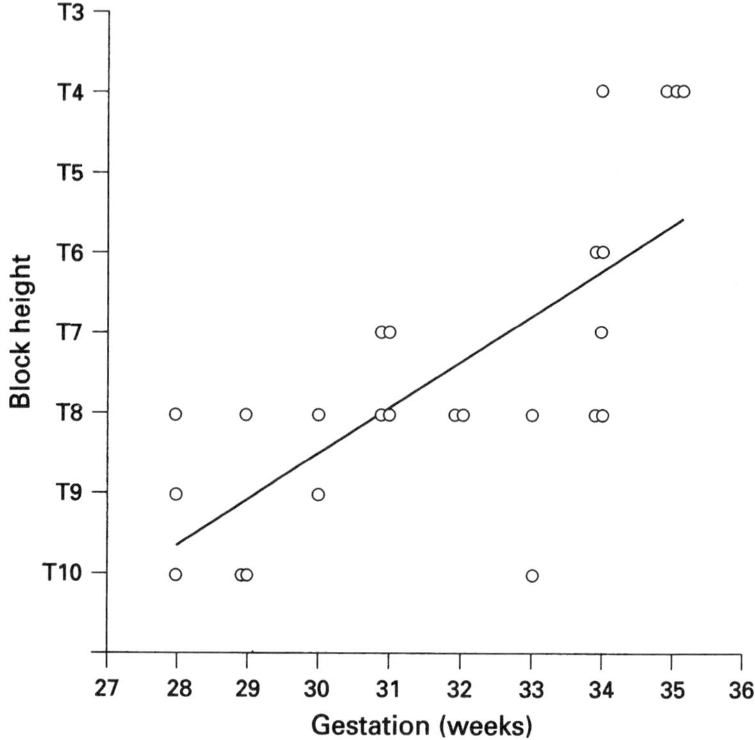

FIGURE 1.—Correlation between maximum sensory block height achieved with subarachnoid anesthesia alone and gestational age. (Reprinted with permission of the BMJ Publishing Group, from James KS, McGrady E, Patrick A: Combined spinal-extradural anesthesia for preterm and term Caesarian section: Is there a difference in local anaesthetic requirements? *Br J Anaesth* 78:498–501, 1997.)

Time to achieve a sensory block was significantly longer in the preterm women than in the term group (15 minutes vs. 5 minutes). Blocks heights were significantly higher in the term than in the preterm group even after administration of supplementary anesthesia to the latter group (T4 vs. T3). The preterm group experienced significantly less hypotension than did the term group.

Conclusion.—Subarachnoid administration of 2.25 mL of 0.5% hyperbaric bupivacaine did not provide a suitable sensory block in 84% of preterm women undergoing cesarean section. Gestation was correlated with a higher block.

▶ The incidence of preterm delivery in the United States now exceeds 10%. Further, patients who deliver preterm are more likely to undergo cesarean section than women who deliver at term. Thus it is disappointing that there are few published studies of anesthetic management of preterm parturients. In the present study, the authors administered spinal anesthesia in the sitting position, with a total dose of 11.25 mg of hyperbaric bupivacaine. All women in the term group developed a sensory level of at least T4, but 21

(84%) of the 25 women in the preterm group failed to achieve a T4 sensory level. It is likely that a greater number of women in the preterm group would have developed a T4 sensory level if the spinal anesthetics had been administered with the patients in the lateral position. The authors noted that "It is difficult to predict accurately the dose for an individual preterm patient, and the combined spinal-extradural technique should be used when time allows. . . ."

D.H. Chestnut, M.D.

Intravenous Oxytocin in Patients Undergoing Elective Cesarean Section
Sarna MC, Soni AK, Gomez M, et al (Harvard Med School, Boston)
Anesth Analg 84:753–756, 1997 3–21

Introduction.—Oxytocin is the drug of choice for facilitating uterine contractions during vaginal and operative delivery, but recommended doses for elective cesarean section vary widely. A randomized, double-blind, dose-response study was designed to establish dose requirements of oxytocin during elective cesarean section.

Methods.—Study participants were 40 healthy term parturients scheduled for elective cesarean section. Thirty-two underwent spinal anesthesia and 8 had epidural anesthesia. Randomization was to oxytocin 5, 10, 15, or 20 IU, administered IV at a rate of 1.0 IU/min via an infusion pump. The infusion was started immediately after clamping of the umbilical cord. Uterine tone was assessed by the attending surgeon, using palpation and a linear analogue scale of 0 (completely atonic) to 10 (fully contracted). Evaluations were recorded at 5, 10, 15, and 20 minutes after the start of oxytocin infusion. Also reported were estimated blood loss and the difference in preoperative and postoperative hematocrit. There was no effort to control postoperative administration of additional oxytocin.

Results.—The 4 groups were similar in all recorded demographics, with the exception of height, at study entry. Linear analogue scale assessments of uterine tone were equal in the 4 groups at each of the 4 recorded intervals. Also similar were the quantity of estimated blood loss and the difference between the preoperative and postoperative hematocrit. Findings were similar for the 17 patients undergoing a primary cesarean section and the 23 having a second (18) or third (5) cesarean section. No patient required ephedrine for hypotension after delivery or supplemental oxytocin in the recovery room.

Conclusion.—The smallest dose of oxytocin (5 IU) was as effective as the largest dose (20 IU) in these healthy parturients undergoing elective cesarean section. All 4 doses were associated with a similar degree of uterine contraction, estimated intraoperative blood loss, and decrease in hematocrit. The uterus is extremely sensitive at this stage of gestation, and the minimal effective dose is preferred because of the drug's dose-dependent side effects.

▶ I remain puzzled when my obstetric colleagues request large doses of oxytocin immediately after cesarean delivery. (I know one obstetrician who occasionally asks the anesthesiologist to administer 60–80 units of oxytocin in a liter of crystalloid after cesarean delivery.) These suprapharmacologic doses are not physiologic, and may incur maternal risk. In the present study, the authors observed no evidence of increased uterine tone or decreased blood loss with administration of more than 5 units of oxytocin—at a rate of 1 unit per minute—in women undergoing elective cesarean section with epidural or spinal anesthesia.

D.H. Chestnut, M.D.

Anesthetic Quality During Cesarean Section Following Subarachnoid or Epidural Administration of Bupivacaine With or Without Fentanyl

Olofsson Ch, Ekblom A, Sköldefors E, et al (Karolinska Hosp, Stockholm; Löwenströmska Hosp, Upplands Väsby, Sweden)

Acta Anaesthesiol Scand 41:332–338, 1997 3–22

Introduction.—It has been argued that subarachnoid administration of local anesthetics offers a more profound and effective blockade than epidural anesthesia. It has also been reported that addition of fentanyl to subarachnoid or epidural anesthesia has a potentiating effect. Not all investigations confirm these findings. Perceived pain and discomfort during surgery and postoperative pain were evaluated in 100 women who underwent elective cesarean section and received subarachnoid or epidural anesthesia with or without fentanyl.

Methods.—Twenty-five women each were randomized as follows: group A, bupivacaine 12.5 mg, plus 10 µg fentanyl subarachnoidally; group B, bupivacaine, 12.5 mg, plus saline subarachnoidally; group C, bupivacaine, 100 mg, plus 100 µg fentanyl epidurally; and group D, bupivacaine, 100 mg, plus saline epidurally. A visual analogue scale was used to evaluate pain intensity and discomfort during surgery. Postoperative pain intensity and need for analgesics were recorded for 24 hours after surgery.

Results.—There were no between-group differences in pain intensity and discomfort in the intraoperative period. In the first 6 hours postoperatively, patients who received local anesthetics subarachnoidally had more intense pain and need for analgesics than patients in the epidural groups. There were no significant between-group differences in blood pressure, oxygen saturation, or side effects. Apgar and neonatal adaptive capacity scores were normal in all neonates.

Conclusion.—The addition of fentanyl to subarachnoid or epidural local anesthetics did not significantly improve the quality of these already profound blockades. Patients who received epidural anesthesia reported less pain and required less analgesics than patients with subarachnoid anesthesia in the first 6 postoperative hours.

► I am not surprised that the intrathecal administration of 10 µg of fentanyl did not enhance intraoperative analgesia in women who received spinal anesthesia with 12.5 mg of bupivacaine. Intrathecal injection of 12.5 mg of bupivacaine provides dense anesthesia for cesarean section, and it is unnecessary to add fentanyl. However, I am surprised that the epidural administration of 100 µg of fentanyl did not enhance the intraoperative analgesia provided by epidural administration of 100 mg of bupivacaine. In my experience, epidural administration of 0.5% bupivacaine alone does not consistently provide adequate anesthesia for cesarean section. Epidural administration of bupivacaine also incurs the risk of maternal cardiotoxicity. For these reasons, I rarely use bupivacaine for administration of epidural anesthesia for cesarean section.

D.H. Chestnut, M.D.

Intrathecal Morphine for Caesarean Section: An Assessment of Pain Relief, Satisfaction and Side-effects

Swart M, Sewell J, Thomas D (Singleton Hosp, Swansea, England)

Anaesthesia 52:373–377, 1997 3–23

Introduction.—Pain after cesarean section has been managed with both low-dose intrathecal morphine and IV patient-controlled analgesia (PCA). The side effects of these techniques raise questions about the advantages of giving spinal opioids. In a double-blind trial, the effects of IV combined with intrathecal morphine or intrathecal placebo were assessed.

Methods.—Sixty women undergoing elective cesarean section with spinal anesthesia were studied. Each patient received intrathecal morphine, 0.1 mg, or intrathecal saline. After surgery, each patient received morphine IV PCA. Through 24 hours, pain, nausea, and satisfaction were assessed by visual analogue scales. Morphine consumption, sedation, itching, and vomiting were also assessed.

Results.—At both 4 and 24 hours, patients receiving intrathecal morphine had less pain than those receiving intrathecal placebo. The intrathecal morphine group also used less IV morphine. However, the use of PCA morphine among patients receiving intrathecal morphine was variable—although 50% of patients used less than 10 mg, 13% used more than 40 mg. Pruritus was greater at 4 hours in the intrathecal morphine group, but satisfaction at this time was not significantly different. Side effects at 24 hours were similar in the 2 groups. Satisfaction at 24 hours was greater in the intrathecal morphine group. There was 1 case of respiratory depression in the intrathecal morphine group.

Conclusions.—Giving intrathecal morphine leads to increased pain relief and patient satisfaction in women undergoing cesarean section with the use of spinal anesthesia. The amount of PCA morphine used after low-dose intrathecal morphine varies widely. Although low-dose intrathecal morphine reduces side effects, it may increase pain in some patients.

► The present study illustrates the variable response to intrathecal administration of 0.1 mg of morphine for postcesarean analgesia. Fifteen of the 30 patients in the intrathecal morphine group required less than 10 mg of IV morphine during the first 24 hours, but 4 women used more than 40 mg of morphine. The occurrence of late respiratory depression in 1 patient—14 hours after surgery—illustrates the need for vigilance in these patients, especially those who receive *both* intrathecal morphine and supplemental, patient-controlled IV morphine.

D.H. Chestnut, M.D.

A Randomized, Double-blind, Dose-response Comparison of Epidural Fentanyl Versus Sufentanil Analgesia After Cesarean Section

Grass JA, Sakima NT, Schmidt R, et al (Cleveland Clinic Found, Ohio; Johns Hopkins Univ, Baltimore, Md; Bethesda Naval Hosp, Md)

Anesth Analg 85:365–371, 1997 3–24

Introduction.—Epidural fentanyl and sufentanil have been shown to provide analgesia during cesarean section (C/S), but there are no reports comparing the efficacy and dose-response of fentanyl with those of sufentanil for postoperative C/S epidural analgesia. The dose-response characteristics, speed of onset, and relative potency of single-dose epidural fentanyl (F) and sufentanil (S) for postoperative pain relief were compared in 80 women undergoing C/S.

Methods.—Women were randomly assigned to receive double-blind epidural administration of F (25, 50, 100, or 200 μg) or S (5, 10, 20, or 30 μg) as needed for postoperative pain relief. There were 10 women in each group. Pain and sedation were evaluated at baseline and at 3, 6, 9, 12, 15, 20, 25, 30, 45, and 60 minutes and every 30 minutes until further analgesia was requested, using visual analogue scales (VAS, 0–100 mm). Women were excluded at 30 minutes if adequate analgesia was not realized.

Results.—There was a dose-response for both opioids. Significantly fewer women achieved a VAS score above 10 mm with F 25 μg and S 5 μg, compared to F 100 or 200 μg and S 20 or 30 μg. The latter group of women with higher doses of medication all achieved VAS scores greater than 10 mm, with no differences in time to 50% decrease in VAS and no differences in duration of analgesia. The 50% effective dose values to achieve a VAS score of greater than 10 mm were F 33 μg and S 6.7 μg. For 95% effective dose values, the doses were F 92 μg and S 17.5 μg. Sedation and side effects were similar among groups.

Conclusion.—Both epidural fentanyl and sufentanil give effective analgesia for about 2 hours in patients recovering from C/S. The analgesic potency ratio was nearly 5:1 for single-bolus epidural sufentanil to fentanyl. When equianalgesic doses were administered, there were no differences between opioids in the onset, duration, or effectiveness of analgesia.

▶ This study was carefully performed, and the authors have fine-tuned their technique. However, readers should note that these "optimal" doses of epidural fentanyl (100 μg) and sufentanil (20 μg) provided postcesarean analgesia of only 2 hours' duration.

D.H. Chestnut, M.D.

Cocaine-abusing Parturients Undergoing Cesarean Section: A Cohort Study

Kain ZN, Mayes LC, Ferris CA, et al (Yale Univ, New Haven, Conn)

Anesthesiology 85:1028–1035, 1996 3–25

Background.—In the United States, cocaine use is prevalent among pregnant women from inner-city neighborhoods. A cohort study determined the anesthetic implications of cocaine use in parturients undergoing cesarean section delivery.

Methods.—Data on substance abuse were obtained in interviews with 1,970 women seeking prenatal care. In addition, urine was analyzed for benzoylecgonine, tetrahydracannabinol, benzodiazepines, and opioids. The records of parturients undergoing cesarean delivery were reviewed for anesthetic and obstetric outcomes.

Findings.—Fifty-one women were classified as cocaine abusers. The most common reasons for cesarean delivery in this group were fetal distress in 48% and abruptio placentae in 21%. A multivariate analysis indicated that cocaine abuse before delivery independently predicted preoperative diastolic hypertension. Univariate analysis showed that, immediately after intubation, diastolic blood pressure was significantly greater in cocaine users. Epidural anesthesia was associated with hypotension significantly more often among cocaine users. Parturients abusing cocaine also had a higher rate of perioperative wheezing, although this finding did not persist in multivariate analysis. Operative blood loss was comparable among groups. There were no episodes of ventricular dysrhythmias or cerebrovascular or coronary ischemia.

Conclusions.—Parturients who abuse cocaine are at a greater risk for interim peripartum events, such as hypertension, hypotension, and wheezing episodes. However, such women do not have significantly increased rates of maternal morbidity or death.

Cocaine Screening of Parturients Without Prenatal Care: An Evaluation of a Rapid Screening Assay

Birnbach DJ, Stein DJ, Grunebaum A, et al (Columbia Univ, New York)
Anesth Analg 84:76–79, 1997 3–26

Background.—Because cocaine use can cause life-threatening arrhythmias and interact with anesthetic agents, anesthesiologists would benefit from knowing a high-risk patient's cocaine status before administering anesthesia. However, the methods commonly used to detect cocaine abuse often require 1–3 days for laboratory processing, so they are not useful in emergent situations. A rapid screening assay was studied.

Methods and Findings.—The new rapid latex agglutination assay for urinary metabolites of cocaine—OnTrak Abuscreen (Roche Diagnostic Systems Inc, Branchburg, NJ)—was compared with EMIT (Syva Co, San Jose, Calif), an in vitro enzyme multiplied immunoassay technique used by many hospital laboratories. One hundred fifty-one urine samples from parturients without prenatal care were tested. The prevalence of cocaine abuse in this group was 68%. The latex agglutination results were exactly concordant with the hospital laboratory findings.

Conclusions.—The latex agglutination test is easy to perform on a busy inner-city labor and delivery ward, yielding results almost instantly. Knowledge of cocaine-abuse status can help optimize patient care.

▶ There is an epidemic of cocaine abuse—even among pregnant women—in the United States. In the first study (Abstract 3–25), the authors did not observe an increased rate of maternal morbidity or mortality among cocaine-abusing parturients undergoing cesarean section. However, because perioperative events such as hypertension, hypotension, and wheezing episodes were more common in cocaine-abusing parturients, one wonders whether the authors studied enough patients to exclude an increased risk for maternal morbidity or mortality.

It often is difficult for the physician to identify the parturient who abuses cocaine. This may be a problem when examining the parturient with hypertension. Often, it is important to distinguish between cocaine-induced hypertension and pregnancy-induced hypertension (i.e., preeclampsia), because the treatment may differ depending on the cause of the hypertension. The second study (Abstract 3–26) describes a rapid latex agglutination assay for urinary metabolites of cocaine, which should help obstetricians and anesthesiologists to rapidly identify the parturient who has used cocaine. Of interest, in this study fetuses of cocaine-positive patients had a twofold greater risk of fetal compromise during labor when compared with fetuses of non–cocaine-abusing mothers.

D.H. Chestnut, M.D.

Coagulation Evaluation and Management in Obstetric Anesthesia

Management of Anticoagulation Before and After Elective Surgery
Kearon C, Hirsh J (McMaster Univ, Hamilton, Ont)
N Engl J Med 336:1506–1511, 1997 3–27

Objective.—Questions remain about the perioperative management of patients receiving long-term warfarin therapy. Two competing approaches are an aggressive approach, in which the patient receives IV heparin for 2 days before and after surgery, and a minimalist approach, in which the patients receive no heparin immediately before and after surgery. The expected risks and benefits of these 2 approaches are reviewed.

Stopping Warfarin.—If warfarin is stopped 4 days before surgery and resumed as soon as possible afterward, the patient would be expected to have a subtherapeutic international normalized ratio (INR) for 2 days before and 2 days after surgery. However, there will still be partial protection against thromboembolism while the INR remains somewhat elevated. Thus, the thromboembolism risk of stopping warfarin is equivalent to 1 day without anticoagulation before and after surgery. The thromboembolism risk may also be increased by rebound hypercoagulation caused by cessation of warfarin and the prothrombotic effect of surgery. The risk of preoperative arterial and venous thromboembolism and of postoperative venous thromboembolism is comparable to that expected without anticoagulation. However, the risk of postoperative venous thromboembolism will increase greatly. For patients with previous venous thromboembolisms, major surgery increases the short-term recurrence risk by more than 100-fold. Anticoagulation produces an 80% reduction in the risk of recurrent venous thromboembolism, a 66% reduction in the risk of arterial thromboembolism in patients with nonvalvular atrial fibrillation, and a 75% reduction in the risk of major thromboembolism in patients with mechanical heart valves.

The risk of bleeding is low if IV heparin is given for 2 days before surgery, but it is high if heparin is restarted immediately afterward. Giving IV heparin for 2 days will increase the absolute risk of major postoperative bleeding by about 3%. Death will result from recurrent venous thromboembolism in about 6% of cases, death will result from arterial thromboembolism in 20%, and death will result from major postoperative bleeding in 3%.

Perioperative IV Heparin.—The risk of postoperative venous thromboembolism is very high for patients with acute venous thromboembolisms. Thus, postoperative IV heparin reduces postoperative morbidity in these patients, even though it doubles the risk of bleeding. By 2–3 months after the acute episode, however, the risk has dropped sufficiently that preoperative heparin is no longer justified unless other risk factors are present. Postoperative heparin is still indicated because of the high risk of postoperative venous thromboembolism. When it has been more than 3 months since the acute venous thromboembolism, prophylactic measures that carry a lower risk of bleeding than IV heparin should be considered.

Within 1 month after acute arterial thromboembolism, preoperative IV heparin is indicated. Postoperative heparin is recommended only for patients undergoing minor surgery with a low risk of bleeding. For patients at lower risk of arterial thromboembolism, postoperative IV heparin is more likely to increase morbidity than to reduce it. An alternative approach that has been suggested is outpatient administration of subcutaneous heparin or low molecular weight heparin. However, this may be impractical and may give less predictable results than IV heparin.

Recommendations.—If warfarin is withheld the day before surgery, the authors recommend measuring the INR the day before the operation. This gives the physician the alternative of giving a small dose of vitamin K, if needed. When the INR is less than 2.0, other forms of preoperative or postoperative prophylaxis or both should be considered. If surgery must be performed in the first month after acute venous thromboembolism, IV heparin should be given preoperatively and postoperatively while the INR is below 2.0. Intravenous heparin may be stopped 6 hours before surgery if the activated partial thromboplastin time is in the therapeutic range. After major surgery, heparin should not be restarted for at least 12 hours, and it should not be restarted for longer if there are signs of bleeding. When restarted, heparin should be given at no more than the expected maintenance infusion rate.

► Review articles are rarely presented in this YEAR BOOK, but I must make an exception in this instance. This article succinctly outlines the most optimal methods for providing perioperative protection against venous or arterial thromboembolism for patients being managed with warfarin. Every anesthesiologist and surgeon should become acquainted with the recommendations put forth in this article.

D.M. Rothenberg, M.D.

Thromboelastographic Changes in Healthy Parturients and Postpartum Women

Sharma SK, Philip J, Wiley J (Univ of Texas, Dallas)
Anesth Analg 85:94–98, 1997 3–28

Background.—Thromboelastography is used to monitor whole blood coagulation, evaluate the elastic properties of whole blood, and offer a global assessment of hemostatic function. The technique has been modified as it has become more popular. For example, disposable plastic cups and pins are now being used instead of metal cups and pins. Celite accelerates the coagulation of whole blood by activating coagulation factors and platelets, and is now used as an activator for thromboelastography in nonpregnant patients to produce faster results.

Methods.—Thromboelastography using native whole blood and disposable plastic cups and pins was performed in 17 nonpregnant women, 134 healthy term pregnant women, and 69 postpartum women. Thromboelastography using celite-activated whole blood was performed in 15 nonpregnant women, 38 healthy term pregnant women, and 34 postpartum women.

Results.—Compared to values for nonpregnant women in both groups, the thromboelastographic parameters of reaction time and clot formation time were significantly decreased in pregnant and postpartum women. There was a significant increase in maximum amplitude, elastic shear modulus, and α angles in pregnant and postpartum women, compared to nonpregnant women in both groups. Also compared to nonpregnant women in both groups, the thromboelastography coagulation index was significantly greater in pregnant and postpartum women.

Discussion.—These findings show that pregnancy is a hypercoagulable state. Postpartum women remain in this hypercoagulable state for the first 24 hours after delivery. The use of celite produced more rapid results.

► This study provides further evidence that pregnancy is a hypercoagulable state, and that parturients remain in a hypercoagulable state for the first 24 hours after delivery. Pulmonary thromboembolism remains one of the leading causes of maternal mortality in the United States. Recently in our state, a previously healthy parturient experienced cardiopulmonary arrest and died during labor, approximately 3 hours after administration of epidural analgesia. Autopsy revealed a large saddle pulmonary embolus, and the source was a large clot in the femoral vein.

D.H. Chestnut, M.D.

Other Obstetric Anesthesia Topics

Epidural Analgesia, Intrapartum Fever, and Neonatal Sepsis Evaluation

Lieberman E, Lang JM, Frigoletto F Jr, et al (Harvard Med School; Boston Univ; Massachusetts Gen Hosp, Boston; et al)
Pediatrics 99:415–419, 1997 3–29

Background.—Maternal temperature is monitored during labor, because it can be a sign of infection that can adversely affect both mother and infant. The use of epidural analgesia during labor has been associated with increased maternal temperature. The impact of the use of epidural analgesia during labor on the rate of intrapartum maternal fever and the performance of neonatal sepsis evaluations was analyzed in a large hospital-based population.

Study Design.—The base sample for this study was 1,934 nulliparous women participating in the active management of labor (ACT) trial at Brigham and Women's Hospital from May 1990 through October 1994. The group for the current study included only those women with singleton, term pregnancies, with the infant in a cephalic presentation, and labor that resulted in a live birth. Women were excluded if a maternal fever or

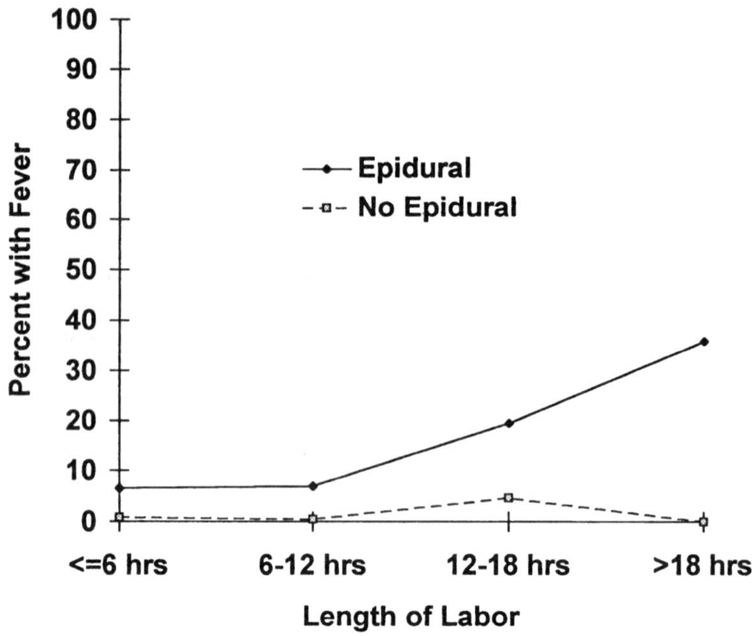

FIGURE 1.—Percent of women with fever greater than 100.4°F according to length of labor and epidural use. (Reproduced by permission of *Pediatrics*, from Lieberman E, Lang JM, Frigoletto F Jr, et al: Epidural analgesia, intrapartum fever, and neonatal sepsis evaluation. *Pediatrics* 99:415–419, copyright 1997.)

infection was present at admission, if they were diabetic, or if birth weight data were missing. The rates of maternal intrapartum temperature greater than 100.4°F, neonatal sepsis evaluation, and neonatal antibiotic treatment were determined, as was the use of epidural analgesia during labor. Rate ratios and confidence intervals (CI) were calculated. Multiple logistic regression was used to explore associations, while controlling for confounding factors.

Findings.—Of the 1,657 women enrolled in this study, intrapartum fever occurred in 14.5% of those who received epidural analgesia, but in only 1.0% of women who did not receive epidural analgesia during labor. In the absence of epidural analgesia, the fever rate was low regardless of labor length, whereas in the presence of the epidural, the rate of fever increased with length of labor (Fig 1). Those neonates whose mothers received epidural analgesia were more often evaluated for sepsis and treated with antibiotics than those whose mothers did not receive this form of analgesia (Fig 3). Although only 63% of the women in this study group had epidural analgesia during labor, 96.2% of intrapartum fevers, 85.6% of neonatal sepsis evaluations, and 87.5% of neonatal antibiotic treatment occurred in the epidural group.

Conclusions.—In this large group of afebrile, nulliparous women, the majority of cases of intrapartum fever, neonatal sepsis evaluations, and neonatal antibiotic treatment was associated with the use of epidural

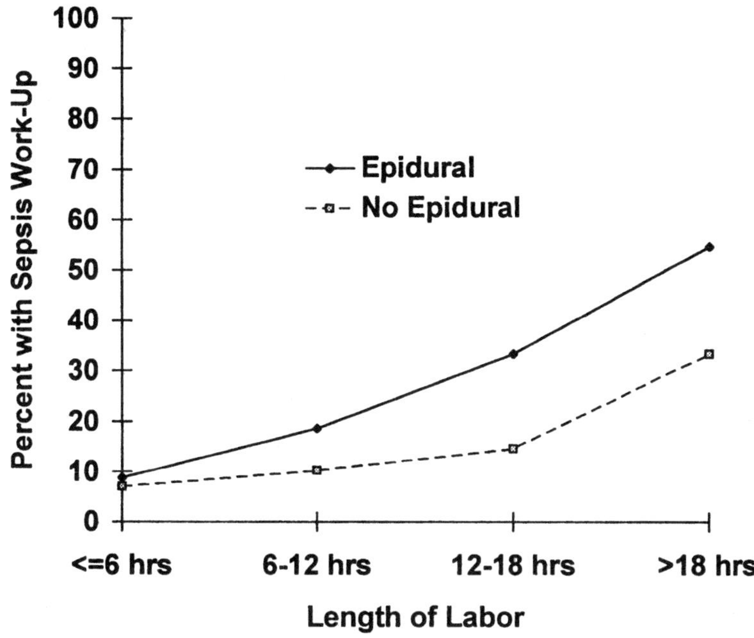

FIGURE 3.—Performance of sepsis evaluations among neonates of afebrile women according to length of labor and epidural use. (Reproduced by permission of *Pediatrics*, from Lieberman E, Lang JM, Frigoletto F Jr, et al: Epidural analgesia, intrapartum fever, and neonatal sepsis evaluation. *Pediatrics* 99:415–419, copyright 1997.)

analgesia during labor. Although most of the intrapartum fevers were not infectious in origin, they resulted in evaluation and treatment of neonates for possible sepsis. These evaluations are associated with cost, risk and pain to newborns. The results of this study suggest that the existing criteria for neonatal sepsis evaluation and antibiotic treatment should be reexamined, methods of limiting epidural-associated temperature elevations should be investigated, and the possible consequences of epidural-associated fevers should be discussed with women and their health care providers when labor analgesia decisions are being made.

► This study has received widespread attention in the lay press. *The New York Times* published a report entitled "Study Associates Fever and Epidurals."[1] Despite the difference between groups in the incidence of maternal fever, there was no difference between groups in the incidence of neonatal sepsis. Thus, Dr. Sheila Cohen suggested an alternative title for the *Times* article: "Study Finds Problems Identifying Infected Babies."

As anesthesiologists, we should not dismiss the implications of this study. Neonatal sepsis evaluations result in pain, risk, and expense for neonates and their families. However, perhaps neonatologists should re-evaluate current standards for evaluation and treatment of infants of febrile mothers who receive epidural analgesia during labor. The authors of the present study stated: "Our results suggest that existing criteria for neonatal sepsis evaluation and antibiotic treatment should be reexamined, perhaps using a higher fever threshold for women with epidural. In addition, there should be additional study of ways to limit epidural-related temperature elevations by adjusting the ambient temperature of the labor room or by cooling the mother by sponging or fan." The present study does not justify a decision to withhold effective pain relief from laboring women.

D.H. Chestnut, M.D.

Reference

1. Gilbert S: Study associates fever and epidurals. *New York Times*. March 12, 1997.

Decreased Thiopental Requirements in Early Pregnancy

Gin T, Mainland P, Chan MTV, et al (Prince of Wales Hosp, Shatin, Hong Kong)

Anesthesiology 86:73–78, 1997 3–30

Objective.—The requirements for inhalant anesthetics are decreased during pregnancy. Whether the requirements for IV anesthetics are similarly reduced has not been examined. The quantal dose-response curves after a bolus dose of thiopental were compared for patients having an elective abortion at 7–13 weeks' gestation and for nonpregnant women having elective gynecologic surgery.

Methods.—Thiopental was administered to 70 pregnant and 70 nonpregnant women, aged 16–45 years. Each group was divided into 7 sets of 10 women each who received 2, 2.4, 2.8, 3.3, 3.8, 4.5, or 5.3 mg of thiopental IV per kilogram. Patients who were able to open their eyes on command 2 minutes after the beginning of anesthesia administration were noted not to be hypnotized. Each patient's dose was calculated using the equation:
lean body mass = 1.07 (total body weight) − 148 (total body weight/height). Differences between groups were compared statistically.

Results.—Six patients were excluded from the study for protocol violations. Although nonpregnant women were significantly older than pregnant women and had significantly higher baseline diastolic and systolic arterial pressures, other characteristics were comparable. The median effective doses for hypnosis and anesthesia for nonpregnant women were 3.1 and 4.9 mg of thiopental per kilogram, respectively, whereas the corresponding values for pregnant women were 2.6 and 4 mg of thiopental per kilogram. The ED_{95}s for hypnosis and anesthesia for nonpregnant women were 4.4 and 6.4 mg of thiopental per kilogram, respectively, whereas the corresponding values for pregnant women were 3.7 and 5.2 mg of thiopental per kilogram. Log dose-response curves showed the pregnant-to-nonpregnant relative median potency to be 0.83 for hypnosis and 0.82 for anesthesia (Fig 2).

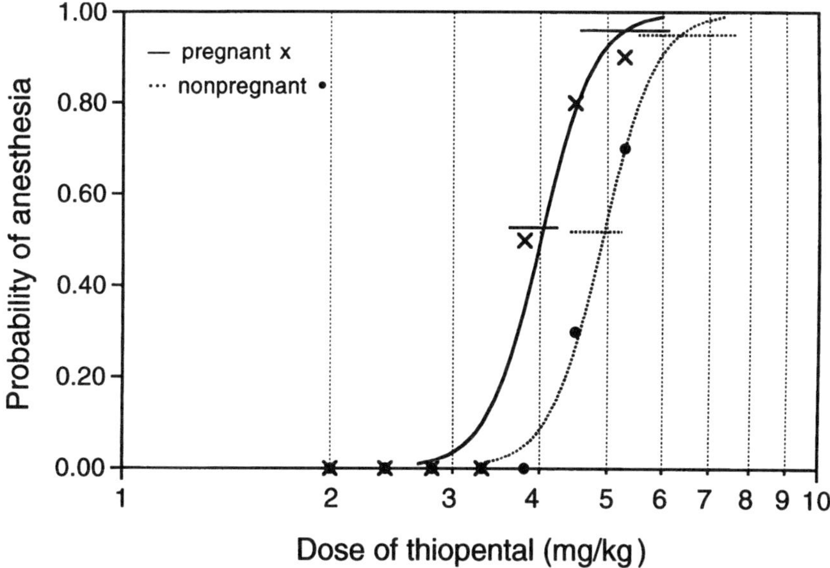

FIGURE 2.—Calculated dose-response curves (log dose scale) for anesthesia in pregnant and nonpregnant women. The 95% confidence intervals for the median effective doses (ED_{50}s) and ED_{95}s also are displayed, slightly offset for clarity. Raw data are shown by X (pregnant group) and (*solid circles*) (nonpregnant group). (Courtesy of Gin T, Mainland P, Chan MTV, et al: Decreased thiopental requirements in early pregnancy. *Anesthesiology* 86:73–78, 1997. Copyright American Society of Anesthesiologists, Inc. Used with permission of Lippincott-Raven Publishers.)

Conclusions.—Compared with nonpregnant patients, pregnant patients have their thiopental requirement reduced by 17% to 18% based on total body mass and by 19% to 20% based on lean body mass. Although the mechanism for this reduction is not understood, studies in animals have shown that progesterone decreases the anesthetic requirement.

Minimum Alveolar Concentration of Halothane and Enflurane Are Decreased in Early Pregnancy

Chan MTV, Mainland P, Gin T (Prince of Wales Hosp, Shatin, Hong Kong)
Anesthesiology 85:782–786, 1996 3–31

Objective.—Although the minimum alveolar concentration (MAC) of enflurane is known to be decreased in early pregnancy, the changes in MAC for different inhalant anesthetics has not been determined. The MAC of halothane and enflurane in pregnant women scheduled for termination of pregnancy between 8 and 13 weeks' gestation and in nonpregnant women undergoing elective laparoscopic sterilization was determined.

Methods.—Eight pregnant and 8 nonpregnant women received enflurane, and 8 pregnant and 8 nonpregnant women received halothane. Inspired and expired halothane or enflurane, carbon dioxide, and oxygen

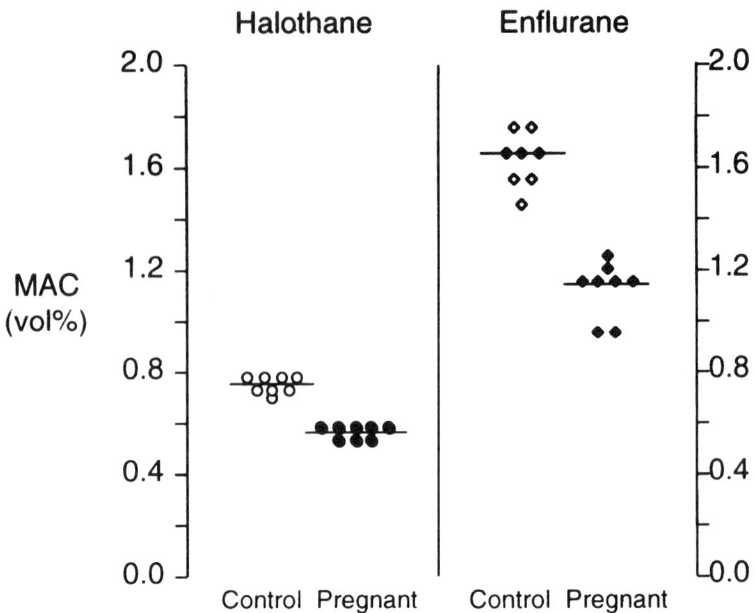

FIGURE 1.—Individual minimum alveolar concentrations (*MAC*) for halothane in pregnant women (*solid circles*) and nonpregnant women (*open circles*), and enflurane in pregnant women (*solid diamonds*) and nonpregnant women (*open diamonds*). (Courtesy of Chan MTV, Mainland P, Gin T: Minimum alveolar concentration of halothane and enflurane are decreased in early pregnancy. *Anesthesiology* 85:782–786, 1996. Copyright American Society of Anesthesiologists, Inc. Used with permission of Lippincott-Raven Publishers.)

were monitored continuously. Minimum alveolar concentration was determined by delivering a standardized transcutaneous electric tetanus of 10-sec, 50-Hz, 80-mamp, 200-μsec square pulses to the ulnar nerve using a constant-current peripheral nerve stimulator. End-tidal concentrations of anesthetics were held constant for at 15 minutes before each stimulus was given. Concentrations of halothane and enflurane were reduced by 0.05 vol% and 0.10 vol%, respectively, to confirm the consistency of 3 responses for each measurement. The MAC for each patient was calculated as the average of the 2 concentrations just permitting and just preventing movement. The percent decrease in MAC between groups was compared statistically.

Results.—Patient characteristics were similar between groups. Minimum alveolar concentration values for both anesthetics were significantly lower for pregnant women than for nonpregnant women (Fig 1). The percentage decrease for halothane averaged 27% (20% to 27%) and for enflurane was 30% (24% to 36%), indicating that pregnancy decreases the MAC more for halothane than for enflurane. The reason for this decrease in humans is unknown, although in animal studies, exogenous progesterone has been shown to lower anesthetic requirements.

Conclusions.—The MAC for both enflurane and halothane in pregnant women was significantly reduced compared with MAC in nonpregnant women. Pregnancy decreased the MAC for halothane more than the MAC for enflurane.

► These 2 studies (Abstracts 3–30 and 3–31) show that the MAC for general anesthetic agents is decreased in women during early pregnancy (i.e., 7–13 weeks' gestation), when compared with MAC in nonpregnant women. Fagraeus et al.[1] earlier observed a greater spread of epidural analgesia in pregnant women during the first trimester than in nonpregnant women.

The mechanism for the decreased anesthetic requirements during pregnancy remains unclear. The authors of these 2 studies call attention to 2 possibilities. First, they note that exogenously administered progesterone reduces anesthetic requirements in animals, although there are no human data that support this hypothesis. Second, they note that increased concentrations of endorphins and dynorphins mediate an increase in pain threshold in pregnant rats, and they speculate that such changes might affect anesthetic requirements.

D.H. Chestnut, M.D.

Reference

1. Fagraeus L, Urban BJ, Bromage PR: Spread of epidural analgesia in early pregnancy. *Anesthesiology* 58:184–187, 1983.

Laparoscopy During Pregnancy: A Survey of Laparoendoscopic Surgeons

Reedy MB, Galan HL, Richards WE, et al (Texas A&M Univ, Temple; Scott & White Mem Hosp, Temple, Tex; Univ of Texas Health Sciences Ctr, Houston; et al)

J Reprod Med 42:33–38, 1997 3–32

Objective.—Laparoscopy during pregnancy has been performed for cholecystectomy, appendectomy, ovarian torsion, and surgery for adnexal masses. A survey of the Society of Laparoendoscopic Surgeons (SLS) was conducted to establish the safety of using laparoscopy during pregnancy.

Methods.—A questionnaire was mailed to 16,329 laparoscopic surgeons who were asked to fill it out and return it if they had performed laparoscopy on pregnant patients.

Results.—A total of 192 surveys were returned of which 189 (413 laparoscopies) met the study criteria. Laparoscopies were performed for cholecystectomy (n = 199), adnexal surgery (n = 116), appendectomy (n = 67), and other procedures (n = 31). In the first trimester 134 laparoscopies were performed; in the second trimester, 224; and in the third trimester, 54. Carbon dioxide was used in all the procedures. There were 5 intraoperative complications, including enterotomy at open laparoscopy, inadvertent intrauterine placement of a Veress needle, laparotomy for severe adhesions or staging of ovarian tumor, and severe upper abdominal pain from carbon dioxide. There were 10 postoperative complications, including 5 spontaneous first-trimester abortions (1.2%); repeat laparoscopy to treat adnexal torsion; pain and stone passed after cholecystectomy; preterm labor, successfully treated after appendectomy in the third trimester; postoperative hemorrhage from a supraumbilical trocar site; and postoperative pancreatitis after cholecystectomy.

Conclusion.—Laparoscopy during pregnancy appears to be safe and carries a low risk of complications.

▶ Of interest is the fact that 54 of the 413 cases were performed during the third trimester. Among those 54 patients, the authors reported no intraoperative complications and only 1 postoperative complication. However, this study suffers from the limitations of such surveys. Respondents are more likely to report good outcomes than bad outcomes. In other words, complications are usually underreported.

D.H. Chestnut, M.D.

Operating on Placental Support: The Ex Utero Intrapartum Treatment Procedure

Mychaliska GB, Bealer JF, Graf JL, et al (Univ of California, San Francisco)
J Pediatr Surg 32:227–231, 1997 3–33

Introduction.—The PLUG (plug the lung until it grows) technique of temporary tracheal occlusion has been used by the authors to treat congenital diaphragmatic hernia in utero. To safely "unplug" the trachea at birth and secure the airway during delivery, the EXIT (ex utero intrapartum treatment) was developed. The technique of the EXIT procedure is reported here, together with results in 8 infants.

Methods.—The EXIT procedure is performed at term if the fetus and mother are doing well, but deterioration of the fetal condition requires operation before term. A multidisciplinary team participates in each procedure. Special instruments are required in addition to those in the usual setup for cesarean section. Fetal heart rate and hemoglobin saturation are monitored continuously, and fetal cardiac sonography is performed periodically. The fetus is usually anesthetized from placental transfer of maternal anesthesia, but paralysis with IM vecuronium may be needed if the fetus is mobile. High doses of inhaled halogenated agents are used to facilitate uterine relaxation. The fetal airway is secured while fetoplacental circulation remains intact. The infant's airway is examined with a bronchoscope and secured with orotracheal intubation or tracheostomy. Surfactant is instilled, the infant is ventilated, and the umbilical cord is divided.

Results.—Six infants had their trachea plugged or clipped in utero for treatment of congenital diaphragmatic hernia, and 2 had prenatally diagnosed cystic hygroma of the neck and oropharynx. Delivery took place at gestational ages ranging from 30 to 39 weeks. All fetuses tolerated the EXIT procedure well, remaining hemodynamically stable during periods of 12–60 minutes on placental support. The mothers also did well, with excellent oxygen saturation and no postpartum bleeding or uterine atony. One infant died in the early postoperative period of severe pulmonary hypoplasia.

Discussion.—The EXIT procedure provides a safe and effective means of treating air obstruction at birth. This approach to problems such as cystic hygroma, hemangioma, laryngeal atresia, and thyroid goiter requires careful planning and monitoring, together with the coordinated efforts of pediatric surgeons, obstetricians, anesthesiologists, sonographers, and neonatologists.

► We recently had our first experience with the EXIT procedure. The pediatric surgeon performed a tracheostomy, and the uterine incision-to-delivery interval was 51 minutes. Uterine relaxation was maintained with isoflurane, and the neonatal outcome was excellent.

D.H. Chestnut, M.D.

Uterine Rupture and Scar Dehiscence: A Five-Year Survey
Lynch JC, Pardy JP (Sutherland Hosp, Caringbah, Australia)
Anaesth Intensive Care 24:699–704, 1996 3–34

Background.—Although uterine rupture is an uncommon event, its associated morbidity and mortality makes it important that at-risk patients be identified. Known risk factors include uterine scars, the use of oxytocics in labor, and breech extraction. When epidural analgesia is given during a trial of labor for patients with previous cesarean section, there is concern that diagnosis of uterine rupture may be delayed. Records from 2 public hospitals were reviewed for cases of uterine rupture.

Methods.—The review covered the years from 1988 to 1992. True rupture of the uterus was defined as the complete separation of the wall of the gravid uterus, with or without expulsion of the fetus. Although a "window" in the uterine muscle is not a rupture, true rupture may occur as an extension of the window. Dehiscence of a previous uterine scar is a separate category.

Results.—There were 31,115 deliveries during the study period and 27 cases (0.086%) of uterine rupture, including 14 in patients with a previous cesarean section. Uterine rupture was more common with increasing gestational age. Seven women had a history of previous uterine infection or gynecologic surgery and 13 received epidural analgesia during labor. In 6 patients diagnosis was made after they experienced vaginal hemorrhage and massive hematuria; 3 had acute massive hemorrhage with hypovolemic shock. The most common site of rupture was in or extending through an existing scar. In 12 patients labor was induced or augmented and 3 were delivered by forceps. There were no cases of maternal mortality, but 5 fetuses died. Fetal death occurred with complete uterine rupture and massive maternal blood loss; in all cases with scar dehiscence, the fetus survived with a high Apgar score at delivery. Five patients carried a later normal pregnancy to 38 weeks and were delivered by elective cesarean section.

Conclusion.—The incidence of uterine rupture in this series was 1:1,162 live births. Most cases occurred in the third trimester in women with a history of cesarean section or uterine surgery. More than half of the women were older than 30 years and 81% were multiparous. Patients with a uterine scar need to be monitored with particular care when given oxytocics or epidural analgesia.

► Uterine rupture is an occasional, albeit uncommon, complication in women who attempt uterine birth after cesarean section. A history of previous cesarean section does not contraindicate the administration of epidural analgesia during labor. Some have suggested that the administration of epidural analgesia—using a dilute solution of local anesthetic—may improve the specificity of abdominal pain as a sign of uterine rupture. Fetal heart rate abnormalities remain the most sensitive sign of uterine rupture.

D.H. Chestnut, M.D.

Normal Saline I.V. Fluid Load Decreases Uterine Activity in Active Labour

Cheek TG, Samuels P, Miller F, et al (Univ of Pennsylvania, Philadelphia)
Br J Anaesth 77:632–635, 1996 3–35

Background.—Authorities disagree on the effect of lumbar extradural block on uterine activity and the progress of labor. Intravenous saline, 500–1,000 mL, is commonly administered during preterm labor and inhibits uterine activity in more than 50% of subjects. The effect of a similar fluid load during normal active labor is unknown. If uterine activity is decreased by such a fluid load, this may explain decreased uterine activity after extradural block, which is normally preceded by a similar fluid load.

Methods.—Thirty-four healthy women in spontaneous labor were randomly assigned to 1 of 3 groups: group A given no fluid load, group B given normal saline 500 mL, or group C given normal saline 1,000 mL. Continued internal measurement of uterine activity was obtained before, during, and after fluid load and extradural block.

Results.—Uterine activity did not change in groups A or B. Uterine activity decreased after the infusion of saline in group C (Fig 1). Uterine activity returned to baseline values during the 20 minutes after the saline infusion. No association was seen between extradural block and uterine activity. In group A, hypotension did not increase.

Discussion.—In these patients in spontaneous labor, an IV fluid load before regional block resulted in a transient decrease in uterine activity. This study controlled for variables such as aortocaval compression, maternal hypotension, beta-agonist activity from low-dose adrenaline in the local anesthetic, and local anesthetic effects on the myometrium.

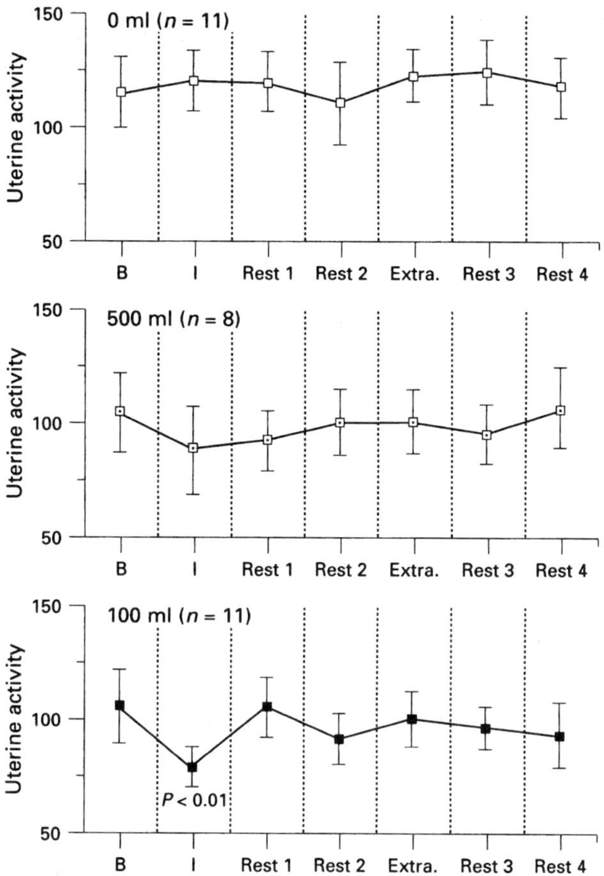

FIGURE 1.—Uterine activity (mean, SD) after no fluid preload (0 mL), and after IV infusion of 500 mL and 1,000 mL saline. *Abbreviations*: *B*, baseline; *Extra.*, extradural injection; *I*, infusion. (Reprinted with permission from the BMJ Publishing Group, from Cheek TG, Samuels P, Miller F, et al: Normal saline i.v. fluid load decreases uterine activity in active labour. *Br J Anaesth* 77:632–635, 1996.)

► This study suggests that acute IV hydration may result in a transient decrease in uterine activity before administration of epidural analgesia in laboring women. However, the effect is transient and likely has little clinical significance. Of interest, women who received no fluid load did not have a greater incidence or severity of hypotension than women who received 1,000 mL of crystalloid. This observation does not dissuade me from giving 500–700 mL of crystalloid before administration of epidural analgesia in laboring women.

D.H. Chestnut, M.D.

Intravenous Nitroglycerin to Relieve Intrapartum Fetal Distress Related to Uterine Hyperactivity: A Prospective Observational Study

Mercier FJ, Dounas M, Bouaziz H, et al (Hôpital Antoine Béclère, Clamart Cedex, France)

Anesth Analg 84:1117–1120, 1997 3–36

Background.—Some complicated obstetric situations require rapid, transient uterine relaxation. Although studies of nitroglycerin (NTG) for such cases have been reported, no one has investigated the use of NTG to relieve intrapartum fetal distress associated with uterine hyperactivity.

Methods.—Twenty-four laboring parturients were injected with 60–90 µg of NTG intravenously 2–5 minutes after the onset of severe fetal distress. In all cases, abnormal fetal heart rates had failed to respond to oxygen administration, left lateral decubitus, and discontinuation of any ongoing oxytocin infusion. When required, a second 60–90 µg dose was administered 2–3 minutes later.

Findings.—The administration of NTG was successful in 22 patients, with fetal distress resolving 4–5 minutes later and normal uterine activity restored. In the remaining 2 patients, fetal distress resolved within 4–5 minutes, but there was residual mild uterine hyperactivity. A second NTG dose was needed in 38% of the patients. In 25% of patients, hypotension developed 2 minutes after the first NTG injection, with a mean nadir of 93.2 mm Hg. Hypotension was reversed rapidly in all patients with a single 4.5–6 mg dose of ephedrine (Figs 1 and 2).

Conclusions.—Small doses of intravenous NTG can resolve severe fetal distress associated with uterine hyperactivity. The adverse effects of NTG administration were negligible.

▶ This study provides further evidence of the efficacy of NTG as a uterine relaxant. Bell[1] reported the use of sublingual nitroglycerin spray to relax the uterus in a patient who had uterine hyperstimulation from intravenous oxytocin. In that case, Dr. Bell documented decreased intrauterine pressure—as measured with an intrauterine pressure catheter—for several minutes after sublingual nitroglycerin administration. In this study, the authors correctly called attention to the need for comparative studies of NTG and β-adrenergic agonists as tocolytic agents.

D.H. Chestnut, M.D.

Reference

1. Bell E: Nitroglycerin and uterine relaxation (letter). *Anesthesiology* 85:683, 1996.

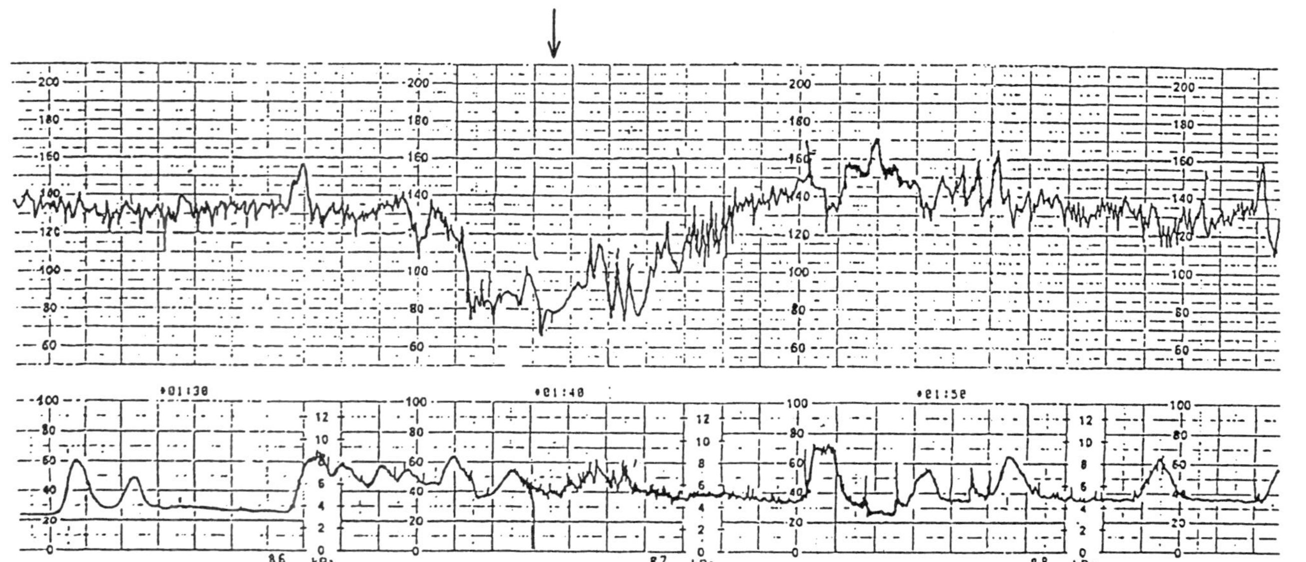

FIGURE 1.—Cardiotocogram (1 cm/min) showing: (1) typical uterine hyperactivity with fetal distress; (2) administration of intravenous nitroglycerin (*arrow*, 90 μg administered); (3) resolution of the hyperactivity with normalization of fetal heart rate; and (4) rapid reappearance of regular uterine activity. (Courtesy of Mercier FJ, Dounas M, Bouaziz H, et al: Intravenous nitroglycerin to relieve intrapartum fetal distress related to uterine hyperactivity: A prospective observational study. *Anesth Analg* 84[5]:1117–1120, 1997.)

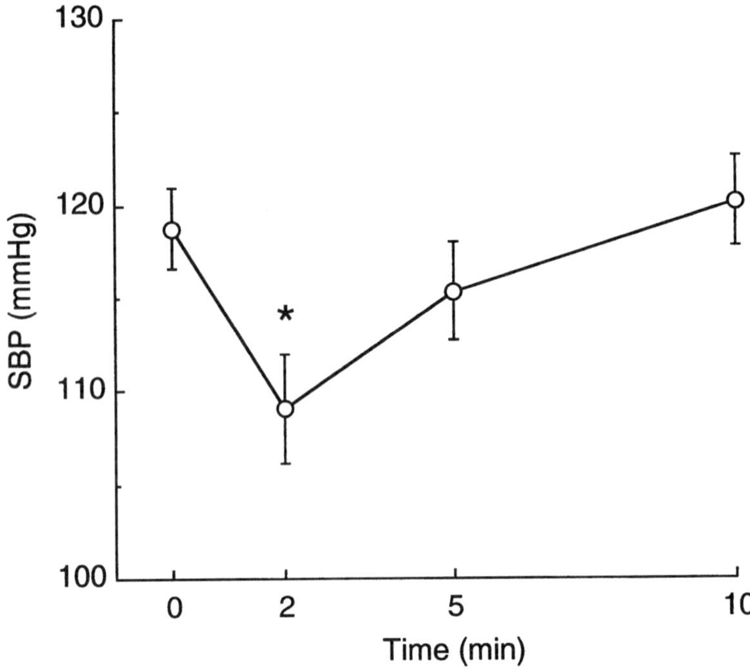

FIGURE 2.—Systolic blood pressure (SBP) changes (mean ± SEM) after a small intravenous bolus (60 μg or 90 μg) of nitroglycerin (NTG) administered to 24 parturients and repeated once within 2–3 min in 9 parturients. The mean decrease in SBP was mild and was only transient 2 min after the first nitroglycerin injection ($P = 0.0009$). At this time, 6 parturients exhibited an SBP of less than 100 mm Hg, which was rapidly normalized by a single 4.5–6 mg intravenous bolus of ephedrine. (Courtesy of Mercier FJ, Dounas M, Bouaziz H, et al: Intravenous nitroglycerin to relieve intrapartum fetal distress related to uterine hyperactivity: A prospective observational study. *Anesth Analg* 84[5]:1117–1120, 1997.)

Ultrasound Examination of the Stomach Contents of Women in the Postpartum Period

Jayaram A, Bowen MP, Deshpande S, et al (Oregon Health Sciences Univ, Portland)

Anesth Analg 84:522–526, 1997 3–37

Introduction.—Previous studies suggest that delayed gastric emptying may increase the risk of aspiration in women in the early postpartum period (within the first 2 hours of delivery), but that this risk is the same as in nonpregnant women from 9 hours postdelivery. Gastric emptying of solids is important, because aspiration of solid food particles is associated with significant mortality. Real-time US imaging was used to examine the stomach contents of women in the postpartum period for solid food particles.

Methods.—The first part of the study involved examination of the stomach contents of 28 women undergoing postpartum bilateral tubal ligation (BTL) and 25 controls scheduled for gynecologic surgery. The interval between the last meal and US examination was required to be at least 6 hours. Patients were examined before induction of anesthesia. Identification of stomach contents was assisted by the entry of nonaerated water and sodium citrate (60–100 mL). The second part of the study included 20 recently delivered women not scheduled for BTL and 21 nonpregnant volunteers of similar body mass index. Gastric emptying after a standardized meal was compared in these 2 groups.

Results.—In the first part of the study, solid food particles were found before surgery in 11 of the 28 patients about to undergo postpartum tubal ligation. No solid food particles were present in the stomachs of the 24 women studied before gynecologic surgery. Similarly, in the second part of the study, all but 1 of 20 women in the postpartum group still had food particles in the stomach 4 hours after the meal. Among nonpregnant volunteers, only 4 of 21 had food particles in the stomach at this time.

Conclusion.—Findings confirm the study hypothesis, that a significant number of women presenting for postpartum sterilization have solid food particles in their stomachs because of a delay in gastric emptying of solids in the postpartum period. Although narcotic medications can delay gastric emptying, they did not appear to make a significant difference in these patients. Obesity might also be a factor, but evidence from other studies is inconclusive.

▶ The timing of postpartum tubal ligation remains a contentious issue. To my knowledge, this is the first study that specifically addressed the gastric emptying of solids in the postpartum period. The authors demonstrated that a significant number of women undergoing postpartum tubal ligation have solid food particles in the stomach, and that the gastric emptying of solids is delayed during the postpartum period. In this study, it appears that the US examination for most of the postpartum patients was performed more than 8 hours after delivery. The study suggests that postpartum patients may be at risk for aspiration of solids as late as 8–16 hours after delivery.

D.H. Chestnut, M.D.

Anaesthesia and the Antiphospholipid Syndrome: A Review of 20 Obstetric Patients

Ringrose DK (St Thomas' Hosp, London)

Int J Obstet Anesth 6:107–111, 1997 3–38

Introduction.—Patients with antiphospholipid syndrome (APS) have autoantibodies to phospholipids, i.e., the lupus anticoagulant and anticardiolipin antibodies. About half of these patients have systemic lupus erythematosus (SLE). Patients with APS commonly have obstetric complications, including intrauterine growth retardation, recurrent miscarriage, fetal death, pre-eclampsia, eclampsia, placental thrombosis, and premature delivery. Because they have a high rate of operative delivery, these patients are commonly encountered by the anesthetist. An experience with the anesthetic management of obstetric patients with APS was reviewed.

Patients.—The 4-year review included 22 women with singleton pregnancies managed at a British national referral center for SLE and APS. Of the 20 patients, 7 had a diagnosis of primary APS and 13 a diagnosis of secondary syndrome associated with SLE. There were many obstetric complications, including 4 cases of intrauterine growth retardation and 2 of placental abruption. Cesarean section was performed in 9 of 19 women whose pregnancies reached the third trimester. Seven pregnancies were associated with prolongation of the phospholipid-dependent coagulation tests secondary to lupus anticoagulant or anticardiolipin antibodies or both. Epidural blockade was successfully administered to 4 of these patients, with no sequelae. The patients were paradoxically hypercoagulable, with estimated blood loss of no greater than 600 mL. A previous history of thrombosis was present in 11 patients. Even though they received antithrombotic therapy, 2 of the women had thrombotic episodes during pregnancy and 3 had such episodes during the postpartum period.

Discussion.—Pregnant women with APS are at high risk of obstetric complications. Optimal management requires early referral to a tertiary center with appropriate multidisciplinary expertise. Although epidural anesthesia was successfully used in this series, the study cannot validate the safety of epidural placement in obstetric patients with APS.

▶ The term *lupus anticoagulant* is a misnomer, because it has no true anticoagulant activity in vivo. Paradoxically, patients with lupus anticoagulant are at risk for thrombotic events, both arterial and venous. In the absence of an underlying coagulopathy or anticoagulant therapy, a prolonged phospholipid-dependent coagulation test does not suggest a bleeding tendency, and regional anesthesia may be administered in these patients.

D.H. Chestnut, M.D.

Pediatric Anesthesia Topics and Issues

The Safety and Efficacy of Oral Transmucosal Fentanyl Citrate for Preoperative Sedation in Young Children

Epstein RH, Mendel HG, Witkowski TA, et al (Jefferson Med College, Philadelphia; Tri City Anesthesia Consultants, Tempe, Ariz)

Anesth Analg 83:1200–1205, 1996 3–39

Background.—Orally given transmucosal fentanyl citrate (OTFC), a labeled preoperative pediatric sedative, is associated with a high incidence of postoperative nausea and vomiting and occasional respiratory depression at doses exceeding 15 µg of the drug per kilogram. The safety and efficacy of a dose of 15 µg of OTFC per kilogram were studied in children aged 6 years and younger.

Methods and Findings.—Nineteen children aged 2–6 years were randomly assigned to OTFC/IV saline or placebo lozenge/IV fentanyl before surgery. Patients given OTFC became more sedated than those in the

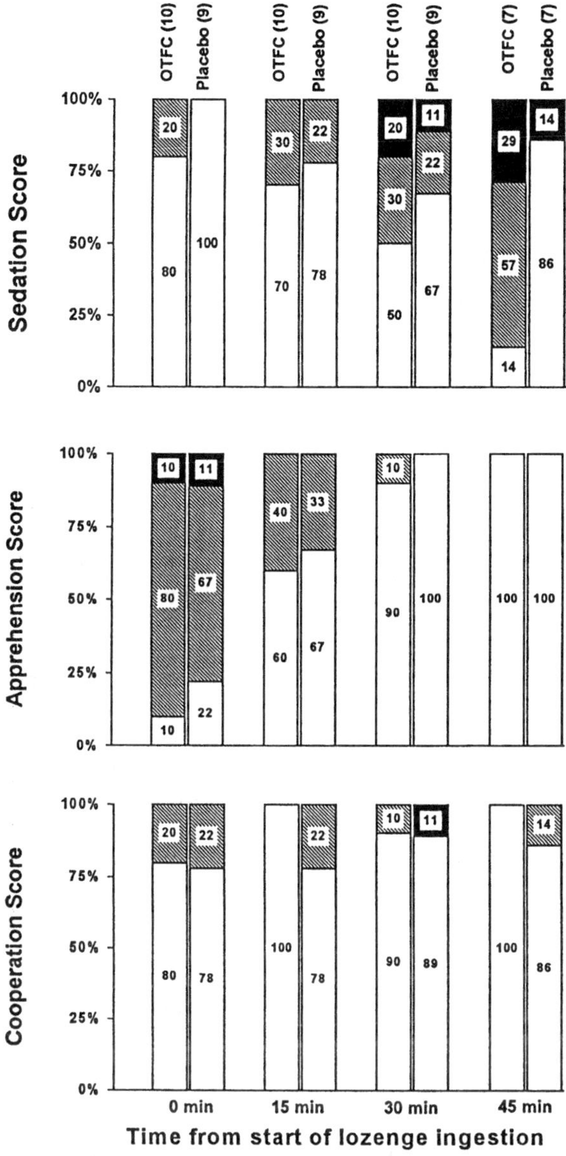

FIGURE 1.—Patient behavior was scored at 15-minute intervals after the start of ingestion of orally given transmucosal fentanyl citrate (*OTFC*) or the placebo lozenge (*open bar* = 1; *striped bar* = 2; *solid bar* = 3). No scores of 4 or 5 were observed in any patient. The *number within each bar segment* represents the percentage of patients with the corresponding score. The value in parenthesis at the top of the graph is the number of patients who could be examined at the indicated time in each group. Apprehension decreased equally over time in both groups (**middle**) and cooperation remained good (**bottom**). There was a significant increase in the level of sedation (**top**) in the OTFC group 45 minutes after the start of ingestion of the lozenge ($P = 0.01$). No other differences reached statistical significance. The mean ingestion time was 13 minutes in the OTFC group and 14 minutes in the placebo group. (Courtesy of Epstein RH, Mendel HG, Witkowski TA, et al: The safety and efficacy of oral transmucosal fentanyl citrate for preoperative sedation in young children. *Anesth Analg* 83[6]:1200–1205, 1996.)

placebo group after 45 minutes. However, the groups did not differ in cooperation, apprehension, parental separation, or induction cooperation scores. None of the children had respiratory depression or oxygen desaturation before surgery. Mild pruritus developed in 9 of the 10 patients given OTFC, and 3 vomited before surgery. Neither complication occurred in the placebo group. The high incidence of preoperative vomiting resulted in protocol termination before the anticipated enrollment of 40 patients was met. General anesthesia was induced by mask, and a propofol infusion was given. One OTFC recipient became rigid during induction. Despite a 50% incidence of postoperative vomiting, emergence and recovery were not delayed by the use of OTFC (Fig 1).

Conclusions.—A 15 μg dose of OTFC per kilogram is not recommended as a routine preoperative sedative in children aged 6 years and younger. This dose is associated with an unacceptably high incidence of vomiting.

▶ The authors noted a 30% incidence of preoperative vomiting in patients who received OTFC, and thus the study was terminated with only 19 patients entered into the study. Orally given transmucosal fentanyl citrate does not appear to have "caught on" as a routine method to produce preoperative pediatric sedation. Studies attempting to better define optimal preoperative sedation in children by drug administration via various routes (preferably painless) are ongoing, and despite an obvious need this area remains a problem.

M. Wood, M.D.

Comparison of Patient-controlled Analgesia With and Without Night-time Morphine Infusion Following Lower Extremity Surgery in Children

McNeely JK, Trentadue NC (Med College of Wisconsin and Children's Hosp of Wisconsin, Milwaukee; Med Ctr of Central Georgia, Macon)

J Pain Symptom Manage 13:268–273, 1997 3–40

Background.—Patient-controlled analgesia (PCA) is commonly used for postoperative pain management in children's hospitals. Some clinicians advocate the use of a supplemental morphine infusion at night to improve the continuity of analgesia for patients who awaken with pain. However, the efficacy and safety of this practice have been questioned. The value of concurrent nighttime morphine infusions with PCA in children was further investigated.

Methods.—Thirty-six school-age children undergoing elective surgery on a lower extremity were assigned randomly to morphine by PCA alone or to PCA with a nighttime infusion of morphine (PCA + BI). After surgery, patients breathed air, and continuous oxygen saturation recordings were obtained for the duration of PCA use.

Findings.—The total morphine requirement was lower in the PCA group than in the PCA + BI group. At all assessments the 2 groups were similar in PCA pump activation, pain recorded on a visual analog scale,

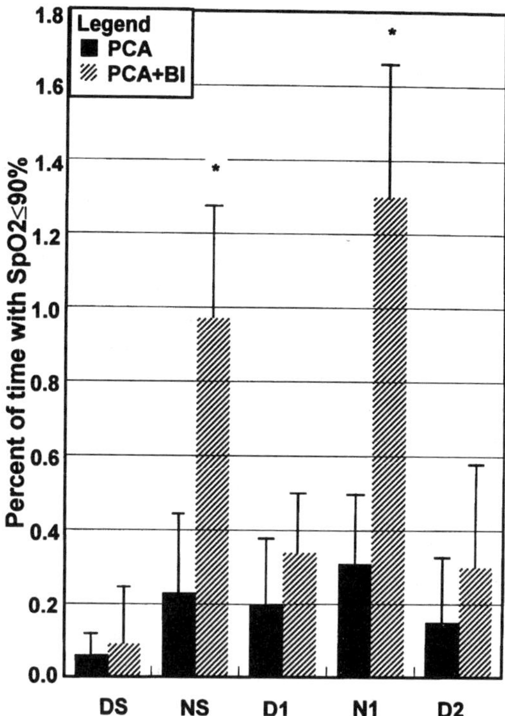

FIGURE 2.—The comparison of mean and SEM percentage of time spent with oxygen saturations at or below 90% between patients in the patient-controlled analgesia (PCA) and PCA + BI groups. $^*P < 0.05$ vs. PCA group. (Reprinted by permission of Elsevier Science, Inc. from McNeely JK, Trentadue NC: Comparison of patient-controlled analgesia with and without nighttime morphine infusion following lower extremity surgery in children. *J Pain Symp Manage* 13:268–273. Copyright 1997 by the U.S. Cancer Pain Relief Committee.)

and sedation scores. Compared with patients given PCA alone, those given PCA + BI spent more time with arterial oxygen saturation (SpO_2) of 90% or less during the nighttime infusion (Fig 2).

Conclusions.—Healthy children undergoing elective lower extremity surgery apparently do not benefit from a nighttime infusion of morphine as a supplement to postoperative PCA morphine analgesia. Patients receiving PCA + BI did not have a reduction in pain scores or PCA activation in the night compared with those given PCA alone.

► This study confirms in pediatric patients the finding shown in several adult studies that basal opioid infusions do not improve analgesia and are associated with a higher incidence of respiratory depression.

S.E. Abram, M.D.

Effect of Pre- vs Postoperative Tonsillar Infiltration With Local Anesthetics on Postoperative Pain After Tonsillectomy

Molliex S, Haond P, Baylot D, et al (Hôpital Bellevue, St Etienne, France)
Acta Anaesthesiol Scand 40:1210–1215, 1996 3–41

Background.—Studies have suggested that pre-incisional peritonsillar infiltrations of local anesthetic solutions decrease postoperative pain after tonsillectomy. The efficacy of preoperative or postoperative local anesthetic infiltration for pain after tonsillectomy was investigated.

Methods.—Sixty-eight patients, aged 8–65 years, were randomly assigned to 1 of 3 groups after induction of general anesthesia. Group 1 received peritonsillar infiltration with 0.25% bupivacaine before incision; group 2, normal saline before incision; and group 3, peritonsillar region infiltration with 0.25% bupivacaine after the completion of surgery but before awakening from anesthesia. In the postoperative period, nonsteroidal anti-inflammatory drugs were given intravenously to adults and rectally to children on patient request. Pain was assessed at 1, 5, 9, 13, 17, 21, and 36 hours after surgery. Swallowing was also assessed during the first postoperative day.

Findings.—In the first 24 hours after surgery, global visual analogue scale pain scores were lower in the groups given bupivacaine infiltration. In the first 9 hours after surgery, supplementary analgesic consumption was lower in group 3 than in group 2. There were no other significant differences among the 3 groups.

Conclusions.—The timing of peritonsillar infiltration with bupivacaine is apparently not clinically important in patients undergoing tonsillectomy. Further research is needed to clarify the significance of preemptive analgesia with local anesthetics on postoperative pain.

► Based on several studies of the timing of local anesthetic infiltration, it appears that there is little or no benefit in terms of postoperative pain levels or analgesic requirements to infiltrating the surgical field *before* incision. There may, however, be some benefit in terms of hemodynamic stability, particularly for hypertensive patients, in providing intraoperative regional blockade.

S.E. Abram, M.D.

Randomized, Single-blinded Trial of Laparoscopic Versus Open Appendectomy in Children: Effects on Postoperative Analgesia

Lejus C, Delile L, Plattner V, et al (Bloc opératoire de Chirurgie Pédiatrique, Nantes, France)
Anesthesiology 84:801–806, 1996 3–42

Introduction.—The most common reason for laparoscopy in children is appendectomy. Laparoscopic cholecystectomy has known benefits in adults, but the results of laparoscopic appendectomy are less clear. The postoperative period after appendectomy was compared in children undergoing a laparoscopic vs. an open procedure.

Methods.—The prospective, randomized trial included 63 children, aged 8–15 years, who were scheduled for appendectomy. Those weighing less than 20 kg were excluded. Participants were randomly assigned in the operating room to open or laparoscopic surgery. The children, parents, and nurses were unaware of which procedure the child had. During laparoscopic appendectomy, intra-abdominal pressure was maintained at less than 12 cm H_2O. The procedure was done through 2 incisions in the right and left lower quadrants. The appendix was removed using a 3.5 endoloop ligature. The open procedures were done through a standard McBurney's incision. Postoperative analgesia was provided with self-administered IV boluses of nalbuphine, 25 $\mu g \cdot kg^{-1}$. The children made pain ratings every 3 hours when awake, on a 10-cm Visual Analogue Scale. The children, parents, and nurses all rated the overall quality of analgesia over the first 3 postoperative days.

Results.—The 2 groups were comparable in demographic characteristics, preoperative dose of opioid analgesia, and delay between the last dose of dextromoramide and the loading dose of nalbuphine. The macroscopic appearance of the appendix also was similar in the 2 groups. Patients undergoing laparoscopy had significantly longer operative and anesthesia times. During the first day, the median patient-controlled analgesia nalbuphine dose was similar: 414 µg of the drug per kilogram kg in the open-surgery group and 562 µg of the drug per kilogram in the laparoscopy group. There was no significant difference on the second day. There were no significant differences in Visual Analogue Scale pain scores during the 3 days after surgery. Shoulder pain occurred in 35% of children in the laparoscopy group vs. 10% in the open-surgery group. No significant differences were found in the children's, parents', and nurses' ratings of analgesia. There were no differences in delays of regular feeding, sedation, nausea, vomiting, or urinary retention.

Conclusions.—Laparoscopic appendectomy in children offers no significant advantages over traditional open appendectomy. There are no differences in pain scores, analgesic usage, or delays in eating or walking. Unlike previous studies—which were neither randomized nor blinded—this trial finds no improvement in the postoperative period with laparoscopic vs. open appendectomy.

► Many clinicians accept that laparoscopic cholecystectomy is of benefit in adults, but the issue is not so clear for other operations—and what about children? Do children recover more quickly than adults, or do they just not complain as much? How can we best assess postoperative pain and recovery in children? Does laparoscopy shorten the duration of hospital stay in children? This study does not provide all the answers, but it does show that laparoscopy does not appear to improve analgesia and postoperative recovery after appendectomy in children.

M. Wood, M.D.

Cardiothoracic Anesthesia Patient Care Issues

Intrathecal Morphine for Coronary Artery Bypass Grafting and Early Extubation

Chaney MA, Furry PA, Fluder EM, et al (Loyola Univ, Maywood, Ill)
Anesth Analg 84:241–248, 1997 3–43

Background.—The current trend in cardiac surgery of early tracheal extubation immediately after operation has been largely driven by economics. Early extubation may cause complications and may not be indicated in some patients. For safe and successful early extubation, patients must have an appropriate sensorium, normothermia, adequate pulmonary function, adequate urine output, minimal chest tube output, and be hemodynamically stable. Pain management is also important. Intrathecal morphine may facilitate early extubation after cardiac surgery because it produces intense and prolonged analgesia by stimulating opioid receptors in the substantia gelatinosa of the posterior spinal cord.

Methods.—In a prospective, randomized, double blind, placebo-controlled trial, patients received intrathecal morphine, 10 µg/kg, or intrathecal placebo after elective coronary artery bypass grafting. Perioperative anesthetic management was standardized and included patient-controlled morphine analgesia.

Results.—There were 19 patients given intrathecal morphine and 21 patients given placebo. Among patients who had early extubation immediately after operation, the mean time from arrival in the ICU to extubation was significantly longer in patients given morphine than in patients given placebo. There was a substantial delay in extubation because of ventilatory depression in 3 patients given morphine. The use of postoperative IV morphine for 48 hours was less in patients who received morphine than in those given placebo, although the difference was not significant.

Discussion.—These findings show that intrathecal morphine is useful in controlling pain after cardiac surgery. The technique appears to be safe when certain precautions are followed. The optimal dose and intraoperative baseline anesthetic that will provide appropriate analgesia, but not delay extubation, have not been determined. Early extubation after cardiac surgery may be delayed by intrathecal morphine until these 2 goals are met.

▶ Early extubation after coronary artery bypass grafting has become a quest and, like any other quest, some folks will approach it with evangelical zeal. I am not accusing the authors of that, but I do ask that we all step back a bit and consider an important aspect of this particular type of therapy. In none of these patients did any bleeding-related complications develop in the neuraxis. Obviously, such complications—including hematomas, obstructions, and infections—are rare, but in fully heparinized patients, do we want to be fiddling around with the neuraxis? How many such rare but devastating complications are you willing to tolerate in order to achieve pain relief that could (arguably) be obtained in some other way?

The authors found that intrathecal morphine does delay their cherished goal of early extubation, yet they still seem to be advocating it with a lame explanation that, somehow, all we need to do is find a better dosage regimen. The curmudgeonly comments above notwithstanding, we should receive applause for our attempts at early extubation, providing we do not do our patients harm.

J.H. Tinker, M.D.

Prevalence of Heparin-associated Antibodies Without Thrombosis in Patients Undergoing Cardiopulmonary Bypass Surgery

Bauer TL, Arepally G, Konkle BA, et al (Thomas Jefferson Univ, Philadelphia; Univ of Pennsylvania, Philadelphia; Children's Hosp, Philadelphia; et al)

Circulation 95:1242–1246, 1997 3–44

Background.—The administration of heparin before cardiopulmonary bypass surgery places patients at risk for heparin-related antibodies and thromboembolic complications. The prevalence of heparin-induced antibodies in patients before and after cardiopulmonary bypass surgery was investigated.

Methods.—Plasma was obtained from 111 patients before and 5 days after surgery. Samples were tested for heparin-dependent platelet-reactive antibodies with a ^{14}C-serotonin–release assay (SRA), and antibodies to heparin–platelet factor 4 complexes with an enzyme-linked immunosorbent assay (ELISA).

Findings.—Postoperative heparin exposure was minimized. Heparin-dependent antibodies were detected preoperatively in 5% of patients with SRA and in 19% with ELISA. By postoperative day 5, the proportion of patients positive by SRA or ELISA was markedly increased to 13% and 51%, respectively. Patients given heparin treatment earlier in their hospital stay were more likely to have a positive ELISA result before surgery and a positive ELISA or SRA result after surgery. However, the prevalance of thrombocytopenia or thromboembolic events between the antibody-positive and antibody-negative groups did not differ.

Conclusions.—Previous heparin exposure results in detectable heparin-induced platelet antibodies before cardiopulmonary bypass surgery in about one fifth of patients. In addition, antibodies develop in many more patients after surgery. The high prevalence of heparin-induced antibodies suggests that these patients may be at risk for complications with additional heparin exposure.

► We are now beginning to understand some aspects of the root causes of thrombotic complications after anesthesia and surgery. I don't think we have appreciated the fact that many (most) of these patients have been on heparin in one context or another previously and would be likely to have antibodies to it. If that's true, then what is the body's response to subsequent heparin administration when these antibodies are present? With the massive dose of heparin used during cardiopulmonary bypass, it may not be obvious when some sort of reaction occurs, but we know that there are subpopulations of patients whose blood becomes hypercoagulable during the first few days after various kinds of major surgery. Perhaps heparin antibodies should be investigated very thoroughly in this context (i.e., thrombotic complications). I think this paper is representative of an exciting series of developments in this important field.

J.H. Tinker, M.D.

Changes in Platelet, Granulocyte, and Complement Activation During Cardiopulmonary Bypass Using Heparin-coated Equipment

Fukutomi M, Kobayashi S, Niwaya K, et al (Nara Med College, Japan)

Artif Organs 20:767–776, 1996 3–45

Introduction.—Even with systemic heparinization, cardiopulmonary bypass (CPB) is associated with activation of the coagulation-fibrinolytic system, which can lead to coagulation abnormalities and excessive postoperative bleeding. Studies suggest that coating artificial surfaces with biologically active heparin could inhibit the deleterious effects of CPB on coagulation. The effects of heparin coating of all CPB components on the platelet, granulocyte, and complement activation of patients undergoing coronary artery bypass surgery were studied.

Methods.—The study included 50 patients undergoing coronary artery bypass grafting. In 30 patients, the procedure was done using a heparin-coated CPB system; in 10 surgery was done with a heparin-coated oxygenator but uncoated CPB circuit; and in 10 the procedure was done with an uncoated CPB circuit. Blood samples were obtained at intervals before and during the procedure for measurement of platelet, granulocyte, and complement activation.

Results.—Ten minutes after protamine administration, patients managed with a heparin-coated oxygenator only had significantly lower plasma C3a concentrations than those managed with an uncoated CPB unit. Platelet and granulocyte counts were similar, however. The patients managed with a heparin-coated CPB system had significantly lower granulocyte elastase concentrations at 120 minutes after the onset of CPB and 10 min after the administration of protamine. At 120 minutes, this group also had a significantly reduced increase in plasma C3a concentration.

Ten minutes after protamine administration, C3a and C4a concentrations were significantly reduced in patients managed with a heparin-coated system than in those managed with an uncoated system. At the same time, platelet counts were significantly higher in patients managed with a heparin-coated system. At 5, 60, and 120 minutes after the start of the procedure, plasma β-thromboglobulin concentration was significantly lower in patients managed with a heparin-coated system. Twelve-hour postoperative blood loss was significantly reduced when a heparin-coated system was used.

Conclusions.—In patients undergoing coronary artery bypass grafting, the use of a heparin-coated oxygenator but an uncoated CPB circuit reduces complement activation but has no effect on platelet and granulocyte activation. All 3 components are significantly reduced when a heparin-coated CPB circuit, with all components making blood contact, is used. This results in reduced postoperative blood loss. The biocompatibility of CPB systems is significantly improved by the use of heparin coating.

► This first study on heparin-coated equipment of all components in the CPB system implies that such a process decreases platelet granulocyte and complement activation, and thus, will decrease postoperative blood loss and the effects of complement activation. The new point in this study is that *all* the equipment in CPB was heparin-coated, not just the oxygenator, which of course comprises 90% of the total of the surface area, but all of the surface area during CPB circuits that make blood contact. These results were not just statistically significant, but there were huge differences in complement levels, in granulocyte activation variables, in clotting variables, and, in fact, correlated with a half-unit decrease in blood transfusion requirement in the postoperative period. Thus, I think the heparin coating may have potential to improve perioperative outcomes of such patients.

M.F. Roizen, M.D.

Anti-Ischemic and Anti-Anginal Effects of Thoracic Epidural Anesthesia Versus Those of Conventional Medical Therapy in the Treatment of Severe Refractory Unstable Angina Pectoris

Olausson K, Magnusdottir H, Lurje L, et al (Sahlgrenska Univ, Göteborg, Sweden)

Circulation 96:2178–2182, 1997 3–46

Objective.—In patients with unstable angina, pain relief can be achieved by means of thoracic epidural anesthesia (TEA) to dilate the stenotic coronary arteries, causing cardiac sympathetic blockade. This treatment also improves the main determinants of myocardial oxygen demand, reducing heart rate, preload, and afterload without altering coronary perfusion pressure. Sympathetic blockade with TEA was evaluated for possible anti-ischemic effects in patients with severe, refractory unstable angina.

Methods.—The randomized trial included 40 patients with unstable angina pectoris that did not respond to standard antianginal therapy. Patients assigned to the intervention group received continuous epidural infusion of bupivacaine, causing blockade of the cardiac sympathetic segments from T1 to T5. The infusion continued for at least 48 hours. The control group received standard antianginal treatments, including β-blockers, calcium antagonists, aspirin, heparin, and nitroglycerin. The

TABLE 2.—Effects of Thoracic Epidural Anesthesia Compared With Conventional Treatment of Holter-Positive Myocardial Ischemia and Anginal Pain During 48 Hours

	Control (n=18)	TEA (n=18)	*P*
Patients with ischemia, n	11	4	<.05
Episodes of ischemia	64	18	
Per patient	3.6±0.9	1.0±0.6	<.05
Episode duration, min	355	69	
Per patient	19.7±6.2	4.1±2.5	<.05
Per patient with ischemia	3.1±0.8	0.8±0.4	<.05
AUC, mm×min	32.2±14.3	6.8±4.3	<.05
Anginal attacks	15	1	
Per patient	0.83±0.21	0.06±0.06	<.01

Note: Data presented are mean ± SEM or number of patients or events.
Abbreviations: TEA, thoracic epidural anesthesia; *AUC,* area under the curve.
(Reproduced with permission of *Circulation* courtesy of Olausson K, Magnusdottir H, Lurje L, et al: Anti-ischemic and anti-anginal effects of thoracic epidural anesthesia versus those of conventional medical therapy in the treatment of severe refractory unstable angina pectoris. *Circulation* 96[7]:2178–2182. Copyright 1997, American Heart Association.)

results were assessed in terms of number of attacks of angina and severity of myocardial ischemia, based on 48-hour ambulatory Holter monitoring.

Results.—The TEA group had a 22% incidence of myocardial ischemia, compared with 61% in the control group. The mean number of ischemic episodes during monitoring was 1.0 vs. 3.6, and the mean duration of episodes was 4 vs. 20 minutes, respectively (Table 2). The TEA group had a mean area-under-the-ST-time-curve of 6.8 mm/min, compared with 32.2 mm/min for the control group. The total number of anginal attacks recorded during monitoring was 1 in the TEA group vs. 15 in the control group, for an average of 0.06 vs. 0.83 per patient.

Conclusion.—In patients with refractory unstable angina, continuous TEA offers better antiischemic and antianginal effects than conventional antianginal therapy (Table 3). This treatment reduces the incidence of myocardial ischemia, the number and duration of episodes of ischemia, and the number of anginal attacks. It also reduces heart rate to a greater extent than that achieved with β-adrenergic blockade, with no effect on arterial blood pressure.

► The discussion section of this paper is worth reading in its entirety, as it mentions several interesting effects of epidural analgesia on platelet aggregation and on coronary vessel diameter in patients with coronary artery disease. The authors' suggestion regarding stabilization of patients with unstable angina with TEA prior to emergency coronary bypass is particularly intriguing.

The role of the anesthesiologist in the management of intractable angina and coronary ischemia may become increasingly important as studies such as this one are published. Another form of treatment that appears promising is the use of dorsal column stimulation in patients with chronic intractable angina. It appears that, as with epidural anesthesia, at least a portion of the

TABLE 3.—Previously Reported Effects of Various Treatments on 48-Hour Holter-Positive Myocardial Ischemia in Severe Unstable Angina Compared With the Outcome of This Study

	Neri Serneri (1990)	Romeo (1995)		Neri Serneri (1995)		Olausson (1997)	
	n=21	n=35	n=27	n=37	n=35	n=18	n=18
Treatment	Heparin IV	Heparin IV	Heparin IV + rTPA	Heparin IV	Heparin SC	Heparin IV	TEA
Ischemic episodes per patient, n	2.0	8.8	2.9	2.3	2.8	3.6	1.0
Episode duration per patient, min	20.1	21	14	24.6	29.6	19.7	4.1
Incidence of ischemia, %	...	89	60	...	...	61	22

Abbreviations: rTPA, recombinant tissue-type plasminogen activator; *SC,* subcutaneous; *TEA,* thoracic epidural anesthesia.

(Reproduced with permission of *Circulation* courtesy of Olausson K, Magnusdottir H, Lurje L, et al: Anti-ischemic and anti-anginal effects of thoracic epidural anesthesia versus those of conventional medical therapy in the treatment of severe refractory unstable angina pectoris. *Circulation* 96[7]:2178–2182. Copyright 1997, American Heart Association.)

analgesic effect of spinal cord stimulation on angina pectoris is related to improvement in coronary flow.

S.E. Abram, M.D.

Postoperative Analgesia Reduces Mortality and Morbidity After Esophagectomy

Tsui SL, Law S, Fok M, et al (Univ of Hong Kong)
Am J Surg 173:472–478, 1997 3–47

Background.—Good pain relief after esophageal cancer surgery can help preserve pulmonary function, minimize increases in sympathetic activity, and control coughing. Various techniques have been used, including epidural and intravenous opioids, intramuscular meperidine, and patient-controlled analgesia (PCA). These investigators examined the morbidity associated with these various analgesic methods in patients after esophagectomy.

Methods.—Over almost a decade, 578 patients underwent a 1-stage resection for esophageal carcinoma. Patients were divided into 2 groups based on whether their postoperative pain was managed by conventional intramuscular meperidine (from 1986 to 1990, $n = 279$) or by an anesthesiology-based acute pain service (from 1989 to 1995, $n = 299$). The acute pain service prescribed and monitored the use of epidural opioids, intravenous opioids, and PCA.

Findings.—Patients receiving care from the acute pain service had significantly fewer complications, a lower hospital mortality, and a shorter hospital stay than those patients managed conventionally (Table 3). In particular, in a subgroup of patients who underwent esophagectomy with thoracotomy, treatment by the acute pain service was associated with significantly fewer pulmonary and lower hospital mortality. Comparisons between the types of analgesia used in the acute pain service (Table 5) showed that epidural morphine was significantly more effective than sys-

TABLE 3.—Overall Postoperative Morbidity, Mortality, and Hospital Stay

	Group APS (n = 299)	Group CON (n = 279)	*P*
Pulmonary complications	39 (13%)	61 (22%)	0.005
Cardiovascular complications	65 (22%)	106 (38%)	<0.001
Tracheostomy	48 (16%)	70 (25%)	0.007
Postoperative mechanical ventilation	77 (26%)	84 (30%)	NS
Anastomotic leakage*	11 (4%)	11 (4%)	NS
Hospital mortality	25 (8%)	38 (14%)	0.043
Mean hospital stay (days ± SD)	21.3 ± 18.9	28.6 ± 33.0	0.001

Note: Figures represent number of patients (percent), unless otherwise stated.
*Including subclinical leakages.
Abbreviations: APS, acute pain service; *CON,* conventional pain treatment; *NS,* not significant.
(Reprinted by permission of the publisher from Tsui SL, Law S, Fok M, et al: Postoperative analgesia reduces mortality and morbidity after esophagectomy. *American Journal of Surgery,* 173:472–478. Copyright 1997 by Excerpta Medica Inc.)

TABLE 5.—Analysis on Postoperative Analgesia in 206 Patients Under Care of Acute Pain Service: Comparison Between Epidural and Systemic Morphine

	All Cases	Epidural Morphine	Systemic Morphine*	P
Number of patients	206	165	41	
Mean dose (mcg/kg/h ± SD)	—	7.3 ± 7.0	30.9 ± 1.8	<0.001
Pain assessment [median NRS score (25%–75% quartile)]				
On day of operation				
At rest	1.0 (0–3.0)	1.0 (0–2.5)	1.5 (0–3.0)	NS
During cough	4.0 (2.0–6.0)	4.0 (2.0–5.5)	5.0 (2.0–6.0)	0.039
First postoperative day				
At rest	0 (0–2.0)	0 (0–2.0)	0 (0–2.0)	NS
During cough	4.0 (2.0–5.0)	4.0 (2.0–5.0)	4.5 (3.0–5.5)	0.045
Second postoperative day				
At rest	0 (0–1.0)	0 (0–1.0)	0 (0–1.0)	NS
During cough	3.0 (2.0–5.0)	3.0 (2.0–5.0)	3.0 (2.0–4.0)	NS
Third postperative day				
At rest	0 (0–0)	0 (0–1.0)	0 (0–0.5)	NS
During cough	0 (0–2.0)	0 (0–1.5)	0 (0–3.0)	NS
Side effects				
Respiratory depression†	3 (2%)	2 (1%)	1 (5%)	NS
Nausea	18 (9%)	12 (7%)	6 (15%)	NS
Pruritus	24 (12%)	23 (14%)	1 (2%)	0.04
Overall satisfaction				
Good	181 (88%)	150 (91%)	31 (76%)	
Fair or unsatisfactory	25 (12%)	15 (9%)	10 (24%)	0.007

*Systemic morphine includes 23 patients with PCA morphine and 18 patients with intravenous morphine.

†Respiratory depression = respiratory rate < 10/min or pulse oximetry reading < 90% for > 1 minute, in 135 spontaneously breathing patients (epidural group 116, systemic group 19).

Abbreviation: NS, not significant.

(Reprinted by permission of the publisher from Tsui SL, Law S, Fok M, et al: Postoperative analgesia reduces mortality and morbidity after esophagectomy. *American Journal of Surgery,* 173:472–478. Copyright 1997 by Excerpta Medica Inc.)

temic morphine (intravenous and PCA morphine results combined) in controlling coughing on the day of operation and on the first postoperative day. Epidural morphine was not associated with any major complications, although pruritus was significantly more likely in these patients.

Conclusions.—The acute pain service plays an important role in reducing postoperative morbidity and mortality after esophagectomy. Epidural morphine provides the best pain relief, probably because epidural administration between T8 and L3 delivers the drug directly to the site of pain. Furthermore, the shortened hospital stay with epidural or systemic morphine compared with conventional meperidine injection leads to reduced health care costs associated with esophageal cancer surgery.

► Unfortunately it is not possible to determine whether the better outcomes associated with inclusion in the acute pain service group were related to better general care and surveillance or to the analgesic technique, since the majority of APS patients received epidural analgesia while the control group received only systemic opioids. The epidural patients had slightly better pain control than the APS patients on systemic opioids, but no other comparisons were made between epidural and systemic opioid patients.

S.E. Abram, M.D.

Anesthesia/Analgesia for Orthopedics

Preemptive Epidural Morphine for Postoperative Pain Relief After Lumbar Laminectomy

Kundra P, Gurnani A, Bhattacharya A (Univ College of Med Sciences, Delhi, India; Guru Teg Bahadur Hosp, Delhi, India)

Anesth Analg 85:135–138, 1997 3–48

Introduction.—Severe pain after lumbar laminectomy may lead to increased postoperative morbidity and complications. Giving a single dose of epidural opioid before surgical opening of the epidural space could provide pain relief while avoiding problems related to catheter placement after the epidural space has been opened. Such preemptive analgesia has been tried in various surgical procedures, to varying effect. Preemptive epidural morphine was studied for use as postoperative analgesia after lumbar laminectomy.

Methods.—The randomized trial included 30 ASA physical status I patients undergoing elective lumbar laminectomy with general anesthesia. Patients in group 1 received preemptive epidural morphine (3 mg) given 60 min before surgery. After surgery, they received epidural placebo. Those in group 2 received epidural placebo preoperatively, with the same dose of epidural morphine as group 1 patients, given after surgery. A visual ana-

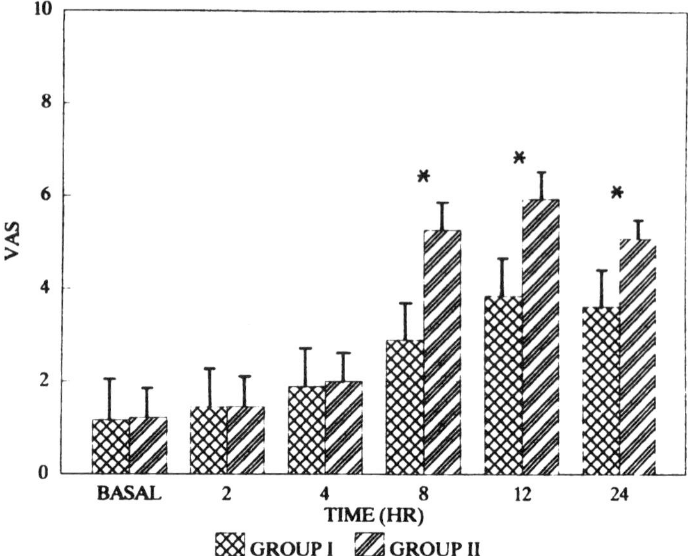

FIGURE 1.—Mean (SD) visual analog scale (*VAS*) pain scores in the 2 groups. *Cross-hatched bars* indicate group 1, the study group. *Striped bars* indicate group 2, the control group. *Asterisk* indicates $P <$ 0.5. (Courtesy of Kundra P, Gurnani A, Bhattacharya A: Preemptive epidural morphine for postoperative pain relief after lumbar laminectomy. *Anesth Analg* 85[1]:135–138, 1997.)

TABLE 2.—Time to First Postoperative Analgesic (TFA) and Opioid Requirement

	Group 1	Group 2
TFA (h) (mean ± SD)	19.9 ± 2.3*	8.5 ± 1.0
Total morphine consumption (mg) (mean ± SD)	9.5 ± 1.7*	30.6 ± 2.5
No. of supplementary doses (median)	1	4*

* $P < 0.05$.

(Courtesy of Kundra P, Gurnani A, Bhattacharya A: Preemtive epidural morphine for postoperative pain relief after lumbar laminectomy. *Anesth Analg* 85[1]:135–138, 1997.)

logue scale was used to rate pain, whereas a 4-point scale was used to rank drowsiness.

Results.—Eight hours postoperatively, patients receiving preemptive analgesia had significantly lower pain scores than those receiving preoperative placebo (Fig 1). The mean time to first postoperative analgesic was 20 hours in group 1, compared with 8.5 hours in group 2 (Table 2). Patients in the control group also required significantly more supplementary analgesia and postoperative morphine. At 12 hours, patients receiving preoperative placebo had significant sedation and a high incidence of nausea and vomiting.

Conclusion.—In patients undergoing lumbar laminectomy, a preemptive dose of epidural morphine significantly reduces postoperative pain. With preemptive morphine, analgesia is better, postoperative opioid requirements are less, and narcotic side effects are less than with postoperative morphine.

▶ Although there are animal data to support the notion that pre-injury epidural opioids are capable of blocking spinal sensitization by noxious stimuli, there has been little clinical evidence of this phenomenon. This study provides such evidence. Unfortunately, there are financial disincentives to initiating epidural analgesia preoperatively, at least in the United States, because reimbursement is less if an epidural is used as part of the intraoperative anesthetic management.

S.E. Abram, M.D.

Intravenous Phentolamine Test: An Aid in the Evaluation of Patients With Persistent Pain After Low-Back Surgery?

Sörensen J, Bengtsson M (Univ Hosp, Linköping, Sweden)

Acta Anaesthesiol Scand 41:581–585, 1997 3–49

Objective.—A subgroup of patients who have had back surgery will continue to have chronic low-back pain after surgery. Pain can be categorized as sympathetically maintained pain (SMP) or sympathetically independent pain (SIP). Systemic administration of phentolamine has been used to diagnose SMP. Phentolamine was used to determine the prevalence of SMP in patients with chronic pain after low-back surgery.

Methods.—Pain intensity was assessed using a visual analogue scale by 37 patients (14 male), aged 31–63 years, with continuous pain after undergoing 1 or more operations (either a lumbar laminectomy, with or without diskectomy, or a posterior fusion, with or without decompression). Patients were classified as placebo responders, phentolamine responders, or nonresponders based on results of an infusion of propranolol (which served as a placebo and provided protection against tachycardia), followed by an infusion of as much as 50 mg of phentolamine (1 mg/kg/hr) until pain intensity was reduced by 50% or more. A lumbar epidural fentanyl blockade was used as the control.

Results.—Baseline visual analogue scale pain scores varied from 39 to 91. Patients were clinically classified as having neuropathic (n = 22), nociceptive (n = 7), or mixed (n = 8) pain. There was 1 responder to the phentolamine test, 34 nonresponders, and 2 placebo responders. There were 9 fentanyl/local anesthetic responders to the diagnostic epidural opioid blockade, 14 local anesthetic responders, 11 nonresponders, and 3 placebo responders.

Conclusions.—Few patients with SMP were identified. Possibly the phentolamine dose was not high enough, the sympathetic nervous system is not involved in chronic spinal pain, or SMP is uncommon.

► Because low-back pain is often relieved temporarily by lumbar sympathetic block does not imply that the pain is maintained by the activity of sympathetic efferent fibers. Much of the sensory innervation of the spinal column (disk, periosteum, ligaments) travels in the sympathetic chain. These fibers leave the chain via the white rami communicantes, have cell bodies in the dorsal root ganglia, and enter the dorsal horn of the spinal cord. Anatomically, they are somewhat analogous to visceral afferents. They are sensory, not autonomic fibers.

S.E. Abram, M.D.

Other Patient Care Issues

Alcohol and Preoperative Management

Wolfort FG, Pan D, Gee J (Harvard Med School, Boston; New England Deaconess Hosp; Johns Hopkins Univ, Baltimore, Md)

Plast Reconstr Surg 98:1306–1309, 1996 3–50

Introduction.—Recent findings that moderate alcohol intake can lower mortality from coronary artery disease has prompted questions regarding alcohol's effect on preoperative platelet aggregation and thus bleeding characteristics of patients. Current research on alcohol and platelet function was reviewed.

Alcohol and Platelet Function.—Alcohol's effect is not on atherogenesis, as was previously thought, but rather on inhibition of platelet aggregation. It may be that alcohol inhibits platelet aggregation by affecting production of thromboxane A_2 or an earlier step of thromboxane A_2 synthesis involving phospholipase A_2. Within 1–2 weeks of acute cessation of drinking, platelets become hyperaggregable. Platelets return to normal levels gradually over several weeks. This rebound effect has been used to explain the rise in sudden cardiac death and stroke in alcoholics after cessation of drinking. Platelet function is particularly decreased with red wine consumption.

Alcohol and Aspirin.—Simultaneous ingestion of alcohol and aspirin has been shown to significantly increase the duration and magnitude of bleeding time, compared with either substance administered alone. The magnitude of response was unpredictable and seemed dependent on an individual's sensitivity to both compounds.

Discussion and Conclusion.—Some reports suggest that alcohol, and probably red wine, have an effect on platelet behavior that could alter bleeding characteristics. It is possible that patients who consume alcohol and take aspirin daily could place themselves at greater surgical risk for bleeding. It may be prudent for surgeons to advocate the cessation of aspirin and alcohol 1–2 weeks before surgery.

▶ The statement, "Therefore, it would be wise for us as physicians to include abstinence from alcohol, and especially the combination of alcohol and aspirin, in our preoperative teaching. It is already standard practice to advocate cessation of aspirin 1–2 weeks prior to surgery, and the same should be done with regard to alcohol," is far from what I think is either accurate or appropriate. Aspirin avoidance 2 days before surgery, if it is 1 aspirin a night, is plenty to have one seventh or more of the platelets functional and bleeding times normalized. Perhaps in plastic or reconstructive surgery, you would want 2 or 3 days, but clearly there is a benefit to aspirin in lowering cardiovascular risks. There also appears to be a benefit from alcohol in lowering these risks. Thus, abstinence for this long a period is recommended without foundation and without scientific evidence saying that there will be a benefit greater than the risk. In fact, without taking into account the rebound hypercoaguable state and potential myocardial infarction in the age-group that is having reconstructive surgery. Thus, I would urge that aspirin only be discontinued for 2 days before surgery. Perhaps we should do similarly with alcohol, although I do not think that we have enough data to recommend either at this time.

M.F. Roizen, M.D.

Glycemic Control and Sliding Scale Insulin Use in Medical Inpatients With Diabetes Mellitus

Queale WS, Seidler AJ, Brancati FL (Johns Hospkins Med Institutions, Baltimore, Md)

Arch Intern Med 157:545–552, 1997 3–51

Introduction.—Suboptimal glycemic control in medical inpatients is associated with serious adverse consequences. Few trials have examined glycemic control in the inpatient setting. Sliding scale insulin regimens have survived, despite years of continuing criticism from diabetic specialists. Predictors of hypoglycemic and hyperglycemic episodes in hospitalized patients with diabetes were prospectively evaluated, with particular attention to sliding scale insulin regimens.

Methods.—One hundred seventy-one adult patients with well-controlled diabetes (as a comorbid condition) on hospital admission were followed up to determine episodes of hypoglycemia and hyperglycemia during hospital stay. Glycemic control regimens were categorized as follows: no standing regimen, oral hypoglycemic agent, or intermediate-acting insulin. Sliding scale insulin regimens were characterized by initial insulin dose, initial glucose level, and increment of insulin per 2.7-mmol/L (50-mg/dL) increments in the glucose level.

Results.—Of 171 patients, 23% had at least 1 episode of hypoglycemia and 40% had at least 1 episode of hyperglycemia during the first 4 hospital days. The overall rate of hypoglycemic episodes was 3.4 per 100 measurements of blood glucose levels; for hyperglycemic episodes, it was 9.9 per 100 capillary blood glucose measurements. Independent predictors of hypoglycemic episodes were African-American race and low serum albumin level. Corticosteroid use was an independent marker of reduced risk of hypoglycemic episodes. Independent predictors of hyperglycemic episodes were female gender, severe diabetic complications, high glucose level on admission, admission for infectious disease, use of a conservative sliding scale regimen, and corticosteroid use. Independent predictors of reduced risk of hyperglycemic episodes were use of either a standing dose of insulin or an oral hypoglycemic agent and dialysis treatment. Patients who were started on either a conservative or aggressive sliding scale regimen without a standing regimen were 3 times more likely to have hyperglycemic episodes, compared with patients who did not begin glycemic control therapy. There was a trend toward reduced hyperglycemic risk in patients treated with oral hyperglycemic agents.

Conclusions.—Suboptimal glycemic control frequently occurs in medical inpatients with diabetes mellitus. Most patients were on sliding scale regimens that were prescribed upon admission and continued throughout hospitalization without modification. Sliding scale regimens were associated with increased risk of hyperglycemia and provided no benefit over the standing glycemic control regimen alone.

► Although this study discounts sliding scale insulin therapy for inpatients with diabetes mellitus, it seems that this arcane practice persists in both the operating room and ICU. I continue to witness physicians, with little understanding of this drug's pharmacokinetic or pharmacodynamic properties, prescribe sliding scale subcutaneous, or worse, sliding scale intravenous insulin for critically ill patients. Although outcome data are lacking, I submit the following "rules of thumb" for the management of the critically ill diabetic patient in the perioperative period:

1. Maintain intravenous insulin infusion until the patient is able to eat.
2. Avoid all forms of subcutaneous insulin in the patient who has clinical evidence of hypoperfusion.
3. Set a minimum goal of avoiding glycosuria, because this will mitigate against electrolyte disturbances and intravascular volume depletion.
4. Resume subcutaneous regular insulin or an oral hypoglycemic agent in anticipation of the patient being discharged from the ICU.

D.M. Rothenberg, M.D.

Comparison of Volume Controlled With Pressure Controlled Ventilation During One-Lung Anaesthesia

Tuğrul M, Çamci E, Karadenîz H, et al (Univ of Istanbul, Turkey)

Br J Anaesth 79:306–310, 1997 3–52

Background.—Volume-controlled ventilation (VCV) is typically used to increase airway pressure in patients undergoing 1-lung anesthesia. An alternative method that is coming into favor is pressure-controlled ventilation (PCV), which distributes inspired gases more uniformly and avoids the barotrauma to the dependent lung often associated with VCV. In this study, VCV and PCV were compared for their effects on airways and hemodynamic parameters in patients undergoing 1-lung anesthesia.

Methods.—All 48 patients were undergoing thoracotomy requiring 1-lung ventilation; no patient had cardiac, hepatic, or renal disease. After tracheal intubation and the insertion of a pulmonary artery catheter, all patients initially received 2-lung ventilation with VCV. Once 1-lung ventilation began, patients were randomized either to receive VCV first and then switch to PCV (n = 24), or to receive PCV first and then switch to VCV (n = 24). Arterial and venous oxygen tensions and saturations were measured at various points, as were airways pressures.

Findings.—The only variables to differ significantly between the 2 ventilation modes were peak airway pressure (significantly lower during PCV, 23.65 vs. 28.3 cm H_2O), inspiratory plateau pressure (significantly lower during PCV, 17.8 vs. 18.5 cm H_2O), the pulmonary shunt (significantly lower during PCV, 36.2% vs. 40.2%), and arterial oxygen tension (significantly higher during PCV, 32.3 vs. 28.4 kPa). The last-mentioned parameter was inversely correlated with pulmonary function tests in that most patients with an improvement in arterial oxygen tension had a forced vital capacity of less than 77% or a forced expiratory volume in 1 second of less than 77%.

Conclusion.—Pressure-controlled ventilation maintained a lower peak airway pressure, lower plateau pressure, and lower pulmonary shunt than VCV, while also keeping arterial oxygen tension higher. These results reflect the lower airways pressures with PCV, which should help avoid barotrauma to the dependent lung. Pressure-controlled ventilation was most beneficial for patients with lower values on pulmonary function testing. Thus, PCV should be considered an alternative to VCV during 1-lung anesthesia, particularly for patients with respiratory disease.

▶ Today's "fad" is PCV. The author chose patients undergoing thoracotomy, specifically with 1-lung ventilation, to provide something close to a "worst case scenario" to see whether PCV is advantageous over conventional VCV. I think these results are dramatic. Peak airway pressure, plateau pressure, and pulmonary shunt were all significantly better during PCV, and arterial partial pressure of oxygen increased in 31 of the 48 patients, compared with VCV. Manufacturers of newer anesthetic equipment are touting its ability to deliver pressure as well as VCV. There are naysayers who scoff at purchasing new anesthesia delivery equipment. Clearly, the old equipment almost never "wears out." Instead, it simply becomes obsolete. It won't be long before inability to deliver PCV may render an anesthesia system obsolete.

J.H. Tinker, M.D.

Intravesical Morphine Analgesia After Bladder Surgery

Duckett JW, Cangiano T, Cubina M, et al (Children's Hosp of Philadelphia)

J Urol 157:1407–1409, 1997 3–53

Objective.—There is no satisfactory method for administering local analgesia to the bladder mucosa to relieve postoperative pain and avoid systemic side effects after ureteroneocystostomy. Because results of a pilot study for evaluating the effect and safety of a morphine drip into the bladder demonstrated efficacy, a prospective randomized study of patients undergoing ureteral reimplantation surgery, using 3 different concentrations of morphine postoperatively, was designed to examine efficacy and determine doses.

Methods.—Intravesical morphine continuous infusion drips were administered to 52 children (14 boys), aged 4.1–13.2 years, who underwent Cohen cross-trigonal reimplantation. Patients were randomly assigned to receive either 0.05, 0.375, or 0.5 mg/mL of intravesical morphine at a rate of 0.04 mL/kg/hr via infusion pump. A Penrose drain remained in place for 48–72 hours or until bladder leakage stopped. Pain was assessed every 4 hours using a Wong-Baker faces scale, and activity and side effects were recorded. Group data were compared statistically using the Kruskal-Wallis and paired *t* tests. Plasma morphine levels were determined by high-pressure liquid chromatography.

Results.—Pain was significantly greater in the group receiving 0.05 mg/mL of morphine than in the other 2 groups during four of six 8-hour shifts. There was no difference between groups on day 3. Plasma levels of morphine were not detectable.

Conclusions.—Bladder morphine infusion is safe and effective in children for treatment of postoperative pain after bladder surgery.

▶ There is growing interest in the peripheral analgesic effects of opiates. This study provides evidence that intravesical application of opioids provides analgesia for postoperative irritation of the bladder mucosa. The obvious benefit is either improved analgesia or reduction in systemic opioids. Although this technique provided improved analgesia, it did not eliminate the need for systemic analgesics, because other sources of nociception were not affected.

S.E. Abram, M.D.

Sevoflurane for Difficult Tracheal Intubation

Mostafa SM, Atherton AMJ (Royal Liverpool Univ, England)

Br J Anaesth 79:392–393, 1997 3–54

Introduction.—Sevoflurane has become a popular choice for induction of anesthesia by inhalation. There have been no reports of the use of sevoflurane in patients with a difficult airway. Three cases in which sevoflurane was used to manage a difficult airway are reported.

Patients.—The patients were 2 men and 1 woman undergoing head and neck surgery, including radical maxillectomy in 2 patients and parathyroidectomy in 1. Tracheal intubation was expected in all patients; however, awake fiberoptic intubation proved infeasible. All patients were premedicated with glycopyrronium (200 μg IV) and temazepam (10 mg orally) or midazolam (3 mg). All received preoxygenation with 100% oxygen for 5 minutes. Anesthesia was then induced with up to 7% sevoflurane in either oxygen or a nitrous oxide/oxygen mix. In 2 of the patients, this produced smooth and fast induction of anesthesia. Airway obstruction developed briefly in 1 patient, but the problem was successfully managed by insertion of a nasopharyngeal airway, without development of hypoxia. None of the patients have an Spo_2 of less than 96%. Pulse oximetry and capnography confirmed satisfactory oxygenation and ventilation throughout induction in 2 of the patients. After induction, fiberoptic or conventional tracheal intubation were performed.

Discussion.—The successful use of sevoflurane for inhalation induction in patients with difficult airways is described. In this situation, sevoflurane provides a greater margin of safety than halothane. Further study of sevoflurane for use in difficult tracheal intubations is warranted.

► Increasingly, around the world, sevoflurane is being used in patients with potentially difficult airways to rapidly induce anesthesia, perform brief examinations with a conventional laryngoscope, then decide what to do while retaining the ability to maintain the airway and awaken the patient rapidly. I think this adds considerably to our armamentarium of techniques in these difficult situations. As everyone who has any experience with fiberoptic gadgetry knows, the latter is by no means the answer in all clinical circumstances of the difficult airway.

J.H. Tinker, M.D.

Comparison of Conventional Anterior Surgery and Laparoscopic Surgery for Inguinal-Hernia Repair

Liem MSL, van der Graaf Y, van Steensel CJ, et al (Univ Hosp Utrecht, The Netherlands; Ikazia Hosp, Rotterdam, The Netherlands; St Clara Hosp, Rotterdam, The Netherlands; et al)

N Engl J Med 336:1541–1547, 1997 3–55

Introduction.—Postoperative recovery for inguinal hernias may be slow, but results of surgical repair often are satisfactory. For postoperative pain and recovery, laparoscopic techniques for the repair of inguinal hernia have proved superior to open repair in small studies. Conventional anterior repair was compared with extraperitoneal laparoscopic repair for recovery, complications, and recurrence rates in patients with primary or first recurrent unilateral hernias in a multicenter, randomized study.

Methods.—Extraperitoneal laparoscopic repair was done in 487 patients and conventional anterior repair in 507 patients. At 1 week, 6 weeks, 6 months, and 1–2 years after surgery, follow-up was conducted to record information about postoperative recovery, complications, and recurrences.

Results.—Wound abscesses were found in 6 patients in the open-surgery group, but in none in the laparoscopic group. A more rapid recovery was seen in the laparoscopic group. Resumption of normal daily activity occurred in a median of 6 days in the laparoscopic group, compared with the open surgery group. The laparoscopic group returned to work at a median of 14 days and the open-surgery group returned to work at a median of 21 days. Athletic activities were resumed at 24 days for the laparoscopic group and at 36 days for the open-surgery group (Fig 2). Those in the laparoscopic group reported less pain after surgery than the open-surgery group (Fig 1). On the day of surgery, 33% of the open-surgery group did not require analgesic drugs for postoperative pain, whereas in the laparoscopic group, 59% did not require drugs. In the open-surgery group, 31 (6%) of the patients had recurrences with a median follow-up of 607 days, whereas there were 17 (3%) of the patients in the laparoscopic group who

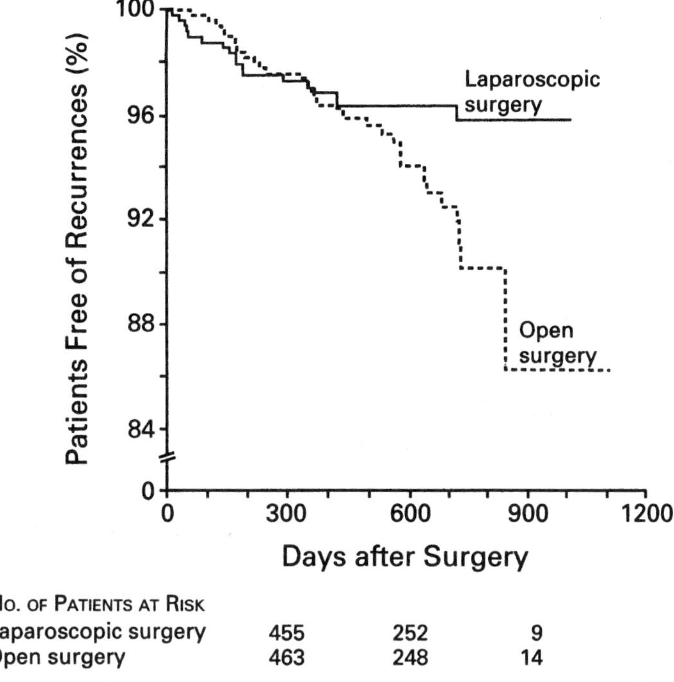

FIGURE 2.—Kaplain-Meier curves for recurrence free survival in the open-surgery and laparoscopic-surgery groups. The median follow-up was 607 days (interquartile range, 369 to 731). The *P* value for the difference in the rates of recurrence between the 2 groups was 0.05 by the log-rank test. (Reprinted by permission of *The New England Journal of Medicine*, from Liem MSL, van der Graaf Y, van Steensel CJ, et al: Comparision of conventional anterior surgery and laparoscopic surgery for inguinal-hernia repair. *N Engl J Med* 336:1541–1547, 1997. Copyright 1997, Massachusetts Medical Society. All rights reserved.)

had recurrences. In the laparoscopic group, all but 3 of the recurrences occurred within 1 year after surgery and were related to surgeon errors. During the first year, 15 patients in the open-surgery group had recurrences and 16 in the second year.

Conclusion.—Patients who have open surgical repair with inguinal hernias recover more slowly and have more recurrences than those who have laparoscopic repair.

▶ This is a well-conducted, multicenter, randomized study that defines outcome after laparoscopic surgery for inguinal hernia repair. Clearly, there are distinct advantages that pertain to laparascopic repair. The authors point out that this study was done by surgeons who *like* and are experienced in laparascopic surgery and that these results may not apply to all surgeons and all hospitals. This is true; however, when looking at outcome, one always has to define the expertise of the surgical team, as has been done for other large, randomized trials, e.g., for incidence of stroke after carotid endarterectomy, for asymptomatic carotid artery stenosis.[1]

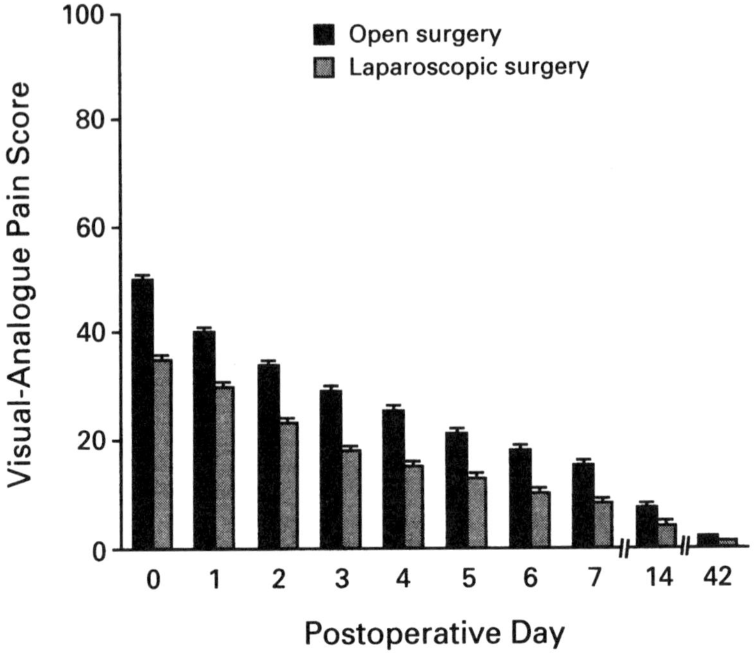

FIGURE 1.—Mean (± SE) Visual Analogue Scores for postoperative pain on the day of surgery, during the first 7 days after surgery, and at 14 and 42 days in patients with inguinal hernias repaired with open or laparoscopic surgery. A score of 0 denotes no pain, and a score of 100, unbearable pain. Postoperative pain was less severe in the laparoscopic-surgery group ($P < 0.001$). (Reprinted by permission of The *New England Journal of Medicine*, from Liem MSL, van der Graaf Y, van Steensel CJ, et al: Comparison of conventional anterior surgery and laparoscopic surgery for inguinal-hernia repair. *N Engl J Med* 336:1541–1547, 1997. Copyright 1997, Massachusetts Medical Society. All rights reserved.)

In this study, when medical management and surgery were compared, the proviso was that the team had to have a 3% perioperative morbidity and mortality.

M. Wood, M.D.

Reference

1. Endarterectomy for asymptomatic carotid artery stenosis. Executive Committee for the Asymptomic Carotid Atherosclerosis Study. *JAMA* 273:1421–1428, 1995.

Treatment of Traumatic Brain Injury With Moderate Hypothermia
Marion DW, Penrod LE, Kelsey SF, et al (Univ of Pittsburgh, Pa)
N Engl J Med 336:540–546, 1997 3–56

Background.—The metabolic processes that result from traumatic brain injury can exacerbate the injury. Evidence suggests that hypothermia may limit some of these responses. The value of moderate hypothermia in patients with traumatic brain injury was determined.

Methods.—Eighty-two patients with closed-head injuries ranging from 3 to 7 on the Glasgow Coma Scale were included in a randomized, controlled study. Patients assigned to hypothermia were cooled to 33°C a mean 10 of hours after injury, remained at about this temperature for 24 hours, and were then rewarmed. The rest of the patients were left normothermic. An examiner unaware of treatment assignments assessed the patients at 3, 6, and 12 months after treatment.

Findings.—Twenty-five survivors (78%) in the hypothermia groups and 29 survivors (88%) in the normothermia group were transferred to a hospital for head injury rehabilitation. The mean length of stay for each group was 69 days. The 2 groups were similar in the rates of incidence of delayed posttraumatic intracranial hematomas; infections; deep venous thrombosis; and pulmonary, renal, and cardiac complications. At the 3-month assessment, 38% of the hypothermia group and 17% of the normothermia group had a Glasgow Outcome Scale score of 4 or 5. At 12 months, 62% in the hypothermia group and 38% in the normothermia group had a score of 4 or 5. Cerebrospinal fluid analysis indicated that, among patients with an initial Glasgow Coma Scale score of 5–7, those in the hypothermia group had a significantly lower mean concentration of interleukin-1β and glutamate compared with the normothermic patients in the first 36 hours after injury.

Conclusion.—Moderate hypothermia (32°C to 33°C) for 24 hours begun shortly after severe traumatic brain injury significantly improves outcomes at 3 and 6 months in patients without flaccidity or decerebrate rigidity on initial assessment. Outcomes at 12 months also appear to be improved.

► The use of moderate hypothermia (33°C) appears to be effective in minimizing neurologic injury after head trauma much as it has been shown to improve neurologic outcome after elective intracranial surgery. This study shows that not all hypothermia is deleterious. (Please note the difference between Glasgow Coma Scale and Glasgow Outcome Scale.)

D.M. Rothenberg, M.D.

► The protective effect of hypothermia during circulatory arrest in preventing organ damage is well recognized, and this technique has been used by anesthesiologists during cardiac surgery and neurosurgery for many years. The fact that moderate hypothermia (32°C to 33°C) for 24 hours may improve outcome in patients with traumatic brain injury is important. The initial Glasgow Coma Score (i.e., the degree of injury) predicated outcome, in that hypothermia did not improve outcome in patients with low scores (3 or 4 on admission). It is of interest that both groups received vecuronium and fentanyl (to prevent shivering in the hypothermia group) and that patients in the normothermia group required passive warming to maintain rectal temperature at 37°C. As for many studies, more questions were raised than answered. When must hypothermia be initiated after brain injury to provide therapeutic effect? Which patients should be selected to be treated with hypothermia? The 2 groups did not differ significantly in terms of age, but does age matter? And what would be the outcome in a pediatric population? This randomized controlled trial raises many questions that intensivists and investigators in the area of brain trauma research will surely address over the next few years.

M. Wood, M.D.

4 Anesthesia-related Pharmacology and Toxicology

Sevoflurane Issues

Serum Glutathione S-transferase Concentrations and Creatinine Clearance After Sevoflurane Anaesthesia

Darling JR, Murray JM, McBride DR, et al (Ulster Hosp, Belfast, Northern Ireland; Queen's Univ of Belfast, Northern Ireland)

Anaesthesia 52:121–126, 1997 4–1

Background.—There is ongoing concern about sevoflurane's potential for organ toxicity, including hepatotoxicity and nephrotoxicity. The body metabolizes sevoflurane to inorganic fluoride, which has been linked to nephrotoxicity in patients receiving methoxyflurane. Sevoflurane and isoflurane were compared for their effects on glutathione S-transferase concentration and creatinine clearance, as markers of hepatic and renal function.

Methods.—The study included 50 adult patients, ASA I–III, scheduled for body surface surgery of 1- to 3-hour predicted duration. They were randomly assigned to receive either sevoflurane or isoflurane in nitrous oxide/oxygen, to an FIO_2 of 0.4. Fluid administration was standardized, and the patients' lungs were ventilated to normocapnia. The systolic arterial pressure was maintained at 70% to 100% of baseline by adjusting the expired concentration of anesthetic.

Results.—Patients in the sevoflurane group received a lower dose of anesthetic, with an MAC-h of 1.0 for sevoflurane vs. 1.5 for isoflurane. The 2 anesthetic groups showed no differences in serum glutathione S-transferase concentration or creatinine clearance (Fig 3). There were no differences in serum or urine osmolality. Serum sodium was significantly higher in the sevoflurane group.

Conclusions.—In patients undergoing body surface surgery, sevoflurane and isoflurane have comparable effects on hepatic and renal function. This occurs despite an increase in serum concentrations of inorganic fluoride.

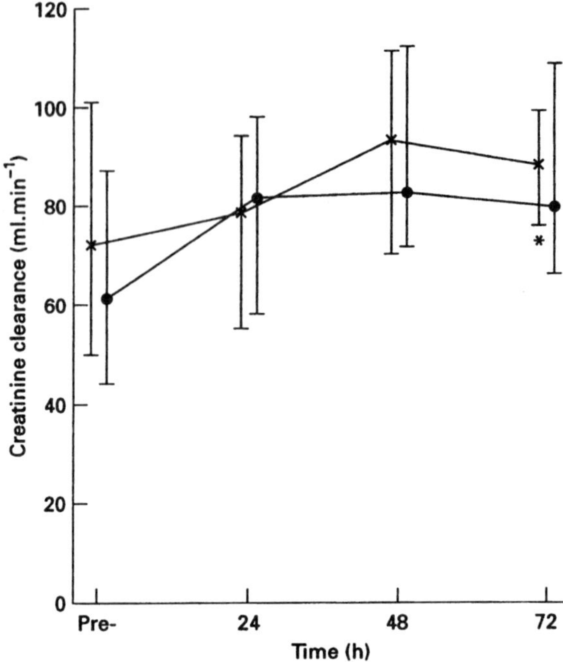

FIGURE 3.—Creatinine clearance (mL·min^{-1}) before and after isoflurane (● [n = 26] or sevoflurane (× [n = 24] anesthesia. Values are median (interquartile range). Normal range: 70–120 mL·min^{-1}. *$P < 0.05$ change from baseline levels using Wilcoxon matched pairs test. (Reprinted from Darling JR, Murray JM, McBride DR, et al: Serum glutathione S-transferase concentrations and creatinine clearance after sevoflurane anaesthesia, *Anaesthesia* 52:121–126. Copyright 1997 by permission of the publisher, WB Saunders Company Limited, London.)

This study finds no differences in serum glutathione S-transferase concentration, creatinine clearance, or serum or urine osmolality between sevoflurane and isoflurane.

▶ Sevoflurane either does or does not impair renal function intraoperatively and postoperatively. One would think that is a straightforward question, but it is not. How to measure renal function seems to be a considerable controversy these days. The standard creatinine clearance rate does not seem to be good enough for some people, so various "modern," but controversial, markers such as glutathione S-transferase are being talked about in various circles. Whichever way you measure it, despite elevated fluoride levels in the sevoflurane group, these markers of renal dysfunction did not show sevoflurane to be productive of same.

J.H. Tinker, M.D.

Compound A Induces Sister Chromatid Exchanges in Chinese Hamster Ovary Cells

Eger EI II, Laster MJ, Winegar R, et al (Univ of California, San Francisco; SRI International, Menlo Park, Calif)

Anesthesiology 86:918–922, 1997 4–2

Objective.—The vinyl ether compound A [$CF_2C{=}C(CF_3)OCH_2F$] is a degradation product of sevoflurane that might be an alkylating agent and therefore a potential carcinogen. To determine if the compound is a genotoxin, its ability to induce sister chromatid exchanges (SCE) was investigated in Chinese hamster ovary cells with and without metabolic activation.

Methods.—Using a modified Galloway et al. protocol, Chinese hamster ovary (CHO) cells were incubated in an 8% carbon dioxide atmosphere with a serum-free medium designed for culturing CHO cells in suspension. Compound A in concentrations of 11–468 ppm was incubated for 2 hours. Then bromodeoxyuridine was added, and the incubation continued for an additional 34 hours. Colcemid was added to arrest growth in metaphase, and chromosome spreads were prepared and stained by the fluorescence plus Giemsa technique. Slides for all exposures were prepared and 50-chromosome spreads were counted in a blind fashion to determine the number of SCEs.

Results.—Concentrations of compound A of 27, 57, 118, 228, and 468 ppm without metabolic activator induced a significant number of SCEs. SCE formation was dose-related. The presence of metabolic activator did not increase the ability of compound A to induce SCEs.

Conclusion.—Compound A appears to induce SCEs in CHOs at concentrations as low as 27 ppm. Additional studies of the possible mutagenic effects of compound A should be conducted in other mammalian cell models.

► This paper invokes a probably disrespectful cartoon of Ted Eger dressed as a nun, namely "Sister Chromatid." As Dr. Eger knows very well, there are many tests for mutagenicity, teratogenicity, and carcinogenicity. Each of these tests has its advocates and detractors. The advocates contend that the particular test in question is the most sensitive or the most predictive of clinically relevant toxicity. In order to get past the FDA, sevoflurane was obviously subjected to several standard tests. This paper is a fairly blatant attempt by a consultant to a competitor to cast aspersions. I can conclude from this paper only one thing, and that is that if I need to anesthetize Chinese hamsters, I would probably have to call Dr. Eger for advice and consultation.

J.H. Tinker, M.D.

Recovery and Kinetic Characteristics of Desflurane and Sevoflurane in Volunteers After 8-h Exposure, Including Kinetics of Degradation Products

Eger EI II, Bowland T, Ionescu P, et al (Univ of California, San Francisco)

Anesthesiology 87:517–526, 1997 4–3

Introduction.—To address the perception that a less soluble anesthetic would better serve the needs of today's anesthesia practitioner, sevoflurane and desflurane were developed. Previous studies with rats have shown that recoveries with desflurane are twice as fast as recovery after anesthesia with sevoflurane; however, these studies had limitations. During administration or elimination of sevoflurane, the kinetics of compound A [CH_2F-O-C(=CF_2)(CF_3)], which are linked to the administration of sevoflurane, have not been adequately defined. Volunteers were given anesthesia at 1.25 minimum alveolar concentration of each anesthetic and at the lowest inflow rate recommended by the U.S. Food and Drug Administration to determine the kinetics, recovery information, and toxicity of desflurane, sevoflurane, and compound A.

Methods.—Volunteers received 1.25 minimum alveolar concentration of desflurane or sevoflurane. Each was given for 8 hours in a fresh gas inflow of 2 L/min. During administration, inspired (F_I) and end-tidal (F_A) concentrations of anesthetic and compound A were measured, and F_A relative to F_{A0} (the last end-tidal concentration during administration) during elimination. Measurements were taken of the index of recovery.

Results.—The F_I/F_A ratio rapidly approached 1.0. The sevoflurane value was 1.11 ± 0.02 and for desflurane, it was 1.06 ± 0.01. For compound A, the F_I/F_A ratio was approximately 0.8. With desflurane, the F_A/F_{A0} ratio decreased slightly more than with sevoflurane. Faster recovery with desflurane was seen, according to objective measures of the initial response to command (14 ± 4 minutes with desflurane vs. 28 ± 8 minutes with sevoflurane) and orientation (19 ± 4 minutes with desflurane vs. 33 ± 9 minutes with sevoflurane). Results of the Digit Symbol Substitution, P-deletion, and Trieger tests showed that recovery was faster with desflurane than with sevoflurane. Less vomiting was produced with desflurane (median of 1 episode) than sevoflurane (median of 5 episodes). For compound A, the F_A/F_{A0} ratio decreased within 5 minutes to a constant value of 0.1.

Conclusions.—The kinetics of desflurane and sevoflurane are consistent with their solubilities. During anesthetic administration, sevoflurane's greater biodegradation probably increases F_I/F_A differences. During elimination, its great biodegradation probably decreases F_A/F_{A0} differences. Because of substantial degradation, there is a 20% difference in F_A for compound A from F_I. Desflurane produces recovery from anesthesia twice as fast when compared with sevoflurane. The slower recovery with sevoflurane is not fully explained by the differences in ventilation, or alveolar or tissue elimination.

▶ I selected this article because it highlights the effects of solubility and metabolism on uptake and elimination of the 2 new inhalational anesthetics. Although recovery from desflurane is faster than that associated with sevoflurane using the protocol described in this study, it is important to recognize that exposure was for 8 hours, whereas in practice these 2 agents are probably used for brief outpatient exposure.

M. Wood, M.D.

Comparison of Induction and Recovery Between Sevoflurane and Halothane Supplementation of Anaesthesia in Children Undergoing Outpatient Dental Extractions

Ariffin SA, Whyte JA, Malins AF, et al (Queen Elizabeth Hosp, Edgbaston, Birmingham, England)

Br J Anaesth 78:157–159, 1997 4–4

Introduction.—A study of 80 children undergoing dental extraction was designed to compare sevoflurane and halothane in terms of induction, maintenance, and recovery from anesthesia. Some previous studies found sevoflurane to have features desirable in this setting, but one report suggests that recovery may not be more rapid with sevoflurane.

Patients and Methods.—The 80 children ranged in age from 5 to 12 years and were not receiving any medication. They were randomly assigned to sevoflurane or halothane supplementation of 66% nitrous oxide in oxygen. Induction employed 2% sevoflurane or 0.75% halothane; maintenance concentrations were 4% or 1.5%, respectively. Recovery from anesthesia was assessed by the time between discontinuation of anesthesia until the children opened their eyes. Also recorded were the presence or absence of nausea, vomiting, shivering, headache, and coughing in recovery and time to return to normal activity and normal appetite.

Results.—The 2 groups were similar in age, weight, number of teeth extracted, duration of administration of anesthesia (less than 4 minutes), and duration of surgery. Children in the sevoflurane group showed a significantly more rapid induction of anesthesia, but were slower to awaken than those in the halothane group. Discharge times from the hospital were similar, and most children had a normal appetite and returned to normal activities on the same day. Complications during induction and maintenance of anesthesia were few in both groups. Nausea after discharge occurred in 10 children in the halothane group vs. 3 in the sevoflurane group.

Discussion.—In contrast to some previous reports, the time to awaken after brief anesthesia for dental extraction was faster for children in the halothane group than for those in the sevoflurane group. Sevoflurane's more rapid induction, however, can be important at a potentially distressing time for children.

▶ Only in Britain would there be operations where the mean duration was less than 4 minutes! Somehow, the children who received sevoflurane were slightly slower to awaken (though only by 65 seconds) than those given halothane. Why? One explanation could be that the more rapid achievement of inspired concentration of sevoflurane, because of its low solublility, may have permitted more rapid induction with it to deeper levels of CNS suppression. I included this article more as an interesting exercise in uptake and distribution than to emphasize the conclusion to which the authors came, namely, that sevoflurane is "acceptable." We already knew that, in spades.

J.H. Tinker, M.D.

Occupational Exposure to Sevoflurane, Halothane and Nitrous Oxide During Paediatric Anaesthesia: Waste Gas Exposure During Paediatric Anaesthesia

Hoerauf K, Funk W, Harth M, et al (Univ Hosp, Vienna)

Anaesthesia 52:215–219, 1997 4–5

Background.—Contamination of the operating room by waste inhalational anesthetic gases is unavoidable. To minimize risk to the operating room staff, the United States and most European public health authorities recommend threshold values of anesthetic gases. The occupational exposure to such gases is higher during anesthesia in children than in adults, although the exact reason is unknown.

Methods.—In a prospective study, concentrations of waste anesthetic gases in the operating room during general anesthesia in 20 children were measured. A highly sensitive, photoacoustic infrared spectrometer was used. Samples were measured from the breathing zones of the anesthetist and circulating nurse, and the data were recorded continuously on a computer system.

Results.—The operating room had 20 changes of air per hour provided by an air conditioning system. The United Kingdom Committee for Occupational Safety and Health recommends threshold values of 100 ppm of N_2O, 50 ppm of isoflurane, and 10 ppm of halothane. These values were briefly exceeded during mask induction in several patients. After tracheal intubation, trace concentrations of sevoflurane, halothane, and N_2O were generally under recommended values and comparable with values during adult anesthesia.

Discussion.—These findings show that the main time of pollution of anesthetic gases during general anesthesia in children is during mask induction. The brief periods of high peak concentrations of anesthetic gases and N_2O had little effect on total occupational exposure, probably because of the effective air conditioning system at this facility. The contribution of mask induction to the overall exposure to waste gases may be greater under substandard conditions.

► Sevoflurane is obviously of benefit in pediatric induction. Mask inductions, in general, are productive of problematic operating room air pollution. On the other hand, it would be expected that a rapidly acting agent, such as sevoflurane, would also allow faster induction and control and, therefore, less operating room air pollution—which is, indeed, precisely what these authors have found. Thus, not only does sevoflurane appear to be an advance in pediatric induction, it seems to have the added benefit of reducing operating room air pollution levels. That certainly cannot be bad, although it may be difficult to prove that it's good.

J.H. Tinker, M.D.

Single-Breath Inhalation Induction of Sevoflurane Anaesthesia With and Without Nitrous Oxide: A Feasibility Study in Adults and Comparison With an Intravenous Bolus of Propofol

Hall JE, Stewart JIM, Harmer M (Univ of Wales, Cardiff)

Anaesthesia 52:410–415, 1997 4–6

Objective.—Sevoflurane offers rapid anesthetic induction and emergence. A previous study in adults found more prolonged induction times with sevoflurane than with propofol. Sevoflurane in nitrous oxide and oxygen was compared for induction with sevoflurane in oxygen alone and propofol infusion in unpremedicated day-case patients.

Methods.—The study included 75 adult patients, all ASA grade 1 or 2, undergoing minor orthopedic or gynecologic surgical procedures. They were randomly assigned to 3 induction groups: propofol 200 mg by IV injection; sevoflurane 8% in oxygen; and sevoflurane 8% in nitrous oxide and oxygen in a ratio of 2:1. Gaseous induction was achieved by a vital capacity technique using a Mapelson A system and a 4 L reservoir bag. Anesthesia was assessed by time to cessation of finger tapping, time to loss of eyelash reflex, time to jaw relaxation, and time to regular settled breathing after insertion of the laryngeal airway mask. The study also monitored blood pressure and pulse rate, adverse airway events, and acceptability of the induction technique.

Results.—Propofol was associated with shorter times to cessation of finger tapping and jaw relaxation. By the final induction stage, these differences were no longer present. Time to regular settled breathing tended to be faster with sevoflurane in nitrous oxide and oxygen, although the difference was not significant. All 3 groups had good cardiovascular stability. Adverse airway events were rare and never caused the oxygen saturation to decline to less than 96%. The patients receiving gaseous induction techniques had more excitation, though this did not cause problems with induction. All groups reported satisfaction with their induction technique.

Conclusions.—Administered by a vital capacity technique, 8% sevoflurane in nitrous oxide and oxygen is a rapid, reliable, and safe method of inducing anesthesia. It may be a useful alternative to IV induction. Induction times are somewhat longer with sevoflurane, but the difference is probably not clinically significant. The cost of sevoflurane in nitrous oxide and oxygen compares favorably with that of propofol.

▶ Whether single-breath induction is particularly important, mask induction with sevoflurane is becoming important for several reasons. First, it seems to be well tolerated by patients and eliminates expensive induction agents. Second, in patients with potentially difficult airways, many anesthesiologists are choosing mask inductions, then have a look with a laryngoscope, examine the "lay of the land" in the back of the patient's pharynx before committing to paralysis. Sevoflurane allows this. In this particular study, in Britain, patient satisfaction with the induction was high. Whether mask induction would produce similarly high patient satisfaction levels in the United States is interesting to think about.

J.H. Tinker, M.D.

Comparison of Inhalation Inductions With Xenon and Sevoflurane

Nakata Y, Goto T, Morita S (Teikyo Univ, Chiba, Japan)

Acta Anaesthesiol Scand 41:1157–1161, 1997 4–7

Objective.—Whereas inhalation induction agents such as sevoflurane and nitrous oxide cause air pollution and have an unpleasant odor, xenon is a colorless gas that is not an environmental hazard and has a low solubility in blood. There is little information comparing inhalation induction with xenon vs. sevoflurane. In a randomized clinical study, the speed of induction, and respiratory and cardiovascular reactions to inhalation induction with xenon compared to equianesthetic concentration of sevoflurane were evaluated.

Methods.—Either xenon with 29% oxygen (n = 12) or sevoflurane with 98% oxygen (n = 12) was administered to 24 adult patients in American Society of Anesthesiologists' class status 1–2 premedicated with midazolam, 0.05 mg/kg. Patients were instructed to take vital capacity breaths until they lost consciousness. Induction time, respiratory rate, tidal volume, inspired minute ventilation, total ventilatory volume until loss of consciousness, end-tidal concentration of anesthetic agents, and any complications were recorded.

Results.—Anesthesia was induced in all patients with the mean induction time significantly shorter in the xenon group than in the sevoflurane group (71 vs. 147 seconds). Total ventilatory volume was similar between groups. Whereas blood pressure was stable in both groups, heat rate increased significantly in the sevoflurane group compared to the xenon group. End-tidal concentration of sevoflurane was significantly higher than end-tidal concentration of xenon after 40 seconds. The incidence of complications and number of complaints of unpleasant odor were similar in the 2 groups.

Conclusion.—Xenon induced anesthesia faster than sevoflurane without complications, with smaller decreases in tidal volume, and a smaller decrease in respiratory rate. Because xenon is environmentally friendly, it represents an acceptable alternative to sevoflurane and other conventional environmentally hazardous inhalation anesthetics.

▶ Although this is a comparison between xenon and sevoflurane, my greater interest is in the fact that xenon is now being tested as a clinically relevant anesthetic. We have long known that it is an anesthetic, albeit a curiosity. If indeed "recycling" methods can be developed that make sense, we may be seeing anesthesia administration systems that actually allow the performance of clinical xenon anesthesia.

J.H. Tinker, M.D.

Haemodynamic and Catecholamine Changes During Rapid Sevoflurane Induction With Tidal Volume Breathing

Nishiyama T, Aibiki M, Hanaoka K (Univ of Tokyo)

Can J Anaesth 44:1066–1070, 1997 4–8

Objective.—The plasma catecholamine concentration changes were compared between rapid inhalation induction of anesthesia with a maximal inspiratory effort using a high concentration of sevoflurane (7%) vs. slow inhalation induction (7 minutes) at a low concentration that is increased gradually to 5% using thiamylal IV induction.

Methods.—Three groups of 8 patients were randomly allocated to receive inhalation induction with sevoflurane 7% (inspiratory concentration) for 3 minutes (group A), inhalation induction with increasing sevoflurane inspiratory concentration rising 0.5% every 2 or 3 breaths to 5% and maintained at 5% for 7 minutes (group B), or thiamylal 5 mg/kg (control group C). Blood pressure, heart rate, and plasma epinephrine and norepinephrine concentration were measured at baseline, after intubation, and at 1, 3, 5, and 10 minutes after intubation. Data were compared statistically.

Results.—Whereas blood pressure increased in the control group, there were no increases in either group A or B. Plasma catecholamine levels decreased similarly in all 3 groups. The control group had a higher rate pressure product at 1 minute after intubation than did either group A or B.

Conclusion.—There were no blood pressure changes before intubation with tidal volume inhalation of sevoflurane 7%. Blood pressure and rate pressure changes after intubation are less with tidal volume induction with sevoflurane 7% than with thiamylal induction.

▶ There is lots of interest these days in rapid induction using sevoflurane for various clinical situations, including difficult airways and in children. The results of this study indicate that, as has been widely believed but not too well documented, sevoflurane, even when induced rapidly, is associated with quite benign hemodynamic changes. This once again confirms the rapidly emerging "user-friendly" nature of this new/old anesthetic.

J.H. Tinker, M.D.

Platelet Aggregation Is Impaired During Anaesthesia With Sevoflurane But Not With Isoflurane

Hirakata H, Nakamura K, Sai S, et al (Kyoto Univ, Japan; Wakayama Med College, Japan)

Can J Anaesth 44:1157–1161, 1997 4–9

Background.—Halothane prolongs bleeding time by suppressing platelet aggregation. The authors have previously shown that sevoflurane suppresses platelet aggregation to a greater extent than halothane. The effects of sevoflurane on platelet aggregation were studied in a clinical setting.

Methods.—The randomized trial included 38 patients undergoing minor elective surgical procedures. Anesthesia consisted of IV thiopentone induction and sevoflurane or isoflurane with nitrous oxide maintenance. Platelet aggregation induced by adenosine diphosphate (ADP) and epinephrine was measured before induction and again 5–10 minutes after tracheal intubation but before the start of surgery. The second measurement was timed for when end-expiratory concentrations of sevoflurane or isoflurane had stabilized at 1–1.5 times the minimum alveolar concentration and mean arterial pressures had reached 80% to 120% of baseline values.

Results.—Primary aggregation was induced by ADP and epinephrine in all samples from patients who had received sevoflurane anesthesia, although secondary aggregation was not. In almost all samples from the isoflurane group, both primary and secondary aggregation were noted. One sample showed abolition of secondary aggregation.

Conclusions.—In clinical use, sevoflurane suppresses platelet aggregation but isoflurane does not. This effect of sevoflurane may occur through suppression of thromboxane A_2. The findings may influence the choice of anesthetics in certain situations; further testing, including patients undergoing more invasive surgery, is needed.

▶ This is an interesting finding from an impeccable group of investigators. I think their discussion is nicely balanced. They talk about how this "might be deleterious in certain clinical situations. . ." including patients who have hemorrhage and platelet disorders and problems of that nature. On the other hand, they contend it might be beneficial in patients who have ischemic heart disease or the potential for myocardial infarction or stroke. The real point, however, is that sevoflurane has never been shown to have any independent clinically relevant effects on blood loss or other platelet-related problems. Nonetheless, this is an interesting effect that needs to be investigated and cataloged. I wonder about combined regional/general anesthetics also.

J.H. Tinker, M.D.

Assessment of Low-flow Sevoflurane and Isoflurane Effects on Renal Function Using Sensitive Markers of Tubular Toxicity

Kharasch ED, Frink EJ Jr, Zager R, et al (Univ of Washington, Seattle; Univ of Arizona, Tucson)

Anesthesiology 86:1238–1253, 1997 4–10

Objective.—Volatile anesthetics are degraded to potentially toxic by-products by carbon dioxide absorbents. One of sevoflurane's degradation products is the nephrotoxin fluoromethyl-2,2-difluoro-1-(trifluoromethyl) vinyl ether (compound A). Although renal function has been monitored by serum creatinine and blood urea nitrogen concentrations to detect low concentrations of compound A, more sensitive markers of renal function are needed. The effects of low-flow sevoflurane and isoflurane on renal tubular function in surgical patients were studied using conventional serum creatinine and blood urea nitrogen concentrations and the more sensitive indices, glucosuria, proteinuria, and enzymuria.

Methods.—With fresh in-line barium hydroxide lime to generate high levels of compound A, either sevoflurane (n = 36) or isoflurane (n = 37) was administered at 1 L/min to patients with normal renal function. Inspiratory and expiratory samples were analyzed for compound A concentrations at 30-minute intervals for the first 2 hours of anesthesia and hourly thereafter. Venous blood and urine samples were analyzed before surgery and at 24 and 72 hours after surgery.

Results.—The highest inspired concentration of compound A was 67 ppm, the mean inspired concentrations ranged from 15 to 30 ppm, and the average maximum was 27 ppm. Compound A concentrations were highest in patients receiving the highest sevoflurane concentrations. Area under the curve total compound A inspiratory and expiratory exposures were 79 and 53 ppm, respectively. The best predictor of both total compound A exposure and deposition was total sevoflurane exposure. Measures of renal and hepatic function were similar between anesthesia groups.

Conclusion.—Conventional and sensitive biomarkers for compound A gave similar results for the renal effects in surgical patients receiving sevoflurane and isoflurane exposed to barium hydroxide lime.

► The flow restriction on the use of sevoflurane, namely, 2 L/min or more, is a nonsensical way to deal with a putative toxin. If you have a potential toxin anywhere else in the realm of toxicology, you set dosage limits for exposure to that toxin! The FDA was convinced to set this flow restriction on the use of sevoflurane by an advocate for a rival pharmaceutical company. The notion behind the flow restriction, and it is simply a notion, is that if you lower the total flows below 2 L, the soda lime will get sufficiently hot that too much compound A will be generated. The motivation behind the argument toward the flow restriction was unfortunately not much toxicologic, but rather mostly commercial. Subsequently, many investigations have been done, including this one, to try to get a handle on the relative safety of sevoflurane in low-flow situations. With one glaring exception, again a study from that same advocate for the commercial company that is competing with sevoflurane's manufacturer, the other low-flow studies don't show that compound A is producing toxicity.

There is enough safety data now to clearly set safe dosage limits before exposure to sevoflurane under low-flow conditions. Setting reasonable exposure limits is the proper way to deal with any potential toxin, not setting flow restrictions. Why are flow restrictions commercial rather than scientific? By setting flow restrictions, the cost of sevoflurane is elevated somewhat. There are few toxicologists who would argue that if one is to be exposed to a potential toxin, then the right way to limit that exposure is by limiting dosage. There is enough human low-flow data today to establish that 6 hours of low-flow (i.e., less than 2 L/min) 1 MAC sevoflurane is safe.

J.H. Tinker, M.D.

Nitric Oxide

The Vasoregulatory Role of Endothelium Derived Nitric Oxide During Pulsatile Cardiopulmonary Bypass

Macha M, Yamazaki K, Gordon LM, et al (Univ of Pittsburgh, Pa)
ASAIO J 42:M800–M804, 1996 4–11

Introduction.—Pulsatile flow stimulates endothelium-mediated vasoregulation, but this function is not well understood. Nonpulsatile flow has been linked to increased vascular resistance and end-organ failure. It has also been shown to decrease nitric oxide (NO) production in vitro. The effects of pulsatile perfusion, with physiologic levels of shear stress, on endothelium-derived NO release were investigated.

Methods.—Cardiopulmonary bypass, with pulsatile or nonpulsatile perfusion, was initiated in anesthetized pigs. Mean aortic flow was kept constant at 1.0–1.3 L/min. The investigators used a method based on the Greiss reaction to test serum samples for nitrate and nitrite, the stable end-products of NO.

Results.—After 1 hour, systemic vascular resistance was 3,713 dyne·sec·cm^{-5} in the nonpulsatile bypass group vs. 2,673 dyne·sec·cm^{-5} in the pulsatile bypass group. This difference was not significant, however. There was a significant difference in NO production: 27% in the nonpulsatile flow group vs. 14% in the pulsatile flow group. Even though relative plasma nitrite/nitrate levels were significantly reduced in the nonpulsatile flow group, mean arterial pressure and systemic vascular resistance were unaffected.

Conclusions.—This study links nonpulsatile flow to reduced endothelial shear stress and reduced endothelial NO production. These effects could play a role in the adverse physiologic sequelae of prolonged nonpulsatile flow. The findings underscore the importance of pulsatile flow as a determinant of basal vasoregulation.

▶ This is a nice study confirming that there is a value to pulsatile cardiac bypass, at least in terms of biochemical markers and production, and in this animal model, vascular resistance. The reader is commended to examine this article, both because of its completeness and its excellent approach to the problem.

M.F. Roizen, M.D.

Inhaled Nitric Oxide Pretreatment But Not Post-treatment Attenuates Ischemia-Reperfusion–induced Pulmonary Microvascular Leak

Chetham PM, Sefton WD, Bridges JP, et al (Univ of Colorado, Denver; Univ of the Health Sciences, Bethesda, Md)

Anesthesiology 86:895–902, 1997 4–12

Background.—Radiographic evidence of reperfusion pulmonary edema is common after lung transplantation. This may be a result of ischemia-reperfusion (I/R), thought to be caused by a leukocyte-dependent, oxidant-mediated mechanism. Conflict exits over whether inhaled nitric oxide (NO) confers protection in I/R-induced microvascuar dysfunction. Ischemia–reperfusion-induced microvascular leak has been reversed and prevented by cyclic adenosine monophosphate (cAMP) agonists. Reversal by inhaled NO has not been tested. The effect of soluble guanylyl cyclase activation in the NO protective effect is unknown.

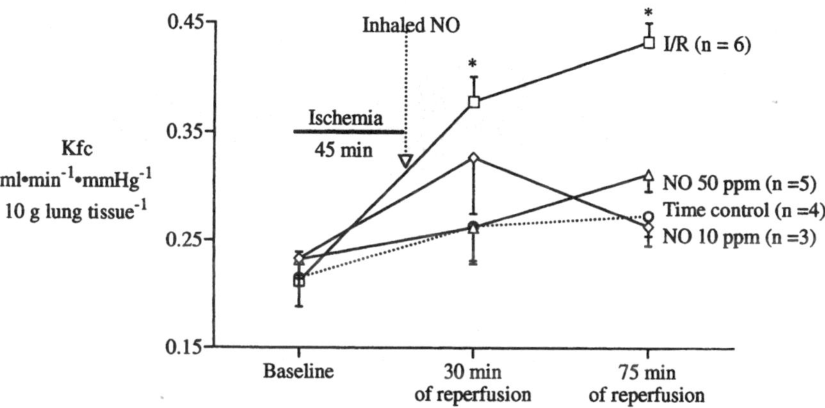

FIGURE 1.—Inhaled nitric oxide (*NO*) attenuates ischemia–reperfusion (*I/R*)-induced microvascular permeability. Capillary filtration coefficients (*Kfc*; permeability) were determined as baseline (before ischemia) and at 30 and 75 minutes of reperfusion. Lungs subjected to I/R demonstrated increased Kfc at both time points. Ventilation of lungs with NO (10 or 50 ppm) on reperfusion blunted I/R-induced microvascular permeability ($P < 0.05$). *Different from time control. (Courtesy of Chetham PM, Sefton WD, Bridges JP, et al: Inhaled nitric oxide pretreatment but not post-treatment attenuates ischemia–reperfusion-induced pulmonary microvascular leak. *Anesthesiology* 86:895–902, 1997. Copyright American Society of Anesthesiologists, Inc. Used with permission of Lippincott-Raven Publishers.)

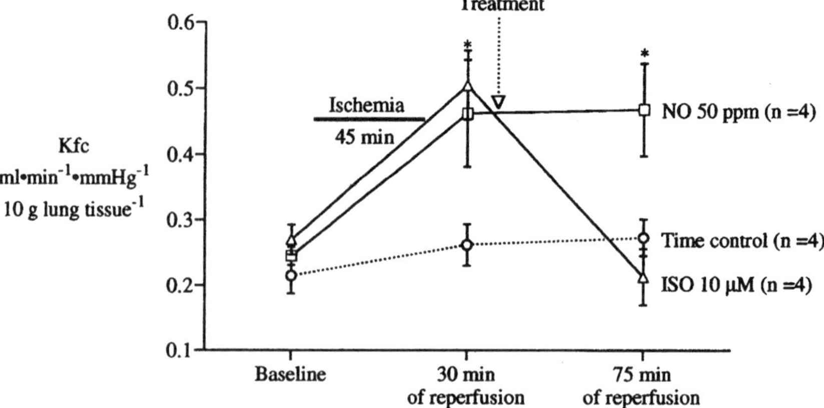

FIGURE 3.—Inhaled nitric oxide (*INO*) does not reverse ischemia–reperfusion-induced microvascular permeability. Capillary filtration coefficients (*Kfc*; permeability) were determined at baseline (before ischemia) and at 30 and 75 minutes of reperfusion. Treatments with either 50 ppm INO or 10 μmol isoproterenol were initiated after the 30-minute Kfc determination. Whereas INO did not reverse Kfc, isoproterenol reduced Kfc to baseline values ($P < 0.05$). *Different from time control. *Abbreviation: ISO,* isoproterenol. (Courtesy of Chetham PM, Sefton WD, Bridges JP, et al: Inhaled nitric oxide pretreatment but not post-treatment attenuates ischemia–reperfusion-induced pulmonary microvascular leak. *Anesthesiology* 86:895–902, 1997. Copyright American Society of Anesthesiologists, Inc. Used with permission of Lippincott-Raven Publishers.)

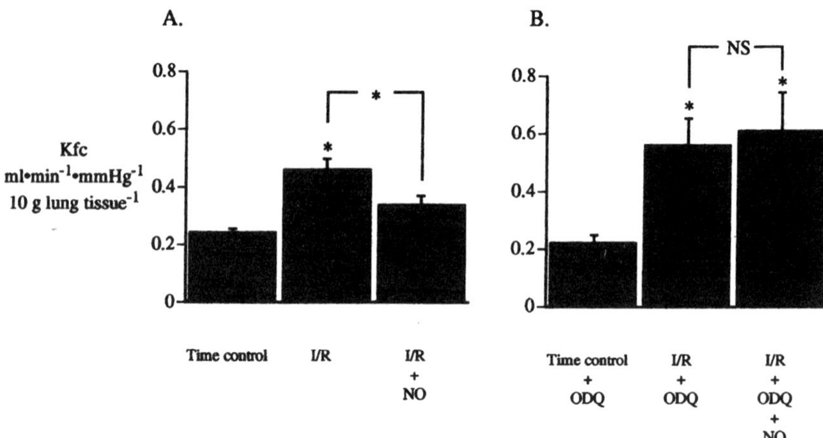

FIGURE 4.—Activation of soluble guanylyl cyclase is required for the protective effect of inhaled nitric oxide (*INO*). Values displayed represent capillary filtration coefficients (*Kfc*) after 30 minutes of reperfusion. **A**, inhaled NO at 50 ppm attenuates ischemia–reperfusion-induced increases in pulmonary microvascular leak ($n = 22$). **B**, inhibition of soluble guanylyl cyclase has no effect on baseline Kfc over time (baseline values not shown). Treatment with 1H-[1,2,4]oxadiazolo[4,3–a]quinoxalin-1-one (*ODQ*) prevented the protective effect of 50 ppm INO after ischemia–reperfusion ($n = 22$). *$P < 0.05$ from time-control and labeled comparison. (Courtesy of Chetham PM, Sefton WD, Bridges JP, et al: Inhaled nitric oxide pretreatment but not post-treatment attenuates ischemia–reperfusion-induced pulmonary microvascular leak. *Anesthesiology* 86:895–902, 1997. Copyright American Society of Anesthesiologists, Inc. Used with permission of Lippincott-Raven Publishers.)

Materials and Methods.—The effects of inhaled NO in the salt solution–perfused rat lung were tested because leukocyte-endothelial cell interactions are a significant mechanism for I/R-induced microvascular leak in this preparation. After perfusion with salt solution, rat lungs were grouped as I/R, I/R with inhaled NO on reperfusion, or time control. At 25 minutes before ischemia and after 30 and 75 minutes of reperfusion, capillary filtration coefficients (Kfc) were estimated. In selected groups, perfusate cell count and lung homogenate myeloperoxidase activity were determined. After 30 minutes of reperfusion, other groups were treated with inhaled NO or isoproterenol. Guanylyl cyclase was inhibited with 1H-[1,2,4] oxadiazolo[4,3-a]quinoxalin-1-one (ODQ), and Kfc was estimated at baseline and after 30 minutes of reperfusion.

Results.—Ischemia–reperfusion induced an increase in pulmonary microvascular permeability. Inhaled NO did not influence pulmonary artery, venous, or capillary pressures, but inhaled NO attenuated the development of I/R-induced permeability when administered at the time of reperfusion (Fig 1). Lung tissue myeloperoxidase activity was increased and found not to be different in either the I/R or NO-treated group compared to controls. This would indicate that lung retention of neutrophils was independent of treatment. Nitric oxide did not reduce Kfc at 75 minutes of reperfusion; isoproterenol reduced Kfc to baseline values (Fig 3), but ODQ had no effect on Kfc (Fig 4). Treatment with 250 μmol 8–bromoguanosine cyclic monophosphate (cGMP) at reperfusion did prevent an I/R-induced increase in Kfc.

Conclusions.—Nitric oxide has been observed to have a protective effect in isolated lung preparations subjected to various chemical forms of oxidant-mediated injury. Inhaled NO was effective if administered at the time of reperfusion but ineffective in reversing established microvascular leak. Prevention of leukocyte adhesion may not be the only way NO protects against I/R-induced microvascular leak. Activation of soluble guanylyl cyclase is required for the protective effect of inhaled NO. Clinically, it would be practical to supplement the NO-cGMP pathway by administering inhaled NO. It was found that isoproterenol increases cGMP, whereas inhaled NO was ineffective in reversing established microvascular leak.

▶ This study in a laboratory animal model further extends the mechanisms whereby inhaled NO might be a useful therapeutic agent in patients with lung disease. Pulmonary edema after lung transplantation is a common clinical entity, and a treatment modality in humans that not only prevents but also reverses established dysfunction would be a major advance.

M. Wood, M.D.

The Role of Nitric Oxide in the Cerebrovascular Response to Hypercapnia

Smith JJ, Lee JG, Hudetz AG, et al (Med College of Wisconsin, Milwaukee)
Anesth Analg 84:363–369, 1997 4–13

Background.—Through unknown mechanisms, increased arterial carbon dioxide leads to increased cerebrocortical blood flow. Some authors believe that the hyperemic response is at least partly related to activation of nitric oxide synthase (NOS). The role of nitric oxide in carbon dioxide-induced cerebrocortical hyperemia was studied in rats using laser Doppler flowmetry.

Methods.—Anesthetized and mechanically ventilated rats were divided into 5 groups. One group received saline infusion, another group received IV infusions of the L-arginine analogue N^{ω}-nitro-L-arginine methyl ester (L-NAME), an inhibitor of NOS; a third group received L-NAME plus the nitric oxide donor sodium nitroprusside to restore cerebrocortical laser Doppler flow (LDF) and mean arterial pressure (MAP) to baseline; a fourth group received phenylephrine infusion intended to restore MAP to the level usually observed after L-NAME; a fifth group received 7-nitroindazole for selective inhibition of brain or nonendothelial NOS. The LDF measurements were used to determine whether nitric oxide acted as a mediator or permissive modulator of carbon dioxide-induced cerebral hyperemia.

Results.—When 5% carbon dioxide was added to the inspired gas at 30 to 45 minutes after treatment, all groups had a significant change in LDF. For the control group, the response to hypercapnia was a 70% increase in LDF. For animals treated with L-NAME, this response was decreased by 36%, resulting in a posttreatment LDF of 25% lower than the pre–L-NAME level. The group receiving L-NAME plus sodium nitroprusside had a 56% response, not significantly different from that of the control group. Rats receiving phenylephrine to increase MAP had a 48% response to hypercapnia, with no change from the pretreatment to posttreatment LDF. Animals receiving 7-nitroindazole had an 8% response to hypercapnia, with a 14% reduction in flow from before to after treatment.

Conclusion.—The cerebrovascular response to hypercapnia is not mediated by endothelial nitric oxide, although nitric oxide may play a permissive role. The response to hypercapnia may involve brain nitric oxide. Inhibition of NOS may lead to increased vascular tone or absence of basal nitric oxide, thus affecting the vasodilator response to hypercapnia.

► In this excellent study by the Wisconsin group, inhibition and selective inhibition of brain and nonendothelial NOS were used to evaluate the role of nitric oxide in the cerebrovascular response to hypercapnia. Although it did not appear that the increased vascular tone was caused by a peripheral response or to peripheral nitric oxide effects, it did appear that nitric oxide neuromodulation, in the CNS, may have a role in this process.

M.F. Roizen, M.D.

A Role for Nitric Oxide in the Vasoplegic Syndrome
Speziale G, Ruvolo G, Marino B (Univ of Rome "La Sapienza")
J Cardiovasc Surg 37:301–303, 1996 4–14

Objective.—Cardiopulmonary bypass (CPB) is often followed by postperfusion syndrome that results from an inflammatory response. Nitric oxide (NO) is a endogenous vasodilator. Changes in NO concentration in 3 patients who experienced vasoplegic syndrome after CPB are reported.

Methods.—NO as nitrite plasma level (NPL) was measured in 95 consecutive patients undergoing normothermic CPB at the Institute of Cardiac Surgery in Rome.

Results.—Compared with baseline values, NO levels were increased significantly 30 minutes after beginning CPB and 10 minutes after discontinuing CPB. Three patients with postperfusion syndrome had NO levels that continued to be elevated significantly at 60, 120, and 240 minutes after discontinuing CPB.

Conclusion.—NO is involved in the hemodynamic disorders that result from postperfusion syndrome after CPB. NO inhibitors might aid in stabilizing vasoplegia.

► The authors report a considerable increase in NPL levels—the breakdown product of nitric oxide—after cardiopulmonary bypass when the vasoplegic syndrome occurs. Whether there is a role for using inhibitors of nitric oxide in these operations is a matter that will remain for future study.

M.F. Roizen, M.D.

Platelet Function Is Inhibited by Nitric Oxide Liberation During Nitroglycerin-induced Hypotension Anaesthesia
Aoki H, Inoue M, Mizobe T, et al (Kyoto Prefectural Univ of Medicine, Japan; Tokyo Univ of Pharmacy and Life Science)
Br J Anaesth 79:476–481, 1997 4–15

Introduction.—The role of organic nitrates, such as nitroglycerin (NTG), is well defined in the treatment of myocardial infarction and angina pectoralis. The inhibitory effects of NTG on platelet function has been described, but trials describing these effects in vitro use concentrations that are higher than what can be achieved in vivo. The effects of NTG on platelet function was assessed in 8 patients undergoing orthopedic surgery. Seven patients undergoing orthopedic surgery of the hip joint with no NTG infusion were also evaluated.

Methods.—Isoflurane and nitrous oxide in oxygen were used as anesthetic agents, with vecuronium as a neuromuscular blocking agent. With isoflurane at 1% and a stable hemodynamic state, NTG solution was administered intravenously at a rate of 1 μg kg^{-1} min^{-1}. The maximum infusion rate was individualized for each patient. Arterial blood samples were taken at baseline and 10 minutes after maximum infusion was achieved for determination of platelet aggregation, intracellular calcium concentration, and intracellular cyclic guanosine monophosphate (cGMP) concentration.

Results.—Continuous infusion with NTG significantly diminished platelet aggregation and significantly increased intracellular $Ca^{2}+$, cGMP, and the concentration of nitrite ion. Seven patients who received nitrous oxide–isoflurane anesthesia without NTG infusion had no inhibition of platelet aggregation. There was an association between the increase in intraplatelet cGMP concentration and the increase in nitrite ion concentration.

Conclusions.—Infusion of a large dose of NTG to induce hypotension resulted in higher intraplatelet cGMP concentrations and inhibition of increases in $Ca^{2}+$ and platelet aggregation. These changes may have been caused by higher concentrations of nitrite ion. Nitric oxide may have an effect in the mechanism of the observed inhibitory effects.

► In patients undergoing total hip replacement, the platelet inhibitory effects of NTG may offer a potential therapeutic effect in decreasing the incidence of postoperative deep venous thrombosis. The use of N-acetylcysteine enhances the effect of NTG by providing thiol groups, thus decreasing tolerance. The formation of the compound N-nitroso-N-acetylcysteine has also been shown to be a potent platelet inhibitor. Future studies need to assess the incidence of deep venous thrombosis and pulmonary embolism when NTG with or without N-acetylcysteine is used for hypotensive anesthesia.

D.M. Rothenberg, M.D.

Propofol

Propofol or Halothane Anaesthesia for Children With Asthma: Effects on Respiratory Mechanics

Habre W, Matsumoto I, Sly PD (Princess Margaret Hosp for Children, Perth, Australia)

Br J Anaesth 77:739–743, 1996 4–16

Objective.—Propofol can cause histamine release. Although propofol has been reported to be safe for individuals with asthma, there is no data on lung function particularly in children. Respiratory mechanics were measured in children undergoing mechanical ventilation during induction of anesthesia with propofol and during maintenance of anesthesia with halothane in children with and without asthma.

Methods.—Airway opening pressure (Pao) and flow (V) were measured in 30 normal children and 30 asthmatic children, aged 2–12, receiving 3 mg/kg propofol, 1 γ/kg fentanyl, and 0.5 mg/kg atracurium as anesthesia before elective surgery. Anesthesia was maintained with an infusion of 10 mg/kg/hr propofol and 50% nitrous oxide in oxygen. Halothane was then administered at a concentration of 1 MAC. Respiratory system compliance (Crs,dyn) and resistance (Rrs) were calculated using a single-compartment model and multilinear regression analysis according to the equation: Pao = V/Crs,dyn + VRrs + PA,EE, where PA,EE represents alveolar pressure, Crs,dyn is respiratory system compliance, and Rrs is resistance from measurements of airway opening pressure.

Results.—Ventilation variables and airway pressure measures were similar between groups. Although tidal volume increased significantly and Rrs decreased during halothane administration in both groups, the changes were not clinically significant.

Conclusion.—Respiratory mechanics after induction of anesthesia with propofol were similar for asthmatic and nonasthmatic children. Changes in tidal volume and Rrs were not clinically significant.

► Although propofol has been anecdotally reported associated with histamine release in both atopic and normal children, I think that most anesthetists would agree that propofol is not known to be contraindicated in asthmatic patients. This is an elegant systematic study of respiratory mechanics in children undergoing either halothane or propofol anesthesia, and although it is a negative study, it is the kind of study that is valuable because it gives us confidence in the use of a drug, namely, propofol, which has proven extraordinarily valuable in our practice. We must rely on these kinds of studies to influence our practice, not anecdotes.

J.H. Tinker, M.D.

Metoclopramide Reduces the Induction Dose of Propofol

Page VJ, Chhipa JH (Hammersmith Hosp, London)

Acta Anaesthesiol Scand 41:256–259, 1997 4–17

Objective.—Although pretreatment with metoclopramide has been shown to reduce the dose of thiopentone required to induce anesthesia, similar studies with propofol have given inconclusive results. The effect of metoclopramide on dose requirements of propofol for induction of anesthesia in a placebo-controlled, randomized, double-blind study are reported.

Methods.—Gynecological, orthopedic, and general surgery patients received either 0.15 mg/kg metoclopramide (group I, $n = 30$) or 0.03 mL/mg 0.9% sodium chloride (group II, $n = 30$) before being injected with propofol at a rate of 1.5 mg/kg over a period of 20 seconds. Anesthesia was reached by definition when patients failed to open their eyes on command after their counting ceased. Doses of propofol required to reach anesthesia were compared statistically between groups.

Results.—Mean induction dose of propofol was 1.86 mg/kg in the control group and a significantly lower 1.41 mg/kg in the metoclopramide group.

Conclusion.—Intravenous metoclopramid significantly reduced the dose of propofol required to induce anesthesia in surgery patients.

▶ I included this paper because a drug like metoclopramide is not normally associated with changing requirements for anesthesia. This finding would have been much more interesting and probably more valid had the authors done a *dose response* curve. As it is, although we may know now that propofol requirement can be reduced by prior treatment with metoclopramide, we do not have much information in this paper as to the time course or dosage by which this might occur. Although this is an interesting paper in terms of notification, considerably more work needs to be done to clarify this issue.

J.H. Tinker, M.D.

Determination of Plasma Concentrations of Propofol Associated With 50% Reduction in Postoperative Nausea

Gan TJ, Glass PSA, Howell ST, et al (Duke Univ, Durham, NC)

Anesthesiology 87:779–784, 1997 4–18

Introduction.—Propofol, used for maintenance of anesthesia, carries a lower incidence of postoperative nausea and vomiting (PONV) than inhalational agents. Studies have shown that, in subhypnotic doses, propofol has direct antiemetic action. However, the doses in these studies were not based on systematic dose-response analysis. A study was performed to establish the plasma propofol concentration capable of managing PONV.

Methods.—Eighty-nine American Society of Anesthesiologists physical status 1 or 2 adult patients undergoing surgery with general anesthesia consented to the study. Fifteen patients met the entry criteria—nausea, retching, or vomiting in the postanesthesia care unit. The nausea had to have a verbal rating score of greater than 5 on a scale of 0–10. A computer-assisted continuous infusion device was used for propofol administration to reach a target plasma concentration of 100, 200, 400, and 800 ng/mL. Every 15 minutes, the propofol concentration was increased until the patients reported a 50% or greater reduction in symptoms. At each interval, an arterial blood sample was obtained to measure plasma propofol concentration. Other measurements included blood pressure, heart rate, respiratory rate, arterial blood saturation, sedation score, and treatment satisfaction.

Results.—Five of the 15 patients were retching or vomiting on entry to the study. A successful response to propofol treatment was achieved in all patients but 1. The remaining patient had no response at a plasma propofol concentration of up to 830 ng/mL. The success rate of propofol as a treatment for PONV was therefore 93%. For the responders, the median plasma propofol concentration at the time of antiemetic response was 343 ng/mL. Propofol caused no change in sedation scores. There were no problems with desaturation, and hemodynamic indices remained stable throughout the study.

Conclusions.—At a nonsedative plasma concentration, propofol is an effective treatment for PONV. It provides an antiemetic effect with few side effects and good patient satisfaction. To reach the target concentration of 343 ng/mL, a bolus 10 mg dose of propofol can be given, followed by infusion at a rate of 10 $\mu g \cdot kg^{-1} \cdot min^{-1}$. This dosing regimen must be individualized to obtain the desired effect.

▶ Propofol in subhypnotic concentrations is effective in reducing postoperative nausea and vomiting. However, the effect of propofol is so short-lived when given by IV bolus that it is not practical to treat postoperative nausea and vomiting unless an infusion is given. The authors found that propofol was effective in 14 of 15 patients; thus propofol does appear to be an effective antiemetic. How propofol exerts this effect remains unknown.

M. Wood, M.D.

Tolerance to Propofol Generally Does Not Develop in Pediatric Patients Undergoing Radiation Therapy

Setlock MA, Palmisano BW, Berens RJ, et al (Children's Hosp of Wisconsin, Milwaukee)

Anesthesiology 85:207–209, 1996 4–19

Background.—When general anesthesia is required in children receiving high-voltage radiation therapy, anesthesia can be induced with small, initial doses of propofol and then maintained with an infusion of propofol. It has been suggested that patients may develop a tolerance to propofol with repeated administration. Deer and Rich reported 1 case of developed tolerance to propofol, but other retrospective and animal studies have not reported such a tolerance. Whether tolerance develops to an induction dose of propofol in children was prospectively determined.

Methods.—There were 6 children who were anesthetized for 159 treatments of high-voltage radiation; their mean age was 2 years. No patient had allergy to propofol, eggs, or soy. An initial bolus of 1 mg/kg of propofol and additional doses of 0.5 mg/kg of propofol as needed every 15–30 seconds were administered. Drug tolerance was determined by linear regression analysis; regression slopes for all patients were pooled. Drug tolerance was defined as a mean slope greater than 0.

Results.—Because the treatment period could not be standardized, total dose and additional boluses administered during treatment were not examined because this would have been related to inconsistencies in treatment procedure, not drug tolerance. In 5 of the 6 patients, the slopes correlating induction dose to treatment number were negative. In 1 patient, the induction dose increased slightly during the course of 22 treatments; induction dose and treatment number did not correlate. For all patients, daily variation in induction dose was observed but was unrelated to treatment number. Because an increase in induction dose of propofol was not needed with repeated administration, tolerance to an induction dose did not develop.

Conclusions.—In these patients receiving high-voltage radiation therapy, tolerance to an induction dose of propofol did not develop. Daily variation in dose occurred but was unrelated to treatment number or pretreatment anxiety. These findings do not support the theory that patients develop a tolerance to propofol with repeated treatment.

▶ A nice case report outlining a common problem—tolerance to drugs administered to pediatric patients receiving radiation therapy. Tolerance has been reported to ketamine in this clinical setting. Ketamine is metabolized to a number of metabolites, some of which are long acting. It is possible that 1 of the metabolites might exert agonist/antagonist effects, and hence be the cause of tolerance.

M. Wood, M.D.

Propofol and Bradycardia: Causation, Frequency and Severity

Tramèr MR, Moore RA, McQuay HJ (Oxford Radcliffe Hosp, England)

Br J Anaesth 78:642–651, 1997 4–20

Introduction.—Available since the early 1980s, propofol offers an excellent hemodynamic state for children; however, the drug has been linked to a low heart rate. Even in healthy adult patients, there have been reports of profound bradycardia and asystole with the use of propofol. Long-term propofol sedation has resulted in severe, refractory, and fatal bradycardia in children in the ICU. A meta-analysis was conducted to study the link between propofol anesthesia and bradycardia.

Methods.—A MEDLINE search (1984 through 1995) was conducted to review the literature on bradycardia and propofol anesthesia. There were 65 reports used. National centers participating in a drug-monitoring scheme were contacted for information about spontaneous reports of bradycardic events and propofol, resulting in 187 reports. Relevant data were sought by the manufacturer of propofol, and abstracts from scientific meetings were also reviewed. Any type of report, published and unpublished, was reviewed to determine whether propofol increases the risk of asystole, bradycardia, and death from bradycardic events. With different strengths of evidence, quantitative and qualitative analyses of data were performed.

Results.—A biological basis for propofol-induced bradycardia was seen. Among the 65 published and 187 spontaneous reports to drug-monitoring centers, there were 1,444 bradycardias, 86 asystoles, and 24 deaths. Propofol significantly increased the risk of bradycardia compared with other anesthetics in controlled clinical trials. An asystole was found in 1 of 660 patients receiving propofol anesthesia. During propofol anesthesia, the risk of bradycardia-related death was estimated to be 1.4 in 100,000.

Conclusions.—There is a clinically relevant relationship between bradycardia or asystole and propofol. Bradycardia with potential for major harm was linked to propofol. Future studies should identify subgroups most likely to benefit from the favorable characteristics of propofol, and the subgroups at particular risk of complications. In the presence of conduction abnormalities, heart rate–lowering medications such as β-blockers, procedures with an increased risk of bradycardia, including squint repair, and laparoscopies, as well as in very sick, old, or young patients, indications for propofol should be questioned.

► Since the introduction of propofol into clinical practice, occasional case reports have been published describing an association between propofol and profound bradycardia. This investigation describes a combined analysis of clinical trials and reports using a systematic literature search. This method of analysis has recently become popular; however, the methodology does have limitations, and randomized controlled trials remain pivotal to good clinical research.

M. Wood, M.D.

Disposition and Renal Clearance of Propofol and Its Glucuronide Metabolites After a Short Intravenous Infusion of Propofol

Vree TB, de Grood P-MRM, van Beem HBH, et al (Academic Hosp Nijmegen Sint Radboud, The Netherlands)

Clin Drug Invest 13:145–151, 1997 4–21

Introduction.—The disposition kinetics and renal clearance of propofol and its metabolites were studied in 9 patients scheduled for abdominal surgery.

Methods.—Patients were 5 women and 4 men with a mean age of 46.4 years. The mean IV dose of propofol was 5.96 mg/kg, infused over 30 minutes. Blood samples were obtained immediately before, during, and after the infusion, continuing until 6 hours after infusion. Urine was collected during a 60-hour period for measurements of volume and pH. High-performance liquid chromatography was used to determine plasma concentrations of propofol and its metabolites. Pharmacokinetic parameters of propofol were calculated by using a 3-compartment model; a 2-compartment model was used to determine the pharmacokinetic parameters of the metabolites propofolglucuronide and 1,4-quinolconjugate. The percentage of the dose excreted was calculated as the amount of drug in the urine (mmol) divided by the dose given (mmol).

Results.—In the typical patient receiving an IV infusion of propofol, 432 mg over 30 minutes, the agent was eliminated rapidly with a terminal half-life of 80 minutes. Propofol was quickly metabolized in its glucuronide (half-life 270 minutes) and quinolconjugate (half-life 450 minutes) forms (Fig 1). Studies during a 120-minute period revealed that propofolglucuronide appeared earlier in the plasma than the 1,4-quinolconjugate

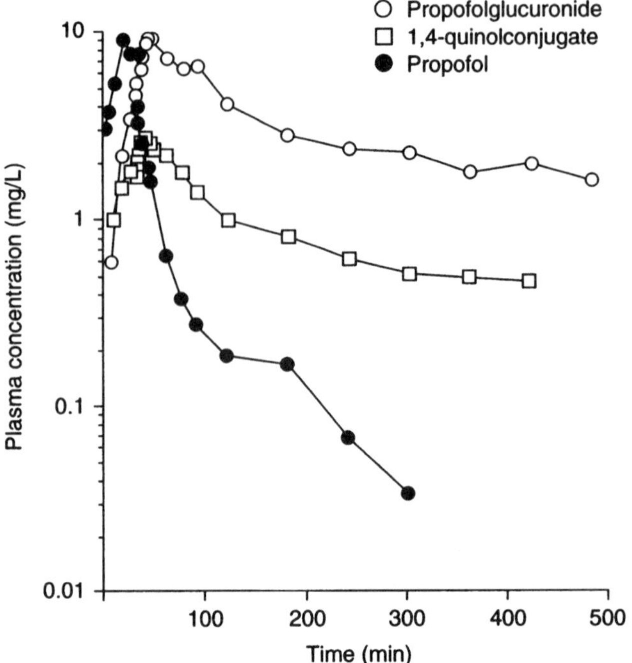

FIGURE 1.—Plasma concentration-time curves of propofol and its metabolites, propofolglucuronide and 1,4-quinolconjugate, in a patient after an intravenous infusion of propofol (432 mg over 30 minutes). (Courtesy of Vree TB, de Grood P-MRM, van Been HBH, et al: Disposition and renal clearance of propofol and its glucuronide metabolites after a short intravenous infusion of propofol. *Clin Drug Invest* 13:145–151, 1997.)

(Fig 2). Two half-life (t½) values were apparent in the elimination of propofol and each of its metabolites. The distribution half-life (t½α) differed significantly from the elimination half-life (t½β) (mean 7.6 vs. 119 minutes, respectively), and the calculated (t½α) and t½β values for each metabolite differed significantly. The apparent $t½_{absorption}$ of both metabolites was similar. Mean total body clearance of propofol was 2.08 L/min. Propofolglucuronide was the main compound in plasma.

Conclusions.—After a short IV infusion of propofol, the metabolites propofolglucuronide and 1,4-quinolconjugate are present in the plasma of surgical patients. Both metabolites are eliminated by renal clearance, and no free propofol is excreted in urine.

▶ It has been known for many years that propofol is metabolized by glucuronidation, and that less than 0.3% of an administered dose is excreted in the urine as the parent compound. However, the sites of metabolism of propofol have long been the subject of investigation, especially because it has been recognized that propofol is metabolized during the anhepatic phase of liver transplantation. Other drugs of importance to anesthesiologists that are known to undergo extrahepatic glucuronidation include midazolam and

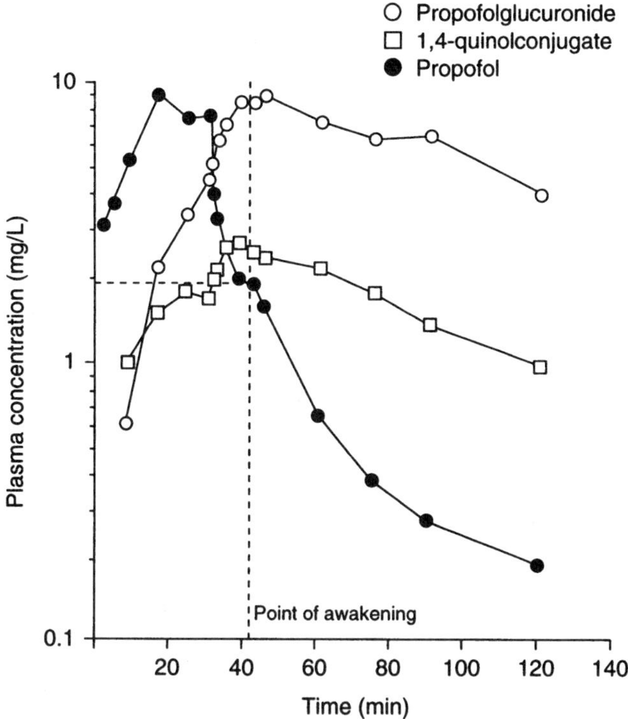

FIGURE 2.—Plasma concentration-time curves of propofol and its metabolites, propofolglucuronide and 1,4-quinolconjugate, in a patient after an intravenous infusion of propofol (432 mg over 30 minutes). The time course has been truncated at 120 minutes to more clearly distinguish the formation of the metabolites. The plasma concentration of propofol at awakening of the patient (1.9 mg/L) is indicated. (Courtesy of Vree TB, de Grood P-MRM, van Been HBH, et al: Disposition and renal clearance of propofol and its glucuronide metabolites after a short intravenous infusion of propofol. *Clin Drug Invest* 13:145–151, 1997.)

morphine. I selected this article, therefore, because it sheds further light on the fate of the metabolites of propofol. Although this paper does not define whether renal conjugation occurs, it does illustrate the fact that when metabolites undergo extensive renal clearance, these metabolites will accumulate in patients with renal failure, but the clearance of the parent compound will be unaltered.

M. Wood, M.D.

Recovery of Consciousness After Thiopental or Propofol: Bispectral Index and the Isolated Forearm Technique

Flaishon R, Windsor A, Sigl J, et al (Emory Univ, Atlanta, Ga; Aspect Med Systems, Natick, Mass)

Anesthesiology 86:613–619, 1997 4–22

Purpose.—There is currently no reliable technique for ensuring adequate anesthesia and unconsciousness in a paralyzed patient. One promising approach is the electroencephalogram-derived bispectral index (BIS). It has shown good correlation with sedation and is a good predictor of patients' response to stimulus. The ability of BIS to predict return of consciousness, as measured by the isolated forearm technique, was evaluated.

Methods.—The study included 40 adult patients scheduled for elective surgery under general anesthesia. With no premedication, 20 patients were anesthetized with 4 mg/kg thiopental and 20 with 2 mg/kg propofol. Electroencephalographic data were recorded for calculation of BIS throughout anesthesia. After induction but before neuromuscular paralysis, the isolated forearm technique was carried out by applying a tourniquet to one arm and inflating it above systolic pressure. This permitted movement of the hand even after the neuromuscular blocking agent was given. Every 30 seconds, the patients were instructed to squeeze the investigator's hand. When the patient responded to this prompt, anesthesia was reinduced and the study was terminated. The ability of the BIS to predict this measure of return to consciousness was determined.

Results.—The propofol and thiopental groups showed no significant difference in BIS at loss of consciousness and recovery of response. The patients were never conscious when the BIS was less than 58. When the BIS was less than 65, the probability of return to consciousness within 50 seconds was less than 5%. At a BIS of 65, nearly all patients responded to the command within several minutes. None of the patients reported any recall during anesthesia.

Conclusions.—Recovery of consciousness after thiopental or propofol anesthesia can be predicted by use of the BIS. Although there is no single BIS value at which consciousness returns, the lower the BIS, the less likelihood of regaining consciousness. The BIS values associated with other anesthetic agents and the chances of return to consciousness in response to surgical stimulus are unknown.

▶ This article is presented because it is a use of the new BIS to try to estimate the point at which loss of consciousness and the point of consciousness occurs, and to use this tool to study drugs in an attempt to get more valid comparisons.

The authors found that patients with certain levels of depression BIS were very likely to be anesthetized and unlikely to recover soon. Can these data be turned around to indicate that the BIS number itself is an assurance of lack of consciousness? I don't think the latter is quite as well established. I am also not sure that these two statements fall logically in line with one another; in fact, I would expect a considerable "hysteresis" in this conscious-anesthetized-conscious scenario. I also think this article is important because it reveals, perhaps inadvertently, just how difficult it is to validate any device that remotely claims to be any sort of monitor of depth of anesthetic depression of the CNS, or consciousness.

J.H. Tinker, M.D.

Conscious Sedation for Interventional Neuroradiology: A Comparison of Midazolam and Propofol Infusion

Manninen PH, Chan ASH, Papworth D (Univ of Toronto)

Can J Anaesth 44:26–30, 1997 4–23

Introduction.—Diagnostic and therapeutic interventional neuroradiologic (INR) procedures are commonly performed in patients with intracranial vascular lesions. Although not painful, the procedures require the patient to remain relatively still and communicative for a prolonged period. Anesthesia thus includes sedative and/or analgesic agents. Two conscious sedation agents—midazolam and propofol—were compared for use during INR procedures.

Methods.—The randomized trial included 40 patients undergoing INR procedures. All patients received midazolam, 15 µg/kg, and fentanyl, 0.75 µg/kg IV. In addition, patients assigned to the midazolam group received an additional 7.5–15.0 µg/kg of midazolam, if required, followed by midazolam infusion, 0.5 µg/kg/min. Patients in the propofol group received a bolus of 0.25–0.5 mg/kg of propofol, followed by a propofol infusion of 25 µg/kg/min. The infusion rates were adjusted to keep the patient in a state of mild sedation, resting comfortably but able to obey commands. The 2 groups were compared for rates of complications and other events requiring intervention, such as respiratory depression, excessive pain, inappropriate movements, and loss of cooperation. The patient and neuroradiologist were asked about their satisfaction with the anesthetic technique.

Results.—The groups were similar in terms of rates and types of complications. Forty percent of the midazolam group and 62% of the propofol group had at least 1 complication, a nonsignificant difference. Patient and neuroradiologist satisfaction scores were similar for the 2 agents.

Conclusion.—In patients undergoing INR procedures, both midazolam and propofol provide satisfactory conscious sedation. The rates and types of complications are similar for the 2 anesthetic regimens.

► This clinical dose study showed that either anesthetic technique is acceptable, as one would expect. The incidence of complications was not great in either patient group and did not differ between groups. Of course, the problem is that one is relying on the experience of the investigators and assuming that these investigators were able to give the drugs at the right dose. In that regard, this is an efficacy study rather then an effectiveness study. For those who believe that effectiveness is the right thing to study—that is, how the drugs do in clinical practice—this is an excellent article except that it uses very few practitioners. A larger study with many different practitioners using the drugs would really indicate their effectiveness.

M.F. Roizen, M.D.

Dexmedetomidine

Effect of Dexmedetomidine on Lumbar Cerebrospinal Fluid Pressure in Humans

Talke P, Tong C, Lee H-W, et al (Univ of California, San Francisco; Bowman Gray School of Medicine, Winston-Salem, NC)
Anesth Analg 85:358–364, 1997 4–24

Introduction.—The selective α_2-adrenoreceptor agonist dexmedetomidine has sympatholytic, sedative, and analgesic properties. It can provide analgesia without respiratory depression, which makes it a useful adjunct to anesthesia during neurosurgical procedures. However, no studies have examined the effects of dexmedetomidine on intracranial pressure (ICP) in humans. Patients undergoing pituitary surgery were studied to determine the effects of dexmedetomidine on lumbar CSF pressure.

Methods.—The randomized trial included 16 patients undergoing transsphenoidal tumor surgery for pituitary tumors. In the postanesthesia care unit, they received either dexmedetomidine, 200 µg/mL, or placebo in a 60-minute infusion administered by a continuous computer-controlled infusion pump. This infusion produced a high clinical plasma dexmedetomidine concentration of 600 pg/mL. The patients received patient-controlled analgesia with morphine for postoperative discomfort. A lumbar intrathecal catheter was used to measure lumbar CSF pressure; intra-arterial blood pressure and heart rate were monitored as well.

Results.—Neither dexmedetomidine nor placebo produced any significant change in lumbar CSF pressure; peak values were 19 and 20 mm Hg, respectively. In patients receiving dexmedetomidine, mean arterial pressure decreased from 103 to 86 mm Hg, heart rate from 77 to 64 beats/min, and cerebral perfusion pressure from 95 to 78 mm Hg during the infusion. These values were unchanged in the placebo group. Patients receiving dexmedetomidine made fewer patient-controlled analgesia attempts.

Conclusion.—In patients with normal ICP undergoing transsphenoidal pituitary surgery, dexmedetomidine does not alter lumbar CSF pressure. This drug does significantly reduce blood pressure, heart rate, and cerebral perfusion pressure. More research is needed to examine the uses of dexmedetomidine for anesthesia during neurosurgical procedures.

► Dexmedetomidine has been around for quite some time and is an interesting drug. It seems to do enough things to some slight extent that it isn't particularly focused and, therefore, has not found a "home," pharmacologically speaking. It seems to be somewhat of an analgetic, but not too much, i.e., it decreases requirements for opioids a bit, and it seems to decrease requirements for inhaled anesthetics as well. The history of drugs would indicate that most drugs that have so many diverse effects really are not very useful. I think that dexmedetomindine may be an interesting drug looking for a clinically relevant use.

J.H. Tinker, M.D.

Reduction of the Minimum Alveolar Concentration of Isoflurane by Dexmedetomidine

Aantaa R, Jaakola M-L, Kallio A, et al (Orion Corp, Turku, Finland; Turku Univ, Finland)

Anesthesiology 86:1055–1060, 1997 4–25

Objective.—Whereas α2-adrenergic agonists have an anesthetic sparing effect, they also are potent sympatholytic agents, which raises concerns about the possibility of patient awareness during anesthesia. The anesthetic interaction of isoflurane and an intravenous infusion of dexmedetomidine was investigated using the minimum steady-state alveolar anesthetic concentration (MAC) of isoflurane as the measure of anesthetic potency.

Methods.—Either a placebo infusion (n = 16) or a 2-stage infusion of dexmedetomidine to achieve a steady-state plasma concentration of 0.3 ng/mL (n = 17) or of 0.6 ng/mL (n = 16) was administered 15 minutes before induction of anesthesia to women undergoing hysterectomy. Anesthesia was induced with 15 γ/kg alfentanil and 2 mg/kg thiopental. The target end-tidal concentration of isoflurane was determined using the "up-down" technique of Dixon and Mood. After a minimum of 15 minutes, the patients' response to skin incision was determined. The MAC of isoflurane was compared in all 3 groups.

Results.—The MAC of isoflurane in the control group was significantly higher than in either dexmedetomidine-treated group, but was not significantly different between dexmedetomidine-treated groups. The low-dose group required an average of 17% less thiopental to induce anesthesia, and the high-dose group required an average of 30% less thiopental. The percentage of end-tidal MAC of isoflurane was 0.85 for the placebo group, 0.55 for the low-dose dexmedetomidine group, and 0.45 for the high-dose dexmedetomidine group. Plasma thiopental and alfentanil concentrations were similar among all groups.

Conclusion.—There is a dose-related and significant reduction of isoflurane MAC in surgery patients receiving dexmedetomidine prior to induction of anesthesia.

► Dexmedetomidine (DEX) is one of several alpha adrenergic agonists. Although this study clearly shows that DEX does reduce MAC with isoflurane, I don't think these authors have eliminated the possibility that despite reduced MAC, there might be an increased level of awareness, since MAC doesn't have all that much to do with awareness as far as we know. DEX is a fascinating compound that may find a place in clinical practice, but in all honesty, I can't, at this juncture, figure out where that place might be.

J.H. Tinker, M.D.

Xenon Anesthesia

The Effect of Xenon on Spinal Dorsal Horn Neurons: A Comparison With Nitrous Oxide

Utsumi J, Adachi T, Miyazaki Y, et al (Kyoto Univ, Japan)

Anesth Analg 84:1372–1376, 1997 4–26

Objective.—Although xenon (Xe) possesses anesthetic properties, its expense limits its use. The introduction of low flow or closed circuit anesthesia techniques has permitted reconsideration of the use of Xe as an anesthesia. The effects of Xe and nitrous oxide (N_2O) on the spinal cord dorsal horn neurons were compared in cats.

Methods.—Anesthesia was induced in 11 cats with 20 mg/kg ketamine and 0.01 mg/kg im atropine. The trachea was intubated. Blood pressure and heart rate were monitored at the right common carotid artery. Drugs were administered via the right jugular vein. Concentrations of N_2O, oxygen, and carbon dioxide were monitored continuously. Anesthesia was maintained with 3.5 mL/kg iv α-chloralose and urethane solution (10 mg/kg α-chloralose and 125 mg/kg urethane). The left superficial peroneal nerve was exposed and connected to an electrode. The activity of the spinal dorsal horn neurons was recorded when the shaved hindpaw was stimulated by pinching it with a serrated forceps or touching it with a paintbrush. N_2O (70% in oxygen) was administered using a nonrebreathing apparatus and Xe (70% in oxygen) was administered using a semi-closed circuit with low flow to each animal for 20 minutes in a random sequence with 30 minutes between sequences. Neuronal responses were measured.

Results.—The response to stimuli was proportional to the strength of the applied stimuli. Responses had returned almost to normal 10 minutes after discontinuing Xe inhalation. Responses to stimuli of 7 of 11 neurons were suppressed by Xe inhalation. Responses to stimuli of 8 of 11 neurons were suppressed by N_2O inhalation. At 20 minutes after inhalation, there were no significant differences in response suppression between Xe and N_2O in the 6 neurons suppressed by both gases.

Conclusion.—Xe and N_2O appear to be equally effective at suppressing the spinal cord dorsal horn neurons in cats.

► The "official" reason for including this in the YEAR BOOK is that it is an elegant study looking at potency in a more sophisticated way than MAC. MAC for Xe has been reported to be about 70%, i.e., somewhat more potent than nitrous oxide at 100%. In this study, the two gases were similar in their ability to suppress spinal cord neurons.

My other reason for including this study is so that I could mention a "rumor," which is circulating in various circles. The rumor is that a major anesthesia machine maker is considering introducing an anesthesia delivery system that uses Xe! The system would probably have to include a recapture circuit, i.e., somehow "scrubbing" the patients' exhaled air, extracting the Xe and reusing it. I can't wait to see how they do that. For example, if the patient had eaten (yesterday, of course) a large dose of garlic, would that be "scrubbable"? Seriously, Xe might make excellent sense if it was sufficiently potent. This study indicates that it might not be. Also, it is fascinating to speculate on exactly why an inert gas is an anesthetic at all.

J.H. Tinker, M.D.

Effects on Haemodynamics and Catecholamine Release of Xenon Anaesthesia Compared With Total I.V. Anaesthesia in the Pig
Marx T, Froeba G, Wagner D, et al (Univ of Ulm, Germany)
Br J Anaesth 78:326–327, 1997 4--27

Background.—The dose-dependent effects of xenon anesthesia on hemodynamic variables and catecholamine release have not been established. Different concentrations of xenon were investigated in a porcine model.

Methods.—Twenty-eight pigs were randomly assigned to 1 of 4 groups: total IV anesthesia with pentobarbitone and buprenorphine, and xenon anesthesia with inspiratory concentrations of 30%, 50%, or 70% supplemented with pentobarbitone. Arterial and Swan-Ganz catheters were used to measure hemodynamic variables. Spectral edge frequency analysis was used to monitor the depth of anesthesia, and high-pressure liquid chromatography was used to determine plasma levels of dopamine, noradrenaline, and adrenaline.

Findings.—All hemodynamic variables and plasma levels of dopamine and noradrenaline were in the normal range. Concentrations of adrenaline were decreased significantly in all groups. The significant reduction of adrenaline levels at inspiratory xenon concentrations of 30% and 50% may be explained by the analgesic effects of xenon below its minimum alveolar concentration value.

Conclusions.—Xenon anesthesia had little effect on the cardiovascular system in this porcine model. This may be an important advantage over other inhalation anesthetics.

▶ There's a rumor that a major anesthesia company is working on producing a xenon administration circuit or special machine to "recycle" the xenon and return it to the patient, creating the first commercially available xenon anesthesia administration system. This animal study utilized a pig, which is a valid cardiovascular model. Clearly, in these animals, xenon produced an excellent degree of cardiovascular stability. I think it will be fascinating to see how or if they figure out how to scavenge and recover "used" xenon. Will we need to obtain permission from our patients to deliver "previously used" anesthesia gas? Will there be unforeseen hazards to doing this? How will they get xenon purified in sufficient quantities? What will its price be?

J.H. Tinker, M.D.

Clonidine

Effects of Clonidine on Prolonged Postoperative Sympathetic Response
Dorman T, Clarkson K, Rosenfeld BA, et al (The Johns Hopkins Med Institutions, Baltimore, Md; Univ of Maryland, Baltimore; Vanderbilt Univ, Knoxville, Tenn)
Crit Care Med 25:1147–1152, 1997 4–28

Introduction.—Each year, approximately 1% to 2% of surgical patients in the United States have major morbidity or mortality. Trauma-induced hormonal changes that produce widespread physiologic responses appear to play an important role in perioperative complications. The ability of

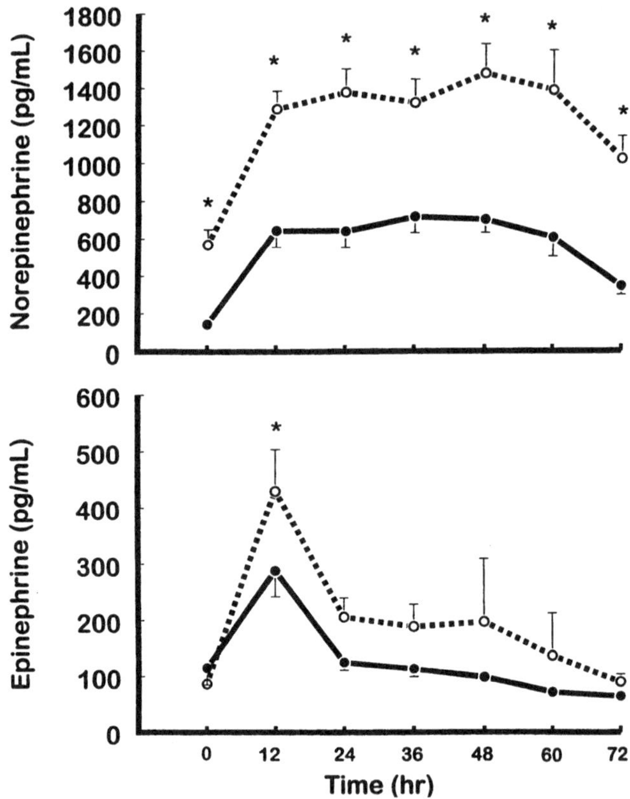

FIGURE 1.—Plasma concentrations of norepinephrine (**top**) and epinephrine (**bottom**). Time zero (0) is just before induction. The clonidine or treatment group (*solid line*) has statistically lower ($P < 0.05$) plasma catecholamines than the placebo group (*dashed line*) at all time points marked with an *asterisk*. (Courtesy of Dorman T, Clarkson K, Rosenfeld BA, et al: Effects of clonidine on prolonged postoperative sympathetic response. *Crit Care Med* 25[7]:1147–1152, 1997.)

clonidine, the α_2 adrenergic-receptor agonist, to attenuate the stress response to surgery was assessed.

Methods.—The 40 adult patients enrolled in the double-blind trial were scheduled for elective pancreatic or biliary major upper abdominal surgery. They were randomly assigned to receive placebo or clonidine, 0.2 mg orally and a clonidine patch the evening before surgery, with 0.3 mg of clonidine administered orally on call to the operating room. Patients received midazolam and/or morphine for preoperative sedation; anesthesia was induced with thiamyal and either isoflurane or enflurane was administered, together with morphine sulfate. No neuraxial opioids or local anesthetics were given. Patients were monitored the day before surgery and for 72 hours postoperatively for heart rate; systemic arterial blood pressure; plasma catecholamine, clonidine, and interleukin-6 concentrations; and 24-hour urine cortisol and nitrogen excretion.

Results.—Therapeutic plasma clonidine concentrations (mean 1.54 µg/mL) were maintained throughout the perioperative period. Mean preoperative epinephrine concentrations were 88 and 116 pg/mL, respectively, in clonidine and control groups. Concentrations peaked 1 hour after ICU admission in both groups, but this peak response was attenuated with clonidine administration (Fig 1). Norepinephrine concentrations were also lower in the clonidine group. Postoperative hypotension occurred with reduced frequency in patients treated with clonidine.

Discussion.—The administration of clonidine attenuated the catecholamine response to surgical stress in these patients undergoing major upper abdominal surgery. Plasma interleukin-6 concentration and the excretion of urine cortisol and nitrogen were not affected. The efficacy and safety of clonidine suggest that it may benefit surgical and critically ill patients.

► This study shows that clonidine reduces epinephrine and norepinephrine concentrations in the postoperative period, thus yielding a prolonged antihypertensive effect. Unfortunately, no other therapeutic end points or outcome parameters were elucidated. I would assume that the same type of effect could be achieved with the administration of intravenous labetalol, with the added benefit of minimizing perioperative myocardial ischemia.

D.M. Rothenberg, M.D.

Dose–Range Effects of Clonidine Added to Lidocaine for Brachial Plexus Block

Bernard J-M, Macaire P (Polyclinique Jean-Villar, Bruges-Bordeaux, France; Clinique du Parc, Lyon, France)

Anesthesiology 87:277–284, 1997 4–29

Introduction.—Depending on the local anesthetic used, analgesia that follows axillary nerve blocks is prolonged by clonidine from 40% to 100%, but there are side effects such as nausea, bradycardia, hypotension, and marked sedation. Studies concerning axillary nerve blocks did not test several dose responses of clonidine. A dose-response relationship for clonidine added to lidocaine for axillary block was defined.

Methods.—Fifty-six outpatients having carpal tunnel release were randomly selected to receive either 400 mg of lidocaine plus saline, or 400 mg of lidocaine plus 30, 90, or 300 μg of clonidine for axillary nerve block. The 4 groups of 14 patients each had blocks evaluated at regular time intervals to determine sensory and motor function in the 5 nerve regions of the hand and forearm. The evaluation also included postoperative pain intensity, side effects, and adequacy of the block for surgery.

Results.—The onset time of sensory block was reduced and the field of adequate anesthesia was extended with each dose of clonidine, compared with saline. In producing sensory blockade, 30 μg of clonidine was more effective than 90 μg of clonidine 10 minutes after injection. Clonidine administered at 30 and 300 μg produced sedation. The use of supplementary intravenous anesthetic agents for surgery was reduced and dose-dependent prolongation of analgesia was produced by clonidine, which reached a mean of 770 minutes for the largest dose. A dose-dependent decrease in systolic arterial pressure of up to −22.5% of baseline was produced by clonidine. Three patients had a mean arterial pressure of less than 55 mm Hg when given 300 μg of clonidine. Episodes of arterial oxyhemoglobin saturation of less than 90% were seen in 4 patients at this same dose, and 2 other patients could not be discharged because of hypotension.

Conclusions.—The quality of the peripheral blocks from lidocaine is enhanced by a small dose of clonidine and the classic α_2-agonist side effects are limited to sedation. Clinically, the best dose to use is between 30 μg and 90 μg. An increased clonidine dose was accompanied by more adverse effects such as decreased blood pressure and an abnormal ventilatory pattern.

► I selected this article to illustrate the increasing use of α_2-adrenergic agonists to produce analgesia and enhance regional blockade.

M. Wood, M.D.

Oral Clonidine Premedication Does Not Alter the Efficacy of Simulated Intravenous Test Dose Containing Low Dose Epinephrine in Awake Volunteers

Tanaka M, Nishikawa T (Univ of Akita, Japan; Univ of Tsukuba, Ibaraki, Japan)
Anesthesiology 87:285–288, 1997 4–30

Introduction.—Increasingly used as an anesthetic adjuvant, clonidine is a selective α2-adrenergic agonistic. Clonidine increases pressor responses to peripherally acting sympathometics such as ephedrine and phenylephrine, and heart rate response to isoproterenol. It also has been shown to reduce intraoperative anesthetic requirements. Few studies have been conducted on modulation by clonidine of hemodynamic responses to intrave-

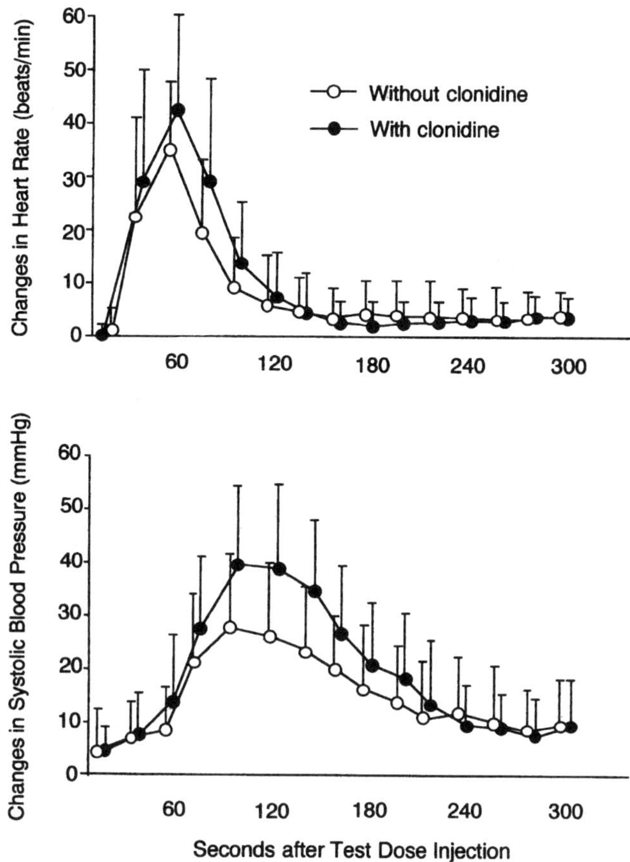

FIGURE 1.—Changes in heart rate (**top panel**) and systolic blood pressure (**bottom panel**) after intravenous injection of an epidural test dose containing 15 μg epinephrine and 45 mg lidocaine with and without clonidine premedication 5 μg/kg. Since heart rates and systolic blood pressure were essentially unchanged after 3 mL saline injection, these data are not presented. Data are mean ± SD. (Courtesy of Tanaka M, Nishikawa T: Oral clonidine premedication does not alter the efficacy of simulation intravenous test dose containing low dose epinephrine in awake volunteers. *Anesthesiology* 87:285–288, 1997. Copyright American Society of Anesthesiologists, Inc. Used with permission of Lippincott-Raven Publishers.)

nously administered epinephrine. The effects of oral clonidine premedication on hemodynamic responses were determined, and the sensitivity, specificity, and positive and negative predictive values were determined.

Methods.—Four series of determinations, separated by at least 72 hours, were performed in random order in 18 healthy volunteers. The 4 series were (1) no premedication followed by 3 mL of IV saline; (2) no premedication followed by IV test dose containing 3 mL of 1.5% lidocaine and 15 μg of epinephrine; (3) oral clonidine (5 μg/kg 1.5 hours before hemodynamic determinations) followed by intravenous saline; and (4) oral clonidine followed by IV epinephrine-containing test dose. Continuous measurements were taken of heart rate and systolic blood pressure, and symptoms associated with CNS toxicity were noted.

Results.—With or without clonidine premedication, heart rate and systolic blood pressure increased after the test dose injections (Fig 1). The maximum heart rate increases with clonidine were 49–61 beats/min, and without clonidine were 44–54 beats/min, indicating that it was not absolutely certain that everyone would have a positive heart rate response. In 18 of 18 volunteers given epinephrine with or without clonidine and in 0 of 18 volunteers given saline, the heart rate increases were 20 beats/min or greater. Based on the conventional heart rate criterion, the calculated sensitivities, specificities, and positive and negative predictive values were all 100% and were not altered by clonidine. Clonidine did not affect subjective symptoms.

Conclusions.—The efficacy of epinephrine-containing test doses used for detecting intravascular injection is not altered by oral clonidine. In healthy awake volunteers, oral clonidine premedication at 5 μg/kg increases heart rate and blood pressure responses to an intravenously administered epinephrine-containing test dose. The efficacy on the heart rate criterion or the incidence of subjective symptoms as a result of test dose injection were not affected by clonidine.

▶ Clonidine is used as an anesthetic adjuvant to produce sedation, reduce anesthetic requirements during surgery, and produce analgesia. It is well recognized that chronic β-adrenergic blockade can alter the hemodynamic response to epinephrine; similarly, clonidine (an α_2-adrenergic agonist) has been shown to modify the pressor response to sympathomimetics. This study demonstrated that clonidine does not alter the sensitivity and specificity of a simulated intravenous test dose of low-dose epinephrine. This may be important because small doses of epinephrine are used in an epidural test dose solution to detect accidental intravascular injection.

M. Wood, M.D.

Sodalime/Baralyme

Rehydration of Desiccated Baralyme Prevents Carbon Monoxide Formation From Desflurane in an Anesthesia Machine

Baxter PJ, Kharasch ED (Univ of Washington, Seattle)
Anesthesiology 86:1061–1065, 1997 4–31

Objective.—Increased intraoperative carbon monoxide (CO), produced by degradation of desflurane, enflurane, and isoflurane in the presence of soda lime or barium hydroxide lime (Baralyme), can result in poisoning. Because CO production increases as water content decreases, results are presented of a study to determine if adding back water to CO absorbent that had become dried could prevent CO formation.

Methods.—Four grams of fresh or desiccated Baralyme and 5 mL desflurane were placed into vials and sealed alone or in the presence of 1.3% or 13% water by weight. Carbon monoxide formation was measured by gas chromatography-mass spectrometry. Experiments were performed in triplicate. A second set of experiments was performed using an anesthesia machine, with a circle circuit, bellows ventilator, gas scavenging system, and an anesthesia gas monitor.

Results.—After 5 hours, total CO formation was 10,700 ppm in the dried Baralyme, 715 ppm in the Baralyme:1.3% water mixture, and less than 100 ppm in the Baralyme:13% water mixture. After 3 hours, complete rehydration of dry Baralyme reduced CO formation from enflurane and isoflurane from an average of 8,400 ppm and 1,240 ppm to essentially zero. In the anesthesia machine, complete rehydration reduced CO formation in the circuit from 2,500 ppm to less than 180 ppm.

Conclusion.—Drying of the carbon dioxide absorbent in anesthesia machines increases the production of CO whereas adding sufficient water to the system to effect 100% rehydration decreases CO production significantly in a cost-effective manner.

► I know of no solid reasons why Baralyme seems to be worse than soda lime, but it does seem to be true. These authors added water by simply pouring it on top of the Baralyme. I don't know if that would work in clinical practice, but I haven't seen any recommendation that we come into our operating rooms on Monday morning with a pitcher of water or a watering can and somehow "water" our Baralyme. In fact, at least in some hospitals, I would imagine that if the nurses saw the anesthesiologist with a watering can, they might call the sheriff. In any event, I included this paper in this year's YEAR BOOK to refresh and educate our readers about this carbon monoxide issue.

J.H. Tinker, M.D.

Amiodarone

Preoperative Therapy With Amiodarone and the Incidence of Acute Organ Dysfunction After Cardiac Surgery
Rady MY, Ryan T, Starr NJ (Cleveland Clinic Found, Ohio)
Anesth Analg 85:489–497, 1997 4–32

Background.—Amiodarone, developed for the treatment of angina pectoris in patients with coronary artery disease, has also proved useful in patients with arrhythmias and congestive heart failure. Several studies have shown that surgical patients receiving amiodarone have an increased incidence of postoperative acute respiratory distress syndrome, cardiac dysfunction, and other forms of organ dysfunction. Because of this, recommendations have called for discontinuation of amiodarone therapy for several weeks before surgery. A matched case-control study was performed to determine the effects of preoperative amiodarone therapy on the incidence of acute organ dysfunction.

Methods.—The subjects were drawn from a series of 11,950 patients admitted for cardiac surgery over a 3.5-year period. Two hundred twenty patients receiving amiodarone before and at the time of surgery made up the case group. The patients received an amiodarone maintenance dose of 200–600 mg/day, with therapy lasting for more than 1 week. They were matched to 220 controls who did not receive amiodarone. The controls were matched by various factors known to affect the incidence of acute organ dysfunction after cardiac surgery: day of surgery, source of admission, demographic characteristics, preoperative intra-aortic balloon pump placement, repeat surgery, emergency surgery, thoracic aorta surgery, and other surgical procedures. The effects of amiodarone therapy on the incidence of postoperative acute organ dysfunction were analyzed.

Results.—Sixty percent of patients in the amiodarone group had a preoperative history of congestive heart failure, compared with 38% in the control group. There were no significant differences in the incidence of acute organ dysfunction, duration of mechanical ventilation, or mortality. Twenty-six percent of patients in the amiodarone group required inotropes, compared with 17% of those in the control group. Patients receiving amiodarone were also more likely to require vasopressors (66% vs. 55%) and had a higher incidence of nosocomial infections after surgery (12% vs. 6%). These differences lost significance after adjustment for congestive heart failure, however.

Conclusion.—Patients taking amiodarone are at no higher risk of acute organ dysfunction or death after cardiac surgery. Patients taking amiodarone are more likely to need inotropes and vasopressors and have a higher incidence of nosocomial infections, but these are related to the severity of the underlying cardiac disease. The findings suggest that it may not be necessary to stop amiodarone therapy before cardiac surgery.

▶ Amiodarone is so toxic and so long acting (it turns some patients purple) that many of us are almost terrified of it. This paper would indicate that it probably should not be stopped despite the above. The reason for this is that it is pretty much a last-ditch drug. I agree with the authors that it probably should not be stopped, but for a different reason. The half-life of this drug is apparently similar to that of DDT, i.e., it never goes away. Therefore, whether you stop it preoperatively or not, probably doesn't make very much difference!

J.H. Tinker, M.D.

Ondansetron

Cardiac Dysrhythmias Associated With the Intravenous Administration of Ondansetron and Metoclopramide

Baguley WA, Hay WT, Mackie KP, et al (Univ of Washington, Seattle)
Anesth Analg 84:1380–1381, 1997 4–33

Background.—Ondansetron and metoclopramide are commonly administered as prophylaxis when the patient has a high postoperative risk of nausea and vomiting or when severe postoperative nausea and vomiting would harm the patient. The cases of 2 patients with cardiac dysrhythmias associated with ondansetron and metoclopramide are described.

Case Report.—Woman, 37, was scheduled for advancement of a thigh flap after a previous leg injury. At the time of the injury, she had severe postoperative nausea and vomiting treated with ondansetron and metoclopramide. At the time of the current procedure, the patient's hematocrit level was 24%. Intravenous ondansetron and metoclopramide were administered in the prcoperative holding area. The patient complained of light-headedness, nausea, and a headache and vomited once en route to the operating room. An ECG showed bigeminy, which spontaneously converted to a sinus rhythm within 10 sec. The ECG showed significant ST-segment depression. The patient had chest heaviness and a tightness in her throat. Arterial blood pressure remained normal. These symptoms and ECG abnormalities were resolved within 5 minutes. Myocardial infarction was ruled out. A dipyridamole thallium study proved normal.

Discussion.—In the literature, there was 1 letter suggesting an association between ondansetron and cardiovascular complications. The authors of this letter reported 7 cases of cardiac symptoms associated with chemotherapy and ondansetron. No significant effects on blood pressure or heart rate were reported by clinical trials of ondansetron. It is unclear what caused the dysrhythmias in these patients, but a possible confounding factor was the administration of metoclopramide, which has been associated with dysrhythmias on rare occasions. It is recommended that when ondansetron and metoclopramide are administered within a few minutes of each other, the ECG should be carefully monitored.

► Ketanserin, a ($5HT_2$) 5-hydroxy tryptamine receptor antagonist, prolongs the QT interval in a dose-related manner, and ventricular arrhythmias and syncope have been reported.[1] Arrhythmogenic effects are more likely to appear in patients with hypokalemia. Thus, it would not be surprising if ondansetron, a $5HT_3$ receptor antagonist, produced dysrhythmias. In addition, hypokalemia may occur preoperatively and during induction in conjunction with hypocapnia.

M. Wood, M.D.

Reference

1. Brogden RN, Sorkin EM: Ketanserin: A review of its pharmacodynamic and pharmacokinetic properties, and therapeutic potential in hypertension and peripheral vascular disease. *Drugs* 40:903–949, 1990.

Rocuronium

Thiopental-Rocuronium Versus Ketamine-Rocuronium for Rapid-Sequence Intubation in Parturients Undergoing Cesarean Section

Baraka AS, Sayyid SS, Assaf BA (American Univ of Beirut, Lebanon)
Anesth Analg 84:1104–1107, 1997 4–34

Background.—Rocuronium, a monoqueternary, aminosteroidal, nondepolarizing neuromuscular blocking agent with a rapid onset of action may be an alternative to succinylcholine for rapid-sequence induction of anesthesia when the latter agent is contraindicated. The onset of vecuronium neuromuscular block (NMB) and the conditions for tracheal intubation for ketamine-rocuronium and thiopental-rocuronium in RSI of general anesthesia in parturients scheduled for elective cesarean section were studied.

Methods.—Forty women were included. After preoxygenation, anesthesia was induced by thiopental 4 mg/kg in 20 patients and by ketamine 1.5 mg/kg in 20 patients. Rocuronium 0.6 mg/kg was then given. Neuromuscular transmission was assessed every 10 seconds with electromyographic response to train-of-4 stimulation of the ulnar nerve at the wrist.

Findings.—Mean time to 50% block in the thiopental and ketamine groups were 45 and 42 seconds, respectively. Mean onset time was 105 and 101 seconds, respectively. Neither mean was siginificantly different between groups. Tracheal intubation at 50% NMB was performed easily in all patients receiving ketamine but was difficult in three fourths of the patients receiving thiopental (Table 2).

Conclusions.—Ketamine 1.5 mg/kg followed by rocuronium 0.6 mg/kg may be suitable for rapid-sequence induction of anesthesia when succinylcholine is contraindicated in parturients undergoing cesarean delivery. With ketamine, tracheal intubation is performed easily at 50% NMB at a mean of 42 seconds after rocuronium administration.

▶ The authors hypothesized that "rocuronium may provide an alternative to succinylcholine for rapid-sequence induction (RSI) of anesthesia . . . ." Yet

TABLE 2.—Onset and Clinical Duration of Rocuronium Neuromuscular Block

	50% NMB* (s)	Onset time† (s)	Recovery time‡ (min)
Group 1: Thiopental group	45 ± 10	105 ± 35	40 ± 9
Group 2: Ketamine group	42 ± 14	101 ± 35	45 ± 10

* Time from end of injection of rocuronium 0.6 mg/kg until T1/control ratio of 50%.
† Time from end of injection of rocuronium 0.6 mg/kg until maximum NMB.
‡ Time of recovery of neuromuscular transmission to 25% of the control value.
Abbreviation: NMB, neuromuscular block.
(Courtesy of Baraka AS, Sayyid SS, Assaf BA: Thiopental-rocuronium versus ketamine-rocuronium for rapid-sequence intubation in parturients undergoing cesarean section. *Anesth Analg* 84[5]:1104–1107, 1997.)

they did not compare rocuronium with succinylcholine. In this study, both groups of patients received rocuronium. The independent variable in this study was the induction agent. The correct conclusion of this study is that the choice of induction agent (i.e., thiopental versus ketamine) did not affect the response to rocuronium.

D.H. Chestnut, M.D.

Ropivacaine/Bupivacaine

Double-blind Comparison of Epidural Ropivacaine 0.25% and Bupivacaine 0.25%, for the Relief of Childbirth Pain

Muir HA, Writer D, Douglas J, et al (Dalhousie Univ, Halifax, NS; Univ of British Columbia, Vancouver, BC; McGill Univ, Montreal)

Can J Anaesth 44:599–604, 1997 4–35

Background.—Ropivacaine is a local anesthetic, structurally related to bupivacaine, but associated with less motor blockade and a shorter elimination half-life. The efficacy of ropivacaine 0.25% administered epidurally for the relief of labor pain was examined and compared to that of bupivacaine 0.25%.

Methods.—A multicenter, prospective, randomized, double-blind study was performed. The study group consisted of 60 ASA I or II women in active labor between the ages of 16 and 40 years, with full-term singleton fetuses. Either ropivacaine or bupivacaine was administered by intermittent top-up epidural analgesia during labor. Maternal blood pressure, heart rate, analgesia, degree of motor block, and visual analogue pain scores were assessed by the nurse before and at regular intervals after administration of the analgesic. Total analgesic dose, labor duration, delivery method, and maternal or neonatal side effects were recorded. The infant was evaluated by the nurse with fetal heart tracing, Apgar 1- and 5-minute scores, and neonatal neurobehavioral evaluations at 2 and 24 postnatal hours.

Results.—Ropivacaine 0.25% provided effective epidural analgesia during labor. There was no significant difference between ropivacaine and bupivacaine in any of the variables measured in this study. There was no significant difference between these 2 drugs in the number of patients with motor blockade or method of delivery.

Conclusions.—Epidural analgesia during labor with ropivacaine 0.25% was effective and similar in efficacy to that of bupivacaine 0.25%. Further studies with a larger population will be necessary to determine whether the trend toward less motor blockade with ropivacaine will have an effect on obstetric outcome.

► During labor, the major potential advantage of epidural ropivacaine is that it may result in less motor block than epidural bupivacaine. Most parturients dislike the motor block that results from epidural analgesia. Further, some have speculated that decreased motor block with ropivacaine might result in an increased likelihood of instrumental vaginal delivery. In the present study, the number of patients who experienced motor block "differed numerically" between the 2 groups (i.e., 21% vs. 42%), but this difference was not statistically significant. Further, there was no difference between the 2 groups in the method of delivery. In fact, the percentage of spontaneous vaginal deliveries was numerically higher in the bupivacaine group, although the incidence was not statistically significant. Larger studies are needed to determine whether the choice between bupivacaine and ropivacaine affects obstetric outcome.

D.H. Chestnut, M.D.

Central Nervous and Cardiovascular Effects of I.V. Infusions of Ropivacaine, Bupivacaine and Placebo in Volunteers

Knudsen K, Suurküla MB, Blomberg S, et al (Sahlgrenska Univ, Göteberg, Sweden; Astra Pain Control AB, Södertälje, Sweden)

Br J Anaesth 78:507–514, 1997 4–36

Background.—The most serious side effects of local anesthetics involve the central nervous and cardiovascular systems. They often occur after accidental intravascular or intrathecal injections, or overdose. Ropivacaine is a new, long-acting local anesthetic with a pharmacokinetic disposition similar to that of bupivacaine, but it is less lipid soluble. Ropivacaine caused less CNS and cardiac toxicity than bupivacaine in preclinical studies. Studies that have compared it to bupivacaine have shown that ropivacaine has similar onset, duration, and extent of sensory block, but less intense and shorter motor block.

Methods.—The incidence of CNS symptoms was examined in 12 healthy male subjects in a randomized, crossover, double-blind study. The subjects were given IV ropivacaine, 5 mg/mL^{-1}, bupivacaine 5 mg/mL^{-1}, and placebo.

Results.—The maximum tolerated dose for CNS effects was higher with ropivacaine in 9 subjects and higher with bupivacaine in 3 subjects. The estimated 95% confidence limits for the difference in mean dose between ropivacaine and bupivacaine were −30 mg and 7 mg. After administration of ropivacaine, the maximum tolerated free arterial plasma concentration was twice as high. More muscular twitching occurred with bupivacaine (Fig 1). Symptoms of CNS toxicity appeared earlier and in more subjects with bupivacaine (Fig 2). Disappearance of all symptoms was more rapid with ropivacaine. The threshold for CNS symptoms was a mean free plasma concentration of 0.6 mg/L^{-1} for ropivacaine and 0.3 mg/L^{-1} for bupivacaine. Compared to placebo and ropivacaine, bupivacaine increased QRS width during sinus rhythm. Compared to placebo, bupivacaine reduced left ventricular systolic and diastolic function, but ropivacaine reduced systolic function only.

Discussion.—In these volunteers, ropivacaine had a higher tolerated dose and free plasma concentration based on shift in dose-response and concentration-response curves for CNS effects. Ropivacaine produced

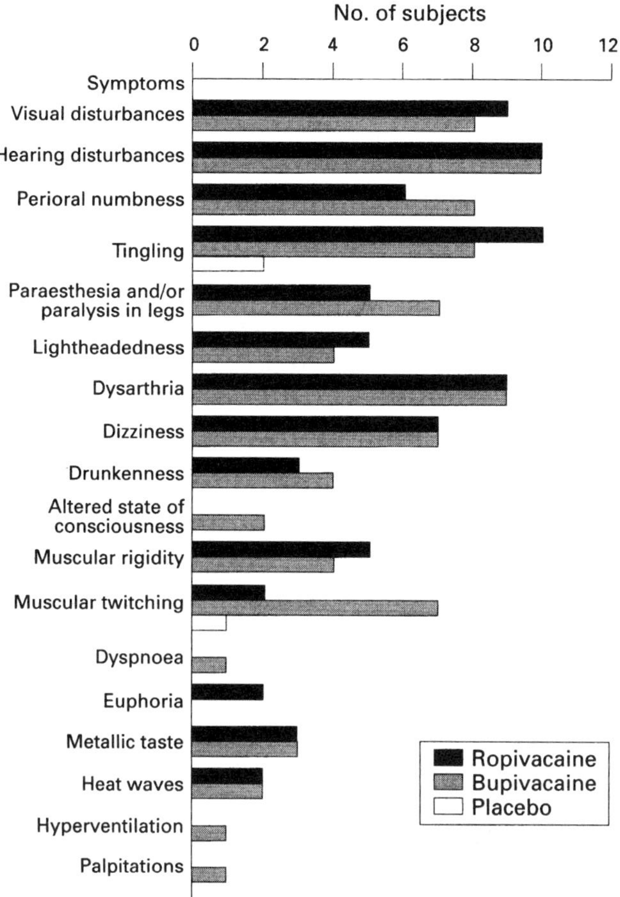

FIGURE 1.—Number of subjects with symptoms, grouped in different categories, during and after IV infusion of ropivacaine and bupivacaine 10 mg/min^{-1} and placebo (saline). Crossover study in 12 volunteers. (Reprinted by permission of the BMJ Publishing Group, from Knudsen K, Suurküla MB, Blomberg S, et al: Central nervous and cardiovascular effects of I.V. infusions of ropivacaine, bupivacaine and placebo in volunteers. *Br J Anaesth* 78:507–514, 1997.)

fewer cardiovascular changes than bupivacaine at doses producing CNS symptoms.

► This is a key study in the evaluation of the relative CNS and cardiovascular effects of the new long-acting, single isomer, local anesthetic, ropivacaine. Bupivacaine and mepivacaine are racemic mixtures; the comparative effects of ropivacaine vs. the enantiomer of bupivacaine (levobupivacaine) will be pivotal in determining the relative toxicity of these 2 local anesthetic isomers.

M. Wood, M.D.

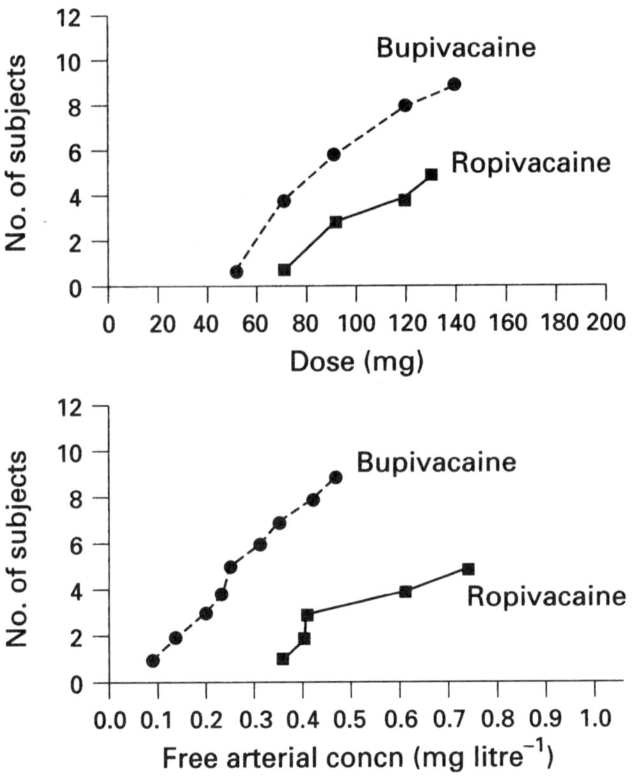

FIGURE 2.—Cumulative number of subjects with muscular twitching or rigidity or both, against dose (**top**) or unbound arterial plasma concentration (**bottom**) at onset of IV infusion of ropivacaine and bupivacaine 10 mg/min^{-1}. Crossover study in 12 volunteers. (Reprinted by permission of the BMJ Publishing Group, from Knudsen K, Suurküla MB, Blomberg S, et al: Central nervous and cardiovascular effects of I.V. infusions of ropivacaine, bupivacaine and placebo in volunteers. *Br J Anaesth* 78:507–514, 1997.)

Plasma Bupivacaine Concentrations Associated With Continuous Extradural Infusions in Babies

Peutrell JM, Holder K, Gregory M (Royal Hosp for Sick Children, St Michael's Hill, Bristol, England)

Br J Anaesth 78:160–162, 1997 4–37

Introduction.—Compared to older children and adults, infants have an increased potential for local anesthetic toxicity because the free fraction of drug is increased. There have been no specific reports of blood concentrations of bupivacaine during extradural infusions during the first year of life. A study of 8 babies with a mean age of 33 weeks was designed to measure venous plasma concentrations of both total and free bupivacaine during continuous infusion of the drug.

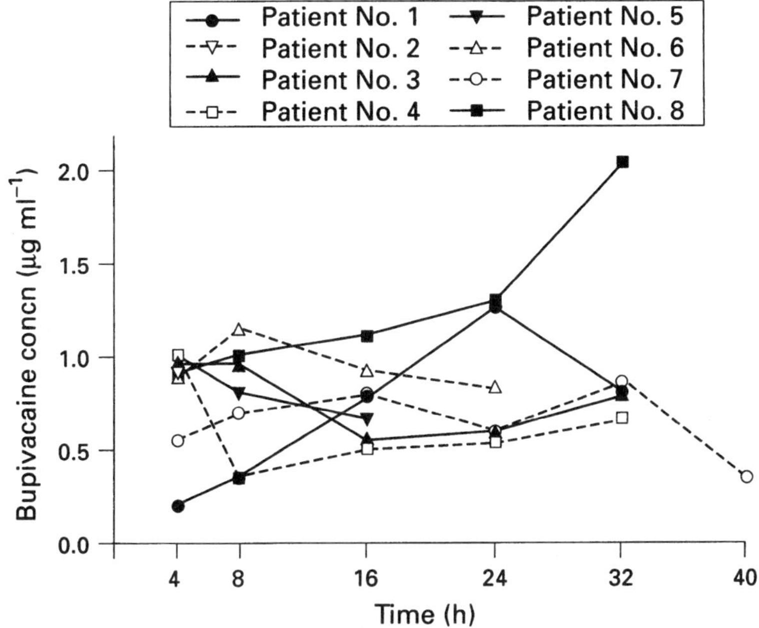

FIGURE 1.—Venous plasma concentrations of total bupivacaine during continuous extradural infusion, measured at 4, 8, 16, 24, 32, and 40 hours. (Reprinted by permission of the BMJ Publishing Group, from Peutrell JM, Holder K, Gregory M: Plasma bupivacaine concentrations associated with continuous extradural infusions in babies. *Br J Anaesth* 78:160–162, 1997.)

Methods.—All infants were ASA I or II and undergoing major abdominal operations. After induction of general anesthesia and intubation, a 23-gauge lumbar extradural catheter was inserted using a 19-gauge Tuohy needle (Portex Minipack System). After a mean initial dose of 1.2 mg/kg^{-1}, bupivacaine was infused at a mean rate of 0.38 mg/kg^{-1}/ hr^{-1} for a mean of 31 hours for postoperative pain relief. Blood samples were obtained from a venous sampling cannula at 4, 8, 16, 24, 32, and 40 hours after starting the infusion. High pressure liquid chromatography was used to measure total plasma bupivacaine concentration.

Results.—One baby experienced distress, attributed to colic, after surgery and was treated with an infusion of morphine. Postoperative assessments of the remaining 7 infants yielded hourly pain scores of "no pain" in most cases; no score was higher than "mild pain." One infant was difficult to arouse at the first assessment, but all others were either "awake and alert" or "drowsy but easy to arouse." Total bupivacaine plasma concentrations were generally less than 2 μg/mL^{-1} (Fig 1), but 1 baby had a concentration of 2.02 μg/mL^{-1} at 32 hours and showed clear evidence of accumulation of the drug throughout the extradural infusion. The free fraction of bupivacaine could not be obtained.

Conclusion.—Despite infusion rates below the currently accepted maximum, infants can accumulate bupivacaine and achieve plasma concentrations above the threshold for toxic side effects. Findings indicate that an extradural infusion rate of 0.375 mg/kg^{-1}/hr^{-1} is probably an absolute maximum during the first year of life.

▶ This is an interesting study reporting bupivacaine concentrations in small babies, and makes recommendations regarding extradural infusion rates. The authors obtained blood samples as long as 40 hours after starting the extradural infusion; it is important to recognize that volatile anesthetics can decrease the clearance of bupivacaine and so bupivacaine concentrations are likely to be higher if the extradural infusion is administered during anesthesia with a volatile anesthetic such as halothane.

M. Wood, M.D.

Fetal Heart Rate Changes After Intrathecal Sufentanil or Epidural Bupivacaine for Labor Analgesia: Incidence and Clinical Significance

Nielsen PE, Erickson JR, Abouleish EI, et al (Univ of Texas, Houston)

Anesth Analg 83:742–746, 1996 4–38

Background.—The effects of intrathecal sufentanil (ITS) and epidural bupivacaine (EB) on fetal heart rate have not been established definitively. The relative effects of these agents on fetal heart tracing (FHT) characteristics during labor and obstetric outcomes were compared.

Methods.—One hundred twenty-nine patients were enrolled in the trial between April and September 1994. The inclusion criteria were singleton pregnancies, gestational age of 36 weeks or more, and cephalic presentation. Sixty-five patients received epidural anesthesia 60 minutes or more after ITS. The other 64 patients received EB.

Findings.—The incidences of clinically significant FHT abnormalities, including recurrent late decelerations, bradycardia, or both, were comparable in the 2 groups, being 21.5% in the ITS group and 23.4% in the EB group. The rates of hypotension in the 2 groups were 18.5% and 17.2%, respectively, not significantly different. The risk of cesarean section was significantly greater in both groups in patients whose previously normal FHT became abnormal after analgesia, compared with patients without a new-onset FHT abnormality.

Conclusions.—The incidences of clinically significant FHT abnormalities and hypotension are comparable in patients receiving ITS and in those receiving EB within the first hour of administration. Patients should be monitored continuously with FHT during this time, because a new-onset FHT abnormality reveals possible fetal compromise and an increased risk of cesarean delivery.

▶ In this study, the authors observed no difference between the 2 groups in the incidence of "clinically significant" abnormalities of the fetal heart rate. Specifically, the authors observed fetal heart rate abnormalities in 22% of the women in the ITS group and in 23% of the women in the EB group.

I do not agree that all of these abnormalities were "clinically significant." For example, the authors defined fetal bradycardia as a fetal heart rate of less than 120 beats/min for less than 2 minutes. At term, it is not uncommon for a healthy fetus to have a baseline fetal heart rate of approximately 110 beats/min. In the presence of normal fetal heart rate variability, such a rate typically does not signal fetal compromise. Nonetheless, this study calls attention to the importance of fetal heart rate monitoring in patients who receive EB or ITS during labor.

D.H. Chestnut, M.D.

Amrinone

Amrinone Versus Dobutamine in Cardiac Surgical Patients With Severe Pulmonary Hypertension After Cardiopulmonary Bypass: A Prospective, Randomized Double-blinded Trial

Jenkins IR, Dolman J, O'Connor JP, et al (Univ of British Columbia, Vancouver)

Anaesth Intensive Care 25:245–249, 1997 4–39

Background.—It can be difficult to separate patients from cardiopulmonary bypass after cardiac surgery. Two types of drugs are commonly used for this purpose: selective factor III phosphodiesterase inhibitors such as amrinone and inotropes such as dobutamine. These 2 agents were studied for their acute postoperative hemodynamic effects in patients with severe pulmonary hypertension.

Methods.—The prospective, randomized, double-blind trial included 20 patients undergoing elective mitral valve replacement. All had severe pulmonary hypertension, defined as a mean pulmonary artery pressure of greater than 30 mm Hg on cardiac catheterization. During weaning from cardiopulmonary bypass, the patients received either dobutamine, 5 µg/kg/min, or amrinone, a 1.0 mg/kg bolus followed by 10 µg/kg/min. The 2 treatments were compared for their effects on right and left ventricular function and on pulmonary artery pressures. The study protocol continued for 3 hours after weaning from bypass.

Results.—At the time of separation, the mean increase in cardiac index was 1.38 ± 0.95 L/min/m^2 with amrinone vs. 0.69 ± 0.63 L/min/m^2 with dobutamine. The increases in right ventricular ejection fraction were 0.15 ± 0.08 and 0.04 ± 0.11, respectively. Patients receiving amrinone had a 8.0 ± 4.4-mm Hg reduction in pulmonary artery wedge pressure at separation, compared with 0.75 ± 6.6 mm Hg with dobutamine. Amrinone was also associated with greater reductions in pulmonary artery systolic and diastolic pressures. Heart rate, mean arterial pressure, central venous pressure, and right ventricular stroke work index were similar for the 2 groups.

Conclusion.—In patients with severe preoperative pulmonary hypertension while undergoing separation from bypass, amrinone produces a better hemodynamic state than dobutamine. Amrinone produces lower pulmonary pressures with increased right ventricular ejection fraction. It is also associated with greater increases in left ventricular stroke work index and stroke volume index. When pulmonary hypertension is a problem, amrinone is helpful during and after the weaning period.

► I do not see why anyone should be surprised that amrinone can be a pulmonary vasodilator. Dobutamine, as a sympathetic agonist, is extremely unlikely to be a pulmonary vasodilator. If dobutamine is associated with a reduction in pulmonary vascular resistance, it is because of the increase in right ventricular output, not direct pulmonary vasodilation. I do not understand precisely how dobutamine became so widely used in clinical situations in which there is increased pulmonary vascular resistance. If you want to increase the cardiac output in a critical situation, you should use 1 of the potent sympathomimetics, namely, isoproterenol, epinephrine, or norepinephrine. If you want to add amrinone to epinephrine, this makes sense to me. Dobutamine does not.

J.H. Tinker, M.D.

Magnesium

Blood Ionized Magnesium Concentrations During Cardiopulmonary Bypass and Their Correlation With Other Circulating Cations
Aziz S, Haigh WG, Van Norman GA, et al (Univ of Washington, Seattle)
J Card Surg 11:341–347, 1996 4–40

Introduction.—There are unanswered questions regarding variations in the levels of various cations during cardiopulmonary bypass (CPB) and about their physiologic effects. With the use of ion-specific electrodes, it is now possible to measure blood ionized magnesium (iMg)—the bioactive fraction of circulating magnesium—during surgery. Changes in blood iMg during CPB were studied, together with the relationships of iMg to other cations.

Methods.—The study included 30 patients undergoing elective coronary artery bypass grafting. Before, during, and after CPB, blood samples were obtained for measurement of iMg, using an AVL 988–4 Electrolyte Analyzer. Longitudinal patterns of change in iMg were assessed, together with the relationship of iMg to Ca^{2+} (iCa), potassium, pH, sodium, and hematocrit.

Results.—Concentrations of both iMg and iCa were dynamic and varied widely. Seventy-three percent of iMg results were abnormally low, 50% during CPB. Some patients had episodes of high and low levels of ionized magnesemia. Before, during, and after CPB, there was a direct correlation between iMg and potassium, suggesting parallel movement of these 2 cations between tissue and blood. Before CPB, iMg and iCa were directly correlated; after CPB, they were inversely correlated. During bypass, however, iMg and iCa were unrelated to each other. All patients had an inverse correlation between iMg and sodium during the postbypass period. Only during CPB and only in patients with concurrent iMg and iCa association, was there an inverse correlation between iMg and pH and a positive correlation between iMg and hematocrit.

Conclusion.—Patients undergoing CPB frequently experience blood iMg depletion. However, blood iMg concentrations are highly variable and unpredictable. Declines in circulating iMg are of greater clinical concern than increases, although the risks of elevated iMg levels remain to be determined. The authors call for studies of the possible association between intraoperative iMg depletion and postoperative atrial fibrillation.

► As we learn more and more about magnesium, it does make sense to believe that it might be useful in the understanding of various rhythm complications during cardiac anesthesia. Whether routine costly measurements make sense is less sure. With calcium, I have long simply titrated it to desired effect. Can we do the same with magnesium?

J.H. Tinker, M.D.

Mexiletine

Response to Intravenous Lidocaine Infusion Predicts Subsequent Response to Oral Mexiletine: A Prospective Study

Galer BS, Harle J, Rowbotham MC (Univ of Washington, Seattle; Univ of California, at San Francisco)

J Pain Symptom Manage 12:161–167, 1996 4–41

Background.—Lidocaine and mexiletine are class 1B local antiarrhythmics, which have demonstrated anesthetic activity in neuropathic pain disorders. The correlation between response to IV lidocaine (IVL) and subsequent response to oral mexiletine therapy for neuropathic pain was explored in a double-blind study.

Methods.—Ten participants were recruited and 9 completed the study. Participants received 2 IVL infusions at 2 mg/kg and 5 mg/kg for a 45-minute period, double-blind and in random order, separated by at least 1 week. Pain intensity was rated using a visual analogue scale and a Pain Relief Scale. At least 1 week after the second IVL, oral mexiletine therapy for 4 weeks was initiated.

Results.—Both IVL doses significantly reduced visual analogue scale scores, with the higher dose producing a greater response. The subsequent response to oral mexiletine was significantly associated with the average response to the 2 previous IVL doses. Neither dose nor blood levels of mexiletine was associated with pain relief.

Conclusion.—In this study of the usefulness of the response to IVL therapy in predicting subsequent response to oral mexiletine therapy, IVL response was correlated with subsequent response to oral mexiletine therapy for neuropathic pain. This suggests that IVL may be a useful predictive tool for assessing which neuropathic patients would benefit from similar oral medications.

► It was disappointing to discover that this study was not placebo controlled. The ability of IVL infusion to predict response to mexiletine is an important issue, particularly in light of the possible pro-arrhythmic effects of oral sodium channel blockers. Given the high placebo responsiveness of patients with chronic pain, this study may simply illustrate the ability of an IV placebo to predict response to an oral placebo.

S.E. Abram, M.D.

Nitrous Oxide and Vomiting

Nitrous Oxide Does Not Increase Vomiting After Dental Restorations in Children

Splinter WM, Komocar L (Children's Hosp of Eastern Ontario, Ottawa; Univ of Ottawa, Ont)

Anesth Analg 84:506–508, 1997 4–42

Background.—Vomiting is common among children after general anesthesia. Nitrous oxide (N_2O) may be one factor contributing to this emesis. Whether N_2O during halothane anesthetic increases the incidence of postoperative vomiting among children after restorative dental surgery was investigated.

Methods.—Three hundred thirty children undergoing outpatient dental restorations were included in the single-blind, randomized, controlled study. One group of children received N_2O during anesthesia; the other group did not. Inhalation with halothane or IV propofol was used to induce anesthesia.

TABLE 1.—Demographic Data and Incidence of Postoperative Vomiting

	Nitrous oxide	Control
n	165	165
Age (yr)	4.7 ± 1.9	4.6 ± 2.0
Weight (kg)	18 ± 5	19 ± 6
Premedication (midazolam)	84	82
Propofol induction	30	30
Inhalation induction	135	135
Length of anesthesia (min)	82 ± 28	70 ± 24
Spontaneous ventilation	123	130
Oral fluid ingested in DCSU	130	119
In-hospital vomiting		
All	24%	15%*
Propofol induction	24%	13%
Inhalation induction	24%	15%
Vomiting out of hospital (same day)	23%	20%
Vomiting out of hospital (Day 1)	4%	3%
Overall vomiting	35%	30%

Note: Values are listed as mean ± standard deviation or *n*.
*$P = 0.03$, N_2O vs. control group.
Abbreviation: *DCSU*, day care surgical unit.
(Courtesy of Splinter WM, Komocar L: Nitrous oxide does not increase vomiting after dental restorations in children. *Anesth Analg* 84[3]:506–508, 1997.)

Findings.—The incidence of vomiting was similar in the 2 groups. Thirty-five percent of the N_2O recipients and 30% of the control group vomited after anesthesia. However, the control group had significantly less in-hospital vomiting (Table 1).

Conclusions.—Overall, N_2O did not significantly affect vomiting among the children in this study. Unless otherwise contraindicated, N_2O should be used for general anesthesia in children undergoing surgery associated with a low risk of vomiting.

► Many people believe that N_2O is the main "culprit" in the production of postoperative nausea and vomiting. This is not the first paper that has disputed this, but it certainly is interesting, because it is such a large and relatively homogeneous study. The authors did, in fact, have a higher numerical incidence of vomiting in the N_2O group, and as Table 1 indicates, even if it isn't statistically significant. I'm not sure the authors have shown that N_2O added nothing to the vomiting picture. I think they have shown that it did contribute. We have a long way to go in understanding perioperative nausea and vomiting.

J.H. Tinker, M.D.

Aprotinin for Blood Loss in Liver Resection

Aprotinin Reduces Blood Loss in Patients Undergoing Elective Liver Resection

Lentschener C, Benhamou D, Mercier FJ, et al (Université Paris-Sud)

Anesth Analg 84:875–881, 1997 4–43

Background.—Bleeding continues to be a significant risk of liver resection. Aprotinin has proved useful in reducing bleeding in situations with and without extracorporeal bypass. However, the mechanism of this effect is unclear. The effects of aprotinin on blood loss in patients undergoing elective liver resection were studied.

Methods.—The prospective, randomized, double-blind trial included 97 patients undergoing elective liver resection through a subcostal incision. The patients were stratified into 3 diagnostic groups: cancer in cirrhosis, cancer in healthy liver, and benign tumor in healthy liver. They were then assigned to receive either large-dose aprotinin, according to a previously published regimen, or placebo starting after induction of anesthesia. The effects of aprotinin on blood loss and transfusion requirements were assessed. Changes in coagulation after aprotinin administration were assessed in an attempt to understand the mechanisms of its effects.

Results.—Intraoperative blood loss was 1,217 mL in the aprotinin group vs. 1,653 mL in the placebo group. Seventeen percent of patients in the aprotinin group required transfusion, compared with 39% of those in the placebo group; number of red blood cell packs transfused was 30 vs. 77 (Table 2). During surgery, the 2 groups had an identical increase in thrombin-antithrombin III complexes, suggesting similar activation of coagulation. The aprotinin group had less intraoperative hyperfibrinolysis

TABLE 2.—Blood Loss and Transfusion Requirement (Mean ± SD)

	Aprotinin group (n = 48)	Placebo group (n = 49)	P value
Mean blood loss (mL)	1217 ± 966	1653 ± 1221	0.048
(range)	(70–4600)	(215–6300)	
Total RBC transfused per group	30	77	0.015
Transfused patients per group: n (%)	8 (17)	19 (39)	0.02
Total FFP transfused per group	2	22	0.1
Total platelet units transfused per group	0	0	

Abbreviations: RBC, red blood cells; *FFP*, fresh frozen plasma.

(Courtesy of Lentschener C, Benhamou D, Mercier FJ, et al: Aprotinin reduces blood loss in patients undergoing elective liver resection. *Anesth Analg* 84[4]:875–881, 1997.)

than the placebo group. Aprotinin had no apparent adverse drug effects, such as circulatory disturbances, deep venous thrombosis, or increased serum creatinine.

Conclusions.—In patients undergoing elective liver resection, aprotinin is associated with a significant reduction in blood loss and transfusion requirement. Prophylactic aprotinin therapy and other blood-saving approaches may be considered for patients at high risk of intraoperative bleeding during liver surgery. Although the mechanism of aprotinin's effect is unclear, inhibition of fibrinolysis likely results from an antiplasmin effect.

► Hepatic resection has long been associated with the potential for large blood loss. Improved surgical techniques (such as the use of ultrasonic dissectors or hepatic vascular exclusion) have helped, but the potential for blood loss remains.

Aprotinin is a drug that has gained popularity in cardiac surgery for its ability to lessen blood loss. Recently it has been employed in a variety of other procedures. This study demonstrates aprotinin's ability to diminish blood loss and transfusion requirements for hepatic resection. The main thesis is enhanced by the large and well-balanced cohort. The second part of the paper, attempting to elucidate the mechanism for aprotinin's action, is less clear. The study also showed no adverse effects of aprotinin use. The article demonstrates that aprotinin may be a useful adjuvant in reducing blood loss for hepatic resection.

R.S. Finn, M.D.

Hirudin vs. Low–Molecular Weight Heparin

A Comparison of Recombinant Hirudin With a Low-Molecular-Weight Heparin to Prevent Thromboembolic Complications After Total Hip Replacement

Eriksson BI, Wille-Jørgensen P, Kälebo P, et al (Sahlgrenska-Östra Univ Hosp, Göteborg, Sweden; Bispebjerg Hosp, Copenhagen; Goethe Unversität, Frankfurt am Main, Germany; et al)

N Engl J Med 337:1329–1335, 1997 4–44

Introduction.—Various methods have been used to prevent deep-vein thrombosis after total hip replacement. A new development in antithrombotic therapy, recombinant hirudin (desirudin), was compared for efficacy and safety with a standard regimen of low–molecular weight heparin (enoxaparin) in patients scheduled for elective primary total hip replacement.

Methods.—The randomized, double-blind trial enrolled 2,079 adult patients at 31 participating centers in 10 European countries. Both treatments were started preoperatively, with enoxaparin administered on the evening before surgery and desirudin within 30 minutes before surgery. The dosage of enoxaparin was 40 mg subcutaneously once daily; 15 mg of desirudin was given subcutaneously twice daily. Treatment continued for 8–12 days. Of the 2,051 patients who underwent surgery after enrollment, 1,023 were randomly assigned to receive enoxaparin and 1,028 to receive desirudin. The 2 groups were similar in demographic characteristics, risk factors, and types of surgery and anesthesia. Patients were followed up for major thromboembolic events, verified by bilateral venography.

Results.—The primary analysis of efficacy included 785 patients in the enoxaparin group and 802 in the desirudin group. Most of the remaining

TABLE 3.—Thromboembolic Events*

Event	Enoxaparin Group†	Desirudin Group	P Value	Reduction in Relative Risk (95% CI)
	no. (%)			%
Deep-vein thrombosis				
Proximal	59 (7.5)‡	36 (4.5)§	0.01	40.3 (10.7–60.1)
Overall	196 (25.5)¶	142 (18.4)∥	0.001	28.0 (12.8–40.6)
Pulmonary embolism	2 (0.3)	2 (0.2)	—	—
Unexplained death	0	1 (0.1)	—	—

*In the enoxaparin group, 785 patients could be evaluated for the primary outcome, and 768 for the secondary outcome. In the desirudin group, the respective numbers were 802 and 773.

†One patient in this group had both proximal deep-vein thrombosis and pulmonary embolism.

‡The 95% confidence interval for the incidence is 5.8% to 9.6%.

§The 95% confidence interval for the incidence is 3.2% to 6.2%.

¶The 95% confidence interval for the incidence is 22.5% to 28.8%.

∥The 95% confidence interval for the incidence is 15.7% to 21.3%.

Abbreviation: CI, confidence interval.

(Reprinted by permission of *The New England Journal of Medicine*, from Eriksson BI, Wille-Jørgensen P, Kälebo P, et al: A comparison of recombinant hirudin with a low-molecular-weight heparin to prevent thromboembolic complications after total hip replacement. *N Engl J Med* 337:1329–1335.)

patients were excluded from analysis when venography was not performed. Ninety-nine patients (6.2%) had a major thromboembolic event, 4.9% in the desirudin group and 7.6% in the enoxaparin group—a relative reduction in risk of 36.4%. Rates of proximal deep-vein thrombosis showed a similar reduction with desirudin vs. enoxaparin (4.5% vs. 7.5%, a relative reduction in risk of 40.3%) (Table 3). The significant effect of treatment persisted after adjustment for age, sex, type of anesthesia, and other prognostic factors. Safety profiles were similar; blood loss, transfusion, serious bleeding episodes, and deep infections did not differ significantly in the 2 groups.

Discussion.—The thrombin inhibitor, desirudin, was more effective than a low–molecular weight heparin, enoxaparin, when administered preoperatively and postoperatively to prevent deep-vein thrombosis after total hip replacement. Although neither treatment group had cases of thrombocytopenia, desirudin has not been associated with this complication, whereas thrombocytopenia can occur with heparin preparations.

▶ Desirudin is another newer anticoagulant that directly inhibits thrombin, although without immune thrombocytopenia as a side effect. In this study, more than half of the patients underwent regional anesthesia for their total hip replacement. Although the authors validate the benefits of regional anesthesia in preventing deep-venous thrombosis in patients undergoing total hip replacement, they fail to comment upon the incidence of epidural or spinal hematoma in those having received either low–molecular weight heparin or desirudin.

D.M. Rothenberg, M.D.

Heparinase 1 vs. Protamine on Platelets

The Effects of Heparinase 1 and Protamine on Platelet Reactivity

Ammar T, Fisher CF (Mount Sinai Med Ctr, New York)

Anesthesiology 86:1382–1386, 1997 4–45

Background.—Protamine is the most common drug for reversing heparin anticoagulation, in spite of its side effects. Heparinase 1 (heparinase) may be an alternative to protamine. The side effects of heparinase have not been thoroughly examined. One study has shown that heparinase did not cause any significant hemodynamic changes when given IV to anesthetized, heparinized dogs. The effects of equivalent doses of heparinase and protamine on platelet reactivity were evaluated.

Methods.—There were 12 healthy control subjects and 8 patients scheduled for cardiopulmonary bypass. From each control subject, 24 mL of blood was drawn. From each patient, 10 mL of blood was drawn before and after cardiopulmonary bypass. Heparin was neutralized with heparinase or protamine, and platelet reactivity was analyzed by P-selectin expression after stimulating platelets with increasing concentrations of a thrombin receptor agonist peptide.

Results.—In the controls, heparinase 12.5 U/mL or protamine 32.5 µg/mL caused the activated coagulation times of heparinized samples to return to baseline values. In the patients, heparinase 20 U/mL or protamine 50 µg/mL caused the activated coagulation times of the samples to return to baseline values. There were no differences in expression of P-selectin in samples neutralized with heparinase. Samples neutralized with protamine had a marked decrease in P-selectin expression.

Discussion.—These findings show that, in vitro, heparinase and protamine were equally effective in neutralizing heparin anticoagulation, but that heparinase had a minimal effect on platelet reactivity. Protamine significantly inhibited platelet responsiveness. These findings need to be confirmed in prospective, clinical studies.

▶ The search continues for an alternative to protamine because of its well-recognized adverse effects: hypotension, pulmonary artery hypertension, vasodilation, decreased cardiac output, and antiplatelet effects.

M. Wood, M.D.

Pentoxifylline in Cardiopulmonary Bypass

Pentoxifylline Preloading Reduces Endothelial Injury and Permeability in Cardiopulmonary Bypass

Tsang GMK, Allen S, Pagano D, et al (Univ Hosp, Birmingham, England)

ASAIO J 42:M429–M434, 1996 4–46

Objective.—Systemic inflammatory responses in patients undergoing cardiopulmonary bypass (CPB) are thought to result in generalized vascular endothelial injury and can lead to end-organ failure. Because the methylxanthine derivative pentoxifylline (PTX) improves capillary blood flow, it may be beneficial in improving systemic vascular permeability. The effect of PTX on inflammatory mediator release, endothelial injury, and permeability measured by circulating levels of von Willibrand factor (vWf) and urinary albumin excretion was investigated in a double blind, prospective, randomized, placebo controlled, parallel study.

Methods.—Either 400 mg PTX (n = 20) or placebo (n = 20) was administered orally 3 times daily to 40 matched patients for 1 week prior to bypass surgery. All patients received CPB anesthetic and myocardial protection. Blood and urine samples were collected at baseline, 20 minutes after start of CPB; 5 minutes after removal of the aortic cross clamp; and 5 minutes, 2 hours, 6 hours, and 24 hours after termination of CPB. Levels of leukotriene B4 (LTB4), complement fragment C3a, interleukin 6 (IL6), vWf, and urinary albumin excretion to creatinine ratio (ACR) were measured.

Results.—In the placebo group, levels of C3a and LTB4 increased significantly during surgery. IL6 and vWf levels increased significantly, peaking at 6 hours after discontinuation of CPB. In the PTX treatment group, C3a, LTB4, and IL6 levels were similar to those of the placebo group. Baseline values of vWf and ACR and levels at 5 minutes and 6 hours after discontinuation of CPB were significantly lower in the PTX-treated group than in the placebo group.

Conclusion.—CPB triggers multiple inflammatory cascades, the effects of which are reduced in patients pretreated with PTX. PTX pretreatment does not appear to alter levels of circulating inflammatory mediators. Additional studies need to be conducted to determine the clinical relevance of these findings.

▶ Pentoxifylline is a methyl xanthine derivative that inhibits cellular phosphodiesterase activity, thereby increasing intracellular levels of cyclic adenosine monophosphate. It appears to decrease injury, both in this experimental model using patients and in other forms of vascular processes by decreasing leukocyte mediated endothelial injury and permeability. It appears that leukocyte mediated endothelial injury and permeability is a major factor in many forms of arterial "aging." We have recently learned that leukocyte affected arterial injury caused by periodontal disease increases the rate of myocardial injury and of stroke. Thus, the role of the "immune system" and infectious disease in arterial damage is highlighted by this article.

M.F. Roizen, M.D.

Nicardipine vs. Nitroprusside Deliberate Hypotension

Nicardipine Versus Nitroprusside for Controlled Hypotension During Spinal Surgery in Adolescents

Hersey SL, O'Dell NE, Lowe S, et al (Vanderbilt Univ, Nashville, Tenn; Univ of Missouri, Columbia)

Anesth Analg 84:1239–1244, 1997 4–47

Background.—Controlled hypotension during spinal fusion can decrease blood loss and improve surgical visibility. Nicardipine is a dihydropyridine calcium-channel antagonist that causes arterial vasodilation. It has limited chronotropic, dromotropic, and ionotropic effects. It has been used extensively to control hypertension, but its use for intraoperative controlled hypotension is limited.

Methods.—There were 20 consecutive adolescent patients with idiopathic scoliosis. Sodium nitroprusside or nicardipine was administered for controlled hypotension during spinal fusion. Standardized anesthesia was administered to all patients. A target mean arterial pressure of 60 mm Hg was achieved by varying the vasoactive infusion. Moderate hemodilution and blood salvage were used. Hemodynamic variables, blood loss, reflex tachycardia, and reversibility of the hypotensive state were compared.

Results.—There were significant differences in blood loss and reversibility of the hypotensive state between groups. Patients given nicardipine had less blood loss than those given nitroprusside. Patients given nicardipine had longer time to return of baseline mean arterial pressure. The amount of crystalloid administered and urine output were similar in both groups (Table 2). The incidence of reflex tachycardia was higher in patients given nitroprusside, but the difference was not statistically significant (Table 4).

TABLE 2.—Intraoperative Data

	Nitroprusside group (n = 10)	Nicardipine group (n = 10)
Operative time (hrs)	4.4 ± 0.18	4.4 ± 0.27
Urine output (cc/kg/hr)	1.9 ± 0.28	3.0 ± 0.58
Crystalloid (cc/kg/hr)	21.7 ± 3.9	16.6 ± 2.1
Levels fused	11 ± 0.5	9.5 ± 0.5
Estimated blood loss (cc)	1297.5 ± 264	761 ± 199*
Time to restoration of MBP	7.3 ± 1.1	26.8 ± 4.0†
Occurrence of reflex tachycardia	5/10	2/10

Note: Values are expressed as mean ± SEM.
*$P \leq 0.05$.
†$P \leq 0.002$.
(Courtesy of Hersey SL, O'Dell NE, Lowe S, et al: Nicardipine versus nitroprusside for controlled hypotension during spinal surgery in adolescents. *Anesth Analg* 84[6]:1239–1244, 1997.)

Both nitroprusside and nicardipine rapidly achieved stable, controlled hypotension and an acceptable operating field.

Summary.—Nicardipine is safe and effective for controlled hypotension in adolescents during spinal surgery. Nicardipine may also reduce blood loss. A gradual return to baseline mean arterial pressure occurred in these patients with nicardipine, but this did not cause any problems in clinical management.

▶ Often drugs are studied in adults, and then administered to children. It is salutary to see a prospective, randomized controlled study of nicardipine or sodium nitroprusside for the production of controlled hypotension.

M. Wood, M.D.

TABLE 4.—Reflex Tachycardia

Initial heart rate (bpm)	Nicardipine Maximum heart rate (bpm)	% change from baseline	Initial heart rate (bpm)	Nitroprusside Maximum heart rate (bpm)	% change from baseline
82	65	20	98	75	23
95	115*	21	95	120†	26
80	100*	31	100	120†	20
85	110*	29	60	110*	83
83	95	15	95	120†	26
70	90	29	90	120*	33
63	110†	75	100	125†	25
80	120†	50	95	75	21
90	80	11	95	110†	16
75	90	17	83	80	4

*Tachycardia less than 10 minutes, not treated with esmolol according to protocol.
†Tachycardia more than 10 minutes, treated with esmolol.
(Courtesy of Hersey SL, O'Dell NE, Lowe S, et al: Nicardipine versus nitroprusside for controlled hypotension during spinal surgery in adolescents. *Anesth Analg* 84[6]:1239–1244, 1997.)

Isoproterenol in Parturients

Hemodynamic Effects of Intravenous Isoproterenol Versus Saline in the Parturient

Marcus MAE, Vertommen JD, Van Aken H, et al (Westfälischen-Wilhelms Universität, Münster, Germany; Katholieke Universiteit, Leuven, Belgium)

Anesth Analg 84:1113–1116, 1997 4–48

Purpose.—There is debate concerning the ideal drug mixture to use in testing for proper placement of an epidural catheter in a laboring woman. Isoproterenol has been proposed as an alternative to epinephrine, but little is known about its effects on the uterine blood flow (UBF) and umbilical blood flow (UMB). A randomized, double-blind, placebo-controlled trial was performed to study the circulatory effects of IV isoproterenol in nonlaboring pregnant women.

Methods.—The study included 60 women at term but not in labor. They were randomly allocated to receive IV injection of either isoproterenol or saline, 5 µg. All subjects underwent assessment of hemodynamic variables for 5 minutes before and 10 minutes after injection. In addition, color Doppler US was used to assess UBF in 35 patients and UMB in 25. Fifty subjects underwent continuous measurement of maternal heart rate (MHR) and every-minute measurement of mean arterial pressure.

Results.—Whereas saline injection produced no change in MHR, a significant increase occurred after isoproterenol injection. Isoproterenol was also associated with a significant increase in UBF but no change in UMB. The other hemodynamic variables studied did not differ in their response to isoproterenol vs. placebo.

Conclusions.—Intravenous injection of isoproterenol, 5 µg, increases MHR and UBF in pregnant women at term. This may serve as a useful test dose of epidural analgesia in obstetric patients. A study comparing isoproterenol with epinephrine as an IV test dose is required.

▶ The first sentence of the abstract published with this article states the following: "The use of epinephrine as a test dose for epidural analgesia in obstetrics remains controversial." Perhaps controversy existed several years ago (and I confess that I contributed to that controversy), but in my judgment, little controversy exists today. To my knowledge, there is no published report of adverse outcome as a result of the use of 15 µg of epinephrine as an epidural test dose in obstetric patients. In the present study, the authors correctly noted that "the epidural use of isoproterenol is prohibited because no data exist concerning possible neurotoxic side effects."

D.H. Chestnut, M.D.

Sufentanil in Labor

Determination of the Dose-Response Relationship for Intrathecal Sufentanil in Laboring Patients

Herman NL, Calicott R, Van Decar TK, et al (Wilford Hall Med Ctr, Lackland Air Force Base, Texas; New York Hosp, New York; 48th Med Operations Squadron, Royal Air Force Lakenheath, England)

Anesth Analg 84:1256–1261, 1997 4–49

Background.—Sufentanil and other intrathecal opioids are effective and popular analgesics for women in labor. Studies to determine the relative efficacy of various drugs require the use of equipotent doses. However, there are few data on the dose-response relationships in laboring women. The dose-response relationship of intrathecal sufentanil was studied in women in early labor.

Methods.—The study included 60 women in active labor. All received intrathecal sufentanil; the dose given, to groups of 10 patients each, was 2.5, 5.0, 7.5, 10.0, 12.5, or 15.0 µg. At intervals from 0 to 30 minutes, pain scores, fetal heart rate, blood pressure, and heart rate were measured. The measurements were repeated when the patient requested additional analgesia. The analgesia was considered successful if it achieved an absolute visual analogue scale score of 25 mm or less. The data were used to

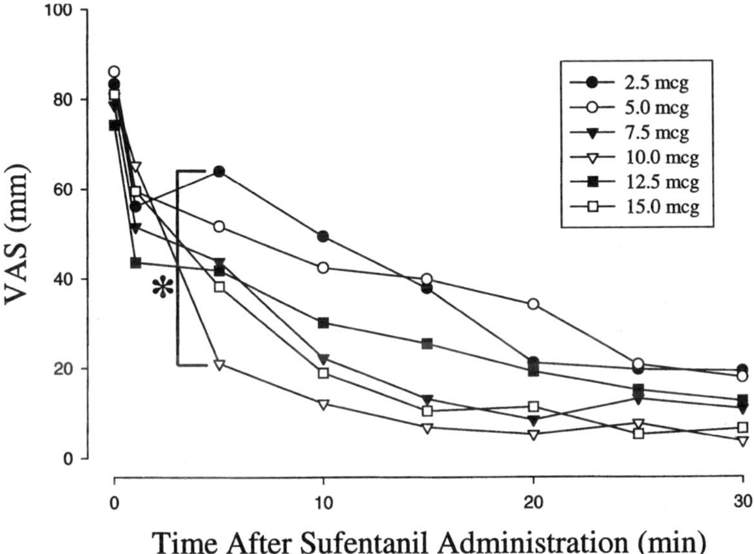

FIGURE 1.—Graph of the changes in visual analogue scale pain scores over time after injection of sufentanil for the 6 different dose groups. Each data point represents $n = 10$. The error bars were large and have been removed to reduce confusion. There was a significant difference between the 2.5 and 10.0 µg groups at 5 minutes; otherwise, there was no significant intergroup differences in visual analogue scores. $*P \leq 0.05$. (Courtesy of Herman NL, Calicott R, Van Decar TK, et al: Determination of the dose-response relationship for intrathecal sufentanil in laboring patients. *Anesth Analg* 84[6]:1256–1261, 1997.)

construct a dose-response curve and to calculate the 50% and 95% effective doses (ED_{50} and ED_{95}).

Results.—Changes in pain scores over time after administration of sufentanil occurred along a family of exponential curves (Fig 1). Intrathecal sufentanil had an ED_{50} of 2.6 μg and an ED^{95} of 8.9 μg. The duration of analgesia tended to increase with increasing dose of sufentanil. There were no differences in side effects among the various groups—pruritus was very common. None of the patients had any apparent change in fetal heart rate, and there was no significant difference in the rates of assisted delivery or cesarean section.

Conclusions.—This dose-response study finds that intrathecal sufentanil provides a rapid onset of analgesia for laboring women. The study sets values for ED_{50} and ED_{95}, which should be helpful in the clinical use of intrathecal sufentanil and for future studies comparing sufentanil with other intrathecal analgesics. The data permit no conclusions about sufentanil's effects on obstetric course and fetal outcome.

▶ In the present study, there was a remarkably wide spread between the ED_{50} (2.6 μg) and the ED_{95} (8.9 μg) for intrathecal sufentanil in laboring women. Knowledge of the ED_{95} is most useful for clinical practice, given the fact that 50% is an unacceptable rate of success when providing analgesia for laboring women. The present study provides support for selecting 10 μg as the dose when giving sufentanil intrathecally in laboring women.

D.H. Chestnut, M.D.

Adenosine-induced Arrhythmia

Adenosine-induced Atrial Arrhythmia: A Prospective Analysis
Strickberger SA, Man KC, Daoud EG, et al (Univ of Michigan, Ann Arbor)
Ann Intern Med 127:417–422, 1997 4–50

Background.—Adenosine has proven to be a safe and effective treatment for paroxysmal supraventricular tachycardia (PSVT). Clinical experience with the compound has suggested that it may induce atrial fibrillation and flutter; however, the existence and frequency of these arrhythmias have not been rigorously explored. The frequency of atrial arrhythmias induced by adenosine, in the treatment of PSVT, was evaluated prospectively.

Methods.—Electrophysiologic evaluation was performed on 200 patients with PSVT to determine the mechanism of the arrhythmia, and 12 mg of adenosine was administered as an intravenous bolus to each patient. Patients were observed for termination of tachycardia and occurrence of additional atrial or ventricular arrhythmias.

Results.—Adenosine administration terminated PSVT in 198 patients (99%), and induced atrial fibrillation in 24 patients (12%), of whom 2 also had atrial flutter. Induced atrial arrhythmias began a mean of 6.3 seconds after PSVT termination and were preceded by atrial premature complexes in 100% of patients who had atrial fibrillation and/or flutter, compared with 58% of patients who did not have induced atrial arrhythmias. Atrial fibrillation or flutter was accompanied by atrioventricular block in 20 patients and a prolonged PR interval in the remaining 4. Pre-excited atrial arrhythmias occurred in 6 patients with accessory pathways capable of anterograde conduction, and 1 patient with atrial fibrillation also had pre-excited atrial flutter. Spontaneous resolution to sinus rhythm occurred in 16 patients, with cardioversion required in 8 patients. Gender, age, cycle length of PSVT, isoproterenol use in PSVT initiation, length of the atrioventricular block cycle, or the RR interval preceding atrial fibrillation were not predictive of induced atrial arrhythmia.

Conclusions.—The intravenous administration of 12 mg of adenosine for termination of PSVT is associated with a 12% incidence of atrial fibrillation. Because PSVT termination was attempted during an electrophysiologic procedure involving a right atrial catheter, the results may not be applicable to patients with PSVT who are treated with adenosine in other clinical settings. Nevertheless, in situations in which the mechanism of PSVT is unknown and Wolff-Parkinson-White syndrome has not been ruled out, adenosine administration should be performed only in settings in which resuscitation equipment is readily available, because of the potential for a rapid, pre-excited ventricular response during atrial fibrillation.

► Adenosine has become a common treatment for PSVT. This article highlights a new finding, namely, that the drug can cause atrial fibrillation. Thus, it should be administered in an area where appropriate equipment is available to treat such arrhythmias.

M. Wood, M.D.

Opiate Detoxification Using Anesthesia

Opiate Detoxification Under Anaesthesia: Enthusiasm Must Be Tempered With Caution and Scientific Scrutiny

Strang J, Bearn J, Gossop M (Maudsley Inst of Psychiatry, London)

BMJ 315:1249–1250, 1997 4–51

Introduction.—A new detoxification treatment for opiate misusers involves provocation of withdrawal by opiate antagonists administered with a general anesthetic. The combination of antagonist provocation with the use of general anesthetic has been deemed controversial, and it is expensive. There is a lack of information on the technique, and the clear-cut benefits that offset its inherent dangers have not been sufficiently proven. The hazards include prolonged general anesthesia and the side effects that result from the pharmacologic bombardment with an opiate antagonist.

History.—This procedure dates back a century to attempts to achieve painless detoxification. The anesthetic provides a means to bypass the distress of withdrawal. To achieve more rapid detoxication, naloxone was used since the early 1970s for an antagonist-precipitated rapid detoxification. During the 1980s, a combination of clonidine and naltrexone was begun, and then in the late 1980s, general anesthesia was introduced to cover the use of naloxone to precipitate detoxification.

Advantages.—Opiate misusers fear detoxification, and this technique helps them avoid the acute withdrawal discomfort and the fatigue, dysthymia, and poor sleep. Better completion rates have also been seen with this procedure. Improved long-term abstinence rates were also seen, but this may result from selection bias, with willing patients paying for the treatment. This procedure has, however, resulted in life-threatening atypical reactions and death, which may be more likely among patients with concurrent dependence on alcohol or benzodiazepines, and among patients with liver disease.

Conclusions.—Until reliable data from controlled studies are available, this technique should not be widely used. Rigorous studies of the benefits and hazards of this technique must be conducted.

▶ I selected this editorial because ultrarapid opiate detoxification during general anesthesia is presently being carried out in special centers, although controversy exists regarding efficacy and safety. Anesthesia-assisted detoxification requires controlled randomized clinical trials with careful statistical analysis on an urgent basis.

M. Wood, M.D.

Halothane in Asthma

Halothane Treatment of Severe Asthma to Avoid Mechanical Ventilation

Padkin AJ, Baigel G, Morgan GA (Royal Cornwall Hosp, Truro, England)
Anaesthesia 52:994–997, 1997 4–52

Background.—In many instances, tracheal intubation and mechanical ventilation are used to treat an acute exacerbation in patients with severe asthma. In this case report, however, both of these measures were avoided by the administration of halothane in 100% oxygen via a face mask.

Case Report.—Woman, 41, with chronic asthma was seen with increasing breathlessness, productive cough, and wheezing. She had been taking terbutaline, ipratropium bromide, salbutamol, and prednisone to control her asthma. At presentation, she was treated with hydrocortisone, aminophylline, terbutaline, antibiotics, and ipratropium bromide, but symptoms were not controlled and she became increasingly exhausted. After the patient was transferred to the ICU, a trial of a subanesthetic dose of 0.5% halothane was administered in 100% oxygen through a close-fitting face mask. Dramatic improvement was seen within 15 minutes of halothane dosing. Pulsus paradoxus improved from 36 to 10 mm Hg, the respiratory rate decreased from 24 to 18 breaths/min, and pulse rate and arterial blood pressure also decreased. Halothane was stopped after 15 minutes, at which point the patient's condition deteriorated. Halothane was reinstituted (at a concentration of 0.2%) and was continued for 4 hours. No complications occurred, and she made a full recovery.

Conclusion.—Halothane caused immediate improvement in respiratory and blood pressure parameters in this patient with acute severe asthma. These effects were seen without any cardiac disturbances, which are reported at halothane concentrations of 1% or greater. Furthermore, the risks of halothane-induced hepatotoxicity (1/25,000) and fulminant malignant hyperthermia (1/175,000) are more than offset by the risks involved with tracheal intubation and mechanical ventilation. Thus, a trial of 0.5% halothane in 100% oxygen via a face-mask should be considered in patients with an acute exacerbation of asthma. However, intubation and ventilation materials should be at hand, just in case they are needed.

► We have long known that halothane is a bronchodilator. Pulmonologists have not been particularly interested; we are insular to a large extent. People just do not feel comfortable with treating patients with "someone else's" drug. Here is a classic example. This patient's bronchospasm resolved "within 15 minutes." Further, after only 1 exacerbation, her bronchospasm did not return during that admission, and she was discharged with a successful outcome. Once again, this is something we anesthesiologists know about, yet we do not use it very often.

J.H. Tinker, M.D.

Platelet Concentrates

Effects of Storage Time on Quantitative and Qualitative Platelet Function After Transfusion

Rosenfeld BA, Herfel B, Faraday N, et al (Johns Hopkins Med Insts, Baltimore, Md)

Anesthesiology 83:1167–1172, 1995 4–53

Objective.—Platelet transfusions are routinely administered to patients with thrombocytopenia before invasive procedures or surgery. However, it is unclear when optimal hemostatic function is achieved. Although reaction mechanisms and energy sources are adversely affected in stored platelets, the time course for platelet recovery of maximal effectiveness has not been well studied. The temporal relationship between platelet number and function after transfusion for 1- and 4-day stored platelets was studied.

Methods.—A total of 25 patients (7 women) with thrombocytopenia as a result of chemotherapy received either 1-day or 4-day stored platelets from single donors over 60 minutes via indwelling central venous catheters. Patients receiving previous platelet transfusions were excluded. Platelet count was measured from whole blood drawn before, after, and at 1, 2, and 24 hours. Platelet function was assessed, and reactivity was determined using agonist-induced platelet aggregation and dense granule secretion.

Results.—Platelet counts for 1- and 4-day platelet groups were increased immediately by 55,000/mm^3 and 45,000/mm^3, respectively, were stable for 2 hours and then decreased by 20% and 27%, respectively. Immediately after transfusion and for 2 hours afterward, agonist-induced platelet aggregation data in both groups showed an increase in 5- and 10-μg collagen-induced and ristocetin-induced aggregation. Agonist-induced dense release data showed an increase in collagen-induced adenosine triphosphate release immediately after transfusion in both groups. The concomitant ristocetin-induced dense granule release was increased after transfusion only in the 1-day platelet group and was maintained for 2 hours. Dense granule release and ristocetin-induced stimulation were increased in 1-day platelets compared to 4-day platelets.

Conclusion.—In patients with thrombocytopenia as a result of chemotherapy, platelet transfusion immediately causes increases in number and function that persist for 2 hours. Because fresh platelets show increased dense granule release and aggregation compared to 4-day platelets, fresh platelets may improve hemostatic function.

► This study by Rosenfeld and colleagues from Hopkins may well prove to be a classic study on quantitative and qualitative function after transfusion. It is clear to me that perhaps we need another test to demonstrate effectiveness, rather than the in vitro tests that were done, but what test that is, is unclear to me.

M.F. Roizen, M.D.

Phenylephrine During Cardiopulmonary Bypass

Regional Perfusion Abnormalities With Phenylephrine During Normothermic Bypass

O'Dwyer C, Woodson LC, Conroy BP, et al (Univ of Texas, Galveston)

Ann Thorac Surg 63:728–735, 1997 4–54

Objective.—Splanchnic organ dysfunction continues to be a problem after cardiopulmonary bypass (CPB). Two factors that may play a role in splanchnic ischemia are hypotension and vasopressors. An experimental model of CPB was used to assess the effects of restoring aortic pressure—by either increasing pump flow or infusing phenylephrine—on visceral, organ, brain, and femoral muscle perfusion.

Methods.—Normothermic CPB was established in 12 anesthetized pigs. Initial measurements were obtained, including assessment of regional blood flow using radioactive spheres. Pump flow was then decreased to reduce aortic pressure to 40 mm Hg for 20 minutes. Aortic pressure then was raised to 65 mm Hg by 2 interventions performed in random order: increasing the pump flow rate and infusing dilute phenylephrine. The effects of restored aortic pressure on regional perfusion of the cerebral cortex, kidneys, splanchnic organs, and skeletal muscle were assessed. The study sought to determine which of these vascular beds were constricted by phenylephrine as perfusion pressure increased.

Results.—Visceral organ and femoral muscle perfusion dropped significantly at an aortic pressure of 40 mm Hg, but brain perfusion was unaffected. When pump flow was increased, perfusion of the pancreas, colon, and kidneys increased significantly. Aortic pressure increased in response to phenylephrine infusion, but splanchnic perfusion was unchanged. As a result, there were significant perfusion differences between pump flow and phenylephrine intervals. Gastrointestinal structures particularly sensitive to changes in pump flow rate, perfusion pressure, and phenylephrine infusion were the gastric mucosa and pancreas. A direct correlation was noted between renal cortical blood flow and pump-flow–regulated perfusion pressure, but not as regulated by phenylephrine infusion.

Conclusions.—Use of phenylephrine rather than increased pump flow to increase systemic pressure during CPB, produces significantly lower splanchnic blood flow values. The results suggest that giving vasoconstrictors during normothermic CPB may lead to substantial but hidden hypoperfusion of splanchnic organs, even though perfusion pressure has been restored. The cerebral circulation is little affected by perfusion pressure in the range studied, independent of pump flow or phenylephrine infusion.

► I have stated many times that my residents in the heart room could use phenylephrine only if they could get the syringe out from under my foot (and there's a lot of weight on that foot, as many of you know). This article indicates substantial underperfusion of various organs when one artificially raises arterial pressure with an α-agonist squeezer like phenylephrine. Certainly there is no surprise here, but this study is well done in animals and quantitates the problem nicely.

J.H. Tinker, M.D.

Steroids for Airway Edema

Upper Airway Edema After Carotid Endarterectomy: The Effect of Steroid Administration

Hughes R, McGuire G, Montanera W, et al (The Toronto Hosp, Western Division)

Anesth Analg 84:475–478, 1997 4–55

Objective.—Upper airway obstruction after carotid endarterectomy (CEA) is a rare but potentially fatal complication. Steroids have been shown to be beneficial in reducing edema and inflammatory response after maxillofacial surgery. The effectiveness of administration of a single bolus dose of steroid, given at induction of anesthesia, on the degree and site of postoperative airway edema associated with CEA was investigated in a randomized, double blind, controlled trial.

Methods.—Of 37 patients (7 females) undergoing elective CEA, 17 received 16 mg dexamethasone and 21 received saline placebo intravenously prior to induction of anesthesia. A CT of the neck was performed on all patients preoperatively and on postoperative day 1. Any edema present was categorized as unilateral, unilateral and retropharyngeal, or bilateral.

Results.—Although edema occurred postoperative, there was no significant difference in upper airway dimensions between groups.

Conclusion.—Steroids administered prior to anesthesia do not reduce edema in the upper airway for CEA patients.

▶ This randomized controlled study approaches a problem logically. In fact, one of my favorite anecdotes that I tell all patients preoperatively who are having thyroid surgery or carotid surgery (for which I am providing anesthesia) is that they will complain of a terribly sore neck afterwards, but it will be the surgeon's fingers and not my endotracheal tube that causes the problem. In any case, like the thyroid surgeons, these vascular surgeons found that there was no relationship between steroids and neck swelling. I believe that the major cause of this neck swelling is the lack of gentleness of the surgeon in handling tissues, and although conticosteroids reduce edema by decreasing capillary endothelium permeability, I believe that the disruption that the surgeon's hands cause when they are not as gentle as the ones I am fortunate to work with are, works by a different mechanism than that which steroids are able to prevent.

One can obviously say that there might be a problem in this study in that a CT scan was used to judge swelling and that this was done early on postoperative day 1. In the defense of this study's protocol, 1 day or earlier is when one is most concerned with airway edema, and thus this appears to be an appropriately designed protocol for the clinical event.

M.F. Roizen, M.D.

Hetastarch vs. Gelatin Colloids

Use of Modified Fluid Gelatin and Hydroxyethyl Starch for Colloidal Volume Replacement in Major Orthopaedic Surgery

Beyer R, Harmening U, Rittmeyer O, et al (Georg-August-Univ of Göttingen, Germany)

Br J Anaesth 78:44–50, 1997 4–56

Objective.—Synthetic colloids, such as dextran, gelatin, and hydroxyethyl starch (HES), are used to stabilize plasma oncotic pressure during blood loss. Few clinical studies have compared the efficiency of these products. Results of a prospective, randomized trial to compare the hemodynamic stabilization comparing the use of 3% modified fluid gelatin (MFG) and 6% hydroxyethyl starch (HES) in the perioperative period during major orthopedic procedures. The effects on fluid balance, transfusion of blood products, blood clotting, plasma oncotic function, renal function, and other laboratory variables were also tested.

Methods.—Hemodynamic variables and fluid input and output were monitored during and after major orthopedic hip surgery in 41 patients, age 21–80. HES was used for volume replacement in 19 patients and MFG in 22.

Results.—Total calcium concentration was significantly higher in the MFG group than in the HES group from 2 hours intraoperative to 12 hours postoperative. Total protein was significantly higher in the MFG group from the end of the operation to 6 hours postoperative. α-Amylase levels were significantly higher in the MFG group from the end of the operation to 24 hours postoperative. There were no significant differences in any other variables. Average colloid volumes infused during surgery and for 24 hours thereafter were 2,500 mL for the HES group and 2,400 for the MFG group.

Conclusion.—Similar volumes of HES and MFG were required to achieve hemodynamic stabilization in patients undergoing major orthopedic surgery. Laboratory and hemodynamic variables were similar for both groups.

► This is a first of a series of studies that I expect to see comparing the modified fluid gelatins with hydroxyethyl starches for use in fluid replacement. While there are limited indications for such colloidal fluid supporting agents, this article looked at a wide range of both physiologic and laboratory findings up to 24 hours following surgery and found no major differences between the two groups. Interestingly in this practice (and I don't know whether it was intended to find a practice where there was a lot of blood loss or not), the blood loss is considerably more than we would expect to experience in the United States during similar surgery in a similar patient population.

M.F. Roizen, M.D.

Oral Methylnaltrexone

The Safety and Efficacy of Oral Methylnaltrexone in Preventing Morphine-induced Delay in Oral-Cecal Transit Time

Yaun C-S, Foss JF, Osinski J, et al (Univ of Chicago)

Clin Pharmacol Ther 61:467–475, 1997 4–57

Background.—Methylnaltrexone, a quaternary opioid antagonist with limited ability to cross the blood-brain barrier, may antagonize the peripherally mediated GI effects of opioids. Volunteer studies have shown that IV methylnaltrexone prevents morphine-induced changes in GI motility and transit without affecting analgesia. The safety, tolerance, and efficacy of oral methylnaltrexone on morphine-induced changes in GI motility and transit in healthy volunteers were reported.

Methods.—In phase A of the study, 14 healthy persons received 3 ascending oral doses of methylnaltrexone. In phase B, the subjects were given oral placebo and IV placebo in a single-blind fashion, followed by oral placebo and IV morphine, 0.05 mg/kg, or oral methylnaltrexone, 19.2 mg/kg, and IV morphine, 0.05 mg/kg, in a randomized, double-blind fashion.

Findings.—Morphine significantly increased oral-cecal transit time from a mean 114.6–158.6 minutes. Morphine-induced increases in oral-cecal transit time were completely prevented by oral methylnaltrexone. Single-blind assessments of descending doses of methylnaltrexone showed that 6.4 mg/kg oral methylnaltrexone significantly attenuated the morphine-induced delay in oral-cecal transit time. A dose-dependent response was obtained. Oral methylnaltrexone effects on transit time were unassociated with drug plasma concentrations, suggesting direct preferential luminal effects of oral methylnaltrexone.

Conclusions.—Oral methylnaltrexone reverses morphine-induced changes in gut motility in healthy persons in a dose-related manner. This effect may be through direct local luminal action of the compound.

▶ Constipation is a major drawback to both acute and chronic opioid administration. Reduced GI transit time caused by opioid analgesics is a major cause for delays in postoperative feeding and the consequent nutritional deficits. While tolerance develops to other opioid side effects, such as sedation and respiratory depression, there appears to be little reduction in GI motility effects over time. The development of drugs that reverse the peripheral effects of opioids while preserving analgesia should have substantial benefits. It is not clear whether other opioid side effects such as urinary retention or pruritis are affected. Intrathecal morphine produces some reduction in GI motility that is unrelated to direct opioid effects on receptors in the GI tract. It remains to be determined whether methylnaltrexone will restore normal transit time in that situation.

S.E. Abram, M.D.

Lorazepam in Cardiac Premedication

Comparison of Lorazepam Alone vs Lorazepam, Morphine, and Perphenazine for Cardiac Premedication

Saccaomanno PM, Kavanagh BP, Cheng DCH, et al (Univ of Toronto)

Can J Anaesth 44:146–153, 1997 4–58

Objective.—Anxiety may contribute hemodynamic changes that increase the risk of myocardial ischemia after coronary artery bypass grafting (CABG). Therefore, standard perioperative procedure at the University of Toronto includes administration of a benzodiazepine, an opioid, and an antiemetic-sedative combination. Because the cardiorespiratory and hemodynamic effects of this regimen are not known, a prospective, randomized, double blind trial was conducted to compare the effects of lorazepam alone versus lorazepam, morphine, and perphenazine on cardiorespiratory variables, sedation, and anxiety in patients prior to CABG.

Methods.—Group 1 patients (n = 38, 12 female) received 0.03 mg/kg lorazepam *sl*, 0.15 mg/kg morphine IM, and 0.05 mg/kg perphenazine IM, and Group 2 patients (n = 28, 2 female) received 0.03 mg/kg lorazepam *s* and 1.5 mL saline IM. Patients were monitored for 1.5 hours before receiving medication and for 2 hours afterward. Arterial hemoglobin saturation, respiration, arterial blood gases, heart rate, and blood pressure, and anxiety and sedation scores were recorded. Medical histories and demographic data were collected. Myocardial ischemia was defined as a greater than 1-mm depression of the ST segment for more than 60 seconds when recorded using a continuous 12-lead ECG real time monitor.

Results.—Sixteen patients had episodes of myocardial ischemia. The number and duration of episodes for both groups was similar. When compared with baseline values, Group 1 patients had significant decreases in pH of arterial blood gases that lasted longer, significant increases in $PaCO_2$, significant decreases in PaO_2, and significantly more hemodynamic events after premedication than did Group 2 patients. After premedication, anxiety scores were low and similar in both groups. Both groups also had higher sedation scores, although Group 1 patients receiving morphine had significantly higher sedation scores than did Group 2 patients.

Conclusion.—Lorazepam alone is an effective premedication for reducing anxiety and producing sedation in patients undergoing CABG. Addition of perphenazine and morphine increases $PaCO_2$, lowers PaO_2, and results in more hemodynamic events that increase the risk of ischemic events.

▶ The authors' likely bias was to do away with premedication for cardiac surgery at least with the old "heavy" premedicants; morphine, perphenazine, and other kinds of "lytic cocktails." Lorazepam itself is a fascinating substance. I selected this paper so that I could comment on my perceptions of Lorazepam. Although it doesn't really produce antigrade amnesia, it seems to have a remarkable ability to blot out perioperative events. I don't think we quite understand why this is so other than its pharmacokinetics (which may or may not be an adequate explanation). With today's "fast tracking," I wonder if lorazepam will continue to fit the picture for cardiac anesthesia.

J.H. Tinker, M.D.

Spinal vs. Epidural Fentanyl on Gastric Emptying in Parturients

A Comparison of the Effect of Intrathecal and Extradural Fentanyl on Gastric Emptying in Laboring Women

Kelly MC, Carabine UA, Hill DA, et al (Queen's Univ of Belfast, Northern Ireland; Royal Group Hosps Trust, Belfast, Northern Ireland)

Anesth Analg 85:834–838, 1997 4–59

Background.—Nausea, vomiting, and delayed gastric emptying are associated with extradural opioid use during labor. These side effects have prompted an interest in the intrathecal administration of opioids, which also provide excellent analgesia. But what are the effects of intrathecal opioids on gastric emptying? These investigators compared gastric emptying after extradural and intrathecal opioids in women during labor.

Methods.—One hundred five women were split into 3 groups of 35 patients each. Group S received intrathecal fentanyl, 25 µg plus bupivacaine; group E received extradural fentanyl, 50 µg plus bupivacaine; and group C received extradural bupivacaine only. All patients received oral ranitidine every 6 hours to prevent gastrointestinal side effects, and additional anesthetic was allowed as needed. A 100-point visual analogue scale was used to assess pain at baseline and at regular intervals thereafter. Oral acetaminophen, 1.5 gm, was taken 15 minutes after the injection, and blood levels were measured from a separate heparinized cannula at baseline and at regular intervals thereafter.

Findings.—Pain scores did not consistently or significantly differ between any of the 3 groups up to 3 hours after drug dosing. Patients in group C required more top-up bupivacaine (mean, 15 mg) than those in group E (mean, 12 mg) and group S (mean, 10 mg, a significant difference compared with group C). The times to reach maximal plasma acetaminophen concentrations were 83, 90, and 120 minutes in groups E, C, and S, respectively (group E was significantly different from group S). Furthermore, the actual plasma acetaminophen concentrations achieved in group S were lower than those in group C and group E (13, 15, and 18 µg/mL, respectively, with group E significantly different from group S). The acetaminophen areas under the curve at 90 and 120 minutes were significantly lower in group S (430 and 649 µg/mL/min, respectively) than in group C (672 and 1,053 µg/mL/min, respectively) and group E (736 and 1,062 µg/mL/min, respectively).

Conclusion.—Gastric emptying of acetaminophen was significantly slower in patients receiving intrathecal fentanyl plus bupivacaine than in patients receiving bupivacaine with and without fentanyl. Thus, although intrathecal fentanyl plus bupivacaine provided the best pain relief, it also had the most substantial effect on delayed gastric emptying. Because delayed gastric emptying may lead to vomiting, this effect is particularly important when general anesthesia is considered for patients in labor.

► When I was a resident 20 years ago, we often argued that epidural analgesia allowed obstetric anesthesiologists to provide pain relief without the adverse effects of systemic opioids (e.g., sedation and delayed gastric emptying). It is ironic that contemporary methods of epidural and spinal opioid analgesia may delay gastric emptying in laboring women. It seems intuitive that epidural administration of fentanyl might delay gastric emptying, because of the rapid systemic absorption of fentanyl when administered by the epidural route. However, published studies have provided conflicting results regarding the effects of epidural opioids on gastric emptying during labor. In reading this study, I was surprised that intrathecal administration of bupivacaine and fentanyl delayed gastric emptying, when compared with epidural administration of bupivacaine, with or without fentanyl. The authors suggested several possible mechanisms for this observation, including the cephalad spread of fentanyl in the subarachnoid space.

D.H. Chestnut, M.D.

5 Anesthesia Techniques and Monitors

"Bispectral" Electroencephalogram Analysis

A Multicenter Study of Bispectral Electroencephalogram Analysis for Monitoring Anesthetic Effect

Sebel PS, Lang E, Rampil IJ, et al (Emory Univ, Atlanta, Ga; Univ of California, San Francisco; Univ of Texas, Dallas; et al)

Anesth Analg 84:891–899, 1997 5–1

Objective.—There are no standards for assessing anesthetic adequacy. Bispectral (BIS) analysis of EEG is a pharmacodynamic measure of anesthetic effects on the central nervous system. The use of BIS as a real-time guide to anesthetic dosing under clinically relevant conditions was examined prospectively in a multicenter study using movement at incision as the primary indicator of inadequate anesthesia.

Methods.—A total of 300 BIS-monitored patients were randomly allocated to receive anesthetic designed to give an approximately 50% movement response rate to skin incision with no action taken by the anesthesiologist (control group) or with the anesthetic concentration altered to decrease BIS to less then 60 (treatment group). EEGs were recorded continuously. Pharmacodynamic drug profiles were calculated retrospectively using STANPUMP software.

Results.—BIS values were lower in the treatment group than in the control group and were significantly lower in the treatment group that used isoflurane with opioids. The movement response rate to incision was significantly less in the treatment group than in the control group (43% vs. 13%). The movement response rate was dampened at sites using opioids. BIS, opioid use, and heart rate were predictors of movement response at skin incision.

Conclusion.—Lowering BIS by increasing anesthesia decreases the movement response rate to incision. Addition of opioids decreases the movement response rate and BIS is no longer a significant predictor of movement response to incision. The use of opioids appears to create a confounding effect with respect to the use of BIS as a measure of anesthetic adequacy.

▶ I have included several papers on bispectral analysis of the EEG in this year's YEAR BOOK because it represents a fascinating new possibility that we might be able to quantify and monitor "level of consciousness." Early reports on bispectral analysis are very enthusiastic. Following the natural course of "Tinker's Law," namely, "beware of enthusiastic early reports," this report is considerably more cautionary. The authors find that conjunctive use of opiates (near universal these days), seems to foul up the bispectral analysis to some extent. Nonetheless, I applaud any and all efforts in this arena to try to get a handle on anesthetic adequacy or "depth." (I like the term "adequacy.")

J.H. Tinker, M.D.

Titration of Volatile Anesthetics Using Bispectral Index Facilitates Recovery After Ambulatory Anesthesia

Song D, Joshi GP, White PF (Univ of Texas, Dallas)

Anesthesiology 87:842–848, 1997 5–2

Objective.—The bispectral (BIS) index is a quantitative measure of the sedative and hypnotic effects of anesthetics. Using a target BIS value to titrate volatile anesthetics may result in more rapid emergence in outpatients receiving desflurane or sevoflurane with nitrous oxide for maintenance of general anesthesia. In a prospective, randomized, controlled study, the effect of BIS monitoring on the utilization of volatile anesthetics and intraoperative hemodynamics and recovery profiles after outpatient surgery was assessed.

Methods.—Sixty women undergoing tubal ligation were randomly allocated to receive 2% to 5% desflurane (groups I and II) or 0.7% to 2% sevoflurane (groups III and IV). Groups II and IV were BIS-titrated to maintain a BIS index of 60. All groups also received nitrous oxide, 1 L/min (65%), in oxygen, 0.7 L/min, and fentanyl, 1 1μg/kg IV. Verbal response, orientation, and home-readiness were assessed at 1-minute and then at 15-minute intervals from discontinuation of anesthetics to discharge.

Results.—After induction of anesthesia with propofol, mean arterial pressure (MAP) decreased by an average of 37% and BIS index values decreased from an average of 97–37. After incision, MAP values increased significantly in all 4 groups, whereas BIS index values were significantly lower in control groups I (44) and III (42) compared with the BIS-titrated groups II (60) and IV (62). During the maintenance period, end-tidal concentrations of anesthesias were significantly lower in BIS-titrated groups I and III compared to control groups II and IV (2.3 vs. 4.2 and 0.9 vs. 1.8, respectively). Dosage requirements for anesthetic drugs were significantly lower in the BIS-titrated groups than for either desflurane (17.3 vs. 25.0 mL) or sevoflurane (8.5 vs. 13.8 mL). Compared to the control groups, verbal responsiveness (min) times were significantly shorter in the BIS-titrated desflurane group (2.8 vs. 6) and in the BIS-titrated sevoflurane (5.0 vs. 7.6).

Conclusion.—Titrating volatile anesthetics to target BIS value uses less anesthetic and results in shorter recovery times in outpatients.

► This is one of many articles recently presented in which the new "bispectral index" monitor is touted as increasing our ability to "titrate" volatile anesthetic administration. The fact that we tend to give relative overdoses of anesthetics is nothing new. Although the caregivers here were blinded to the BIS value in the control groups, they were not blinded to the fact that a study using BIS was going on. Response bias here is likely, namely, any bias in the direction of finding something positive would obviously be in the direction of efficacy for the black box. Therefore, the bias in this study, incredibly difficult to eliminate, is toward the "heavy" side in the control group of patients. Because the other group was being anesthetized by actually watching the numbers on the box, with resultant presumed minimal effective anesthesia, it is hard to argue with my criticism that response bias may have been allowed to creep into this study. As I have said many times before in these pages, "beware of enthusiastic, positive, early results, especially when sponsored at least in part by the company that has invented the drug or equipment." Only time will tell about the usefulness of this new device, and whether in practice it will really result in this large a difference in anesthetic use. Also, if this minimal anesthetic results in more (expensive) neuromuscular blocker use, then perhaps the "cost savings" pitch will prove illusory.

J.H. Tinker, M.D.

Bispectral Analysis Measures Sedation and Memory Effects of Propofol, Midazolam, Isoflurane, and Alfentanil in Healthy Volunteers

Glass PS, Bloom M, Kearse L, et al (Duke Univ, Durham, NC; Univ of Pittsburgh, Pa; Harvard Univ, Boston; et al)

Anesthesiology 86:836–847, 1997 5–3

Background.—Measuring the depth of general anesthesia has been a goal ever since the introduction of drugs that render patients unconscious. The electroencephalogram (EEG) has been extensively evaluated as a tool for measuring anesthetic effect, but research has been hindered by a lack of understanding of the effects of anesthetic drug interactions on the EEG, a lack of agreement on EEG parameters, and the lack of a gold standard of drug effect for comparison. The bispectral index is a value derived from the EEG that may be related to the hypnotic component of the anesthetic state.

Methods.—In a prospective study, 70 healthy volunteers at 4 institutions were given a dose-ranging sequence of isoflurane, midazolam, propofol, or alfentanil to achieve target concentrations. The effects of the drugs on bispectral index score, level of sedation by the observer's assessment of the alertness/sedation scale, and picture/word recall were recorded. Arterial blood samples were drawn and analyzed for drug concentration.

Results.—There was a significantly better correlation between bispectral index score and responsiveness score than between measured propofol concentration and responsiveness score. There was an effective correlation between bispectral index score and the responsiveness score of the observer's assessment of the alertness/sedation scale, and between measured concentrations of midazolam and isoflurane and the responsiveness score. The subjects given alfentanil did not lose consciousness and were excluded from pooled analysis. The pooled bispectral index score at which 50% of subjects lost consciousness was 67, and the score at which 95% of subjects lost consciousness was 50. The prediction probability values for the bispectral index score were 0.885–0.976, giving the bispectral index score excellent predictive performance for indicating probability of loss of consciousness.

Discussion.—In these subjects, the bispectral index score correlated well with the effects of isoflurane, midazolam, and propofol on loss of consciousness and level of responsiveness. The correlation of the bispectral index score to the level of sedation is at least as good as measured drug concentrations. Bispectral index scores less than 50 indicate that a patient is probably unconscious and will have no recall.

▶ The EEG has been multiplied, divided, spectral analyzed, fast Fourier analyzed, and now "bispectral indexed" with secret black-box technology. Our long sought indicator for "level of consciousness" may actually be approximated by the bispectral index score. In this year's YEAR BOOK, I have included several papers on this subject because we may be on the threshold of legitimate level-of-consciousness monitoring. These papers do come under "Tinker's caution," namely, "beware of enthusiastic early reports."

J.H. Tinker, M.D.

Use of Computer-based Technology

The Effect of Electronic Record Keeping and Transesophageal Echocardiography on Task Distribution, Workload, and Vigilance During Cardiac Anesthesia

Weinger MB, Herndon OW, Gaba DM (Univ of California, San Diego; Stanford Univ, Palo Alto, Calif)

Anesthesiology 87:144–155, 1997 5–4

Objective.—Electronic anesthesia record keeping (EARK) is a new innovation that promises to improve performance by reducing workload, enhancing vigilance, or improving the quality of data. Few studies have examined the effects of EARK systems on the performance of anesthetic tasks, however. The impact of EARK on task profile, workload, and vigilance during cardiac anesthesia was assessed. The study also analyzed the effects of routine intraoperative use of transesophageal echocardiography (TEE).

Methods.—Twenty coronary artery bypass grafting patients were randomized to recording with the ARKIVE EARK system or the traditional manual system. Record keeping started at induction of anesthesia and continued until initiation of cardiopulmonary bypass. The activities of senior anesthesia residents were classified into 32 task categories and recorded on computer by a trained observer. "Vigilance latency"—the response time to a randomly activated alarm light—was assessed. Throughout each case, the anesthetist and the observer rated the workload at random intervals. Workload density was calculated as number of tasks per minute × task-specific workload values; task-links, or the relationships between sequential tasks, were assessed as well.

Results.—Before intubation, the EARK and manual cases were comparable in their distribution of tasks. No records at all were made before intubation in 16 of 20 cases. Once the patient had been intubated, time spent keeping records and using TEE were less for the EARK group. However, the EARK group spent more time watching monitors and speaking with the attending physician. In both groups, workload scores were significantly higher before intubation than afterward. Vigilance latency was 57 seconds before intubation vs. 31 seconds afterward. Subjective workload scores, workload density, and vigilance latency were comparable between groups. Vigilance latency was longer during TEE use. Use of TEE was also associated with greater workload density than that during other monitoring or recording tasks.

Conclusion.—During anesthesia for cardiac surgery, the use of an EARK system slightly reduces record keeping during the period after intubation but before bypass. Anesthetist vigilance and indicators of workload are unaffected by EARK. Routine use of TEE appears to increase workload while reducing vigilance.

▶ During routine anesthesia, many anesthesiologists wish to keep busy! In fact, they are so slick and quick at what they do that they need to busy themselves with charting and other routine functions; otherwise what they do looks almost too easy to casual observers, e.g., surgeons, nurses, etc. Therefore, EARK during routine anesthesia has not caught on. Another reason it has not caught on is, I think, because it is *unedited.* Enough said about that. During cardiac anesthesia, when other things are happening, it may make more sense. This study also shows that TEE may reduce vigilance in other areas. I find this a fascinating and elegantly performed iconoclastic study.

J.H. Tinker, M.D.

Anaesthesia and the Internet

Yentis SM, Ooi R (Chelsea & Westminster Hosp, London)

Anaesthesia 51:677–682, 1996 5–5

Objective.—United Kingdom anesthetists discuss the benefits and problems encountered using the Internet to access relevant information.

Access.—Access is available to anyone with a personal computer and modem who subscribes to an Internet provider, via the telephone system to those with portable personal computers, or through academic institutions that are serviced by their own computer networks. Software residing usually on a remote (server) computer makes possible connection to other sites. Individuals can communicate around the world via electronic mail (e-mail) sent to their Internet addresses. Messages can be forwarded or sent simultaneously to a group of people.

General Resources.—Search programs facilitate locating specific information. A list is provided. Most of these programs are available free of charge. Discussion groups and a list of academic courses are also available. There are specific anesthetic sites.

Advantages.—An enormous amount of information is available easily and quickly on the Internet from equipment manufacturers, academic institutions, medical centers, medical journals, and libraries about software, clinical problems, research topics, and specific anesthesia departments. E-mail facilitates communication between organizations and individuals.

Problems and disadvantages.—Information is not screened, and therefore, much of it is poor quality and of unknown authorship in some cases. The quantity of information available is overwhelming, and much of it is unstructured. Security of patient records and e-mail cannot be guaranteed. Costs of upgrading systems may be problematic. During peak user times, transfer of information can be slow. Copyright concerns and legal responsibility for statements and opinions made are areas yet to be resolved.

Conclusion.—The Internet contains a wealth of information that is useful to anesthetists and is easily and quickly obtained. E-mail facilitates communication between individuals and institutions. Much of what is available on the Internet is unregulated, and most communications are not secure.

▶ This is a superb article that details the history of the Internet, useful abbreviations, and a large number of useful locator codes for resources relating to anesthesia. For those just starting out on the Internet, this article is a fantastic starting point.

M.F. Roizen, M.D.

Morphine Patient-controlled Analgesia Is Superior to Meperidine Patient-controlled Analgesia for Postoperative Pain

Plummer JL, Owen H, Ilsley AH, et al (Flinders Med Centre, Bedford Park, Australia)

Anesth Analg 84:794–799, 1997 5–6

Introduction.—The three major reasons for disparity in results of trials evaluating morphine and meperidine for postoperative pain relief are small numbers of patients; in trials where drugs were delivered by patient-controlled analgesia (PCA), a single bolus dose was used for both drugs; and only 3 were blind, randomized controlled trials. The efficacy and side effects of morphine and meperidine were compared when administered by PCA for pain after major abdominal surgery.

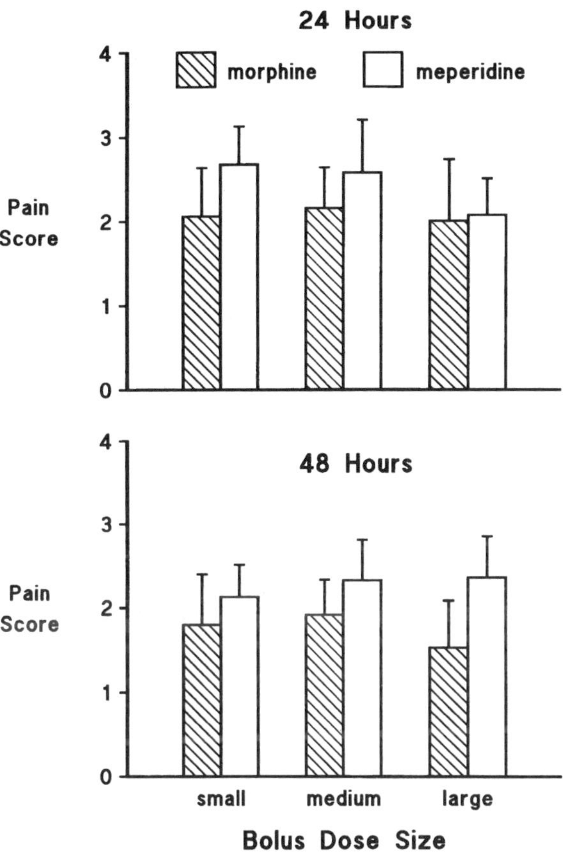

FIGURE 2.—Pain on sitting 24 hours (*upper figure*) and 48 hours (*lower figure*) postoperatively. Data are shown as mean and 95% confidence interval for the mean. (Courtesy of Plummer JL, Owen H, Ilsley AH, et al: Morphine patient-controlled analgesia is superior to meperidine patient-controlled analgesia for postoperative pain. *Anesth Analg* 84[4]:794–799, 1997.)

Methods.—One-hundred two patients were randomized to receive either PCA with morphine (0.75-, 1.0-, or 1.5-mg bolus dose) or meperidine (9, 12, or 18 mg) for pain control after a major abdominal operation. Patients were assessed at 24 and 48 hours after start of PCA for pain at rest and on sitting, nausea, unusual dreams, the Multiple Affect Adjective Check List (to measure mood), and the trailmaking tests A and B (to determine ability to concentrate).

Results.—Pain-at-rest scores significantly decreased from 24 to 48 hours postoperatively, but neither drug nor any bolus size had any effect on these scores. Pain on sitting also diminished significantly from 24 to 48 hours. These scores were not affected by bolus dose size, but were significantly lower in patients receiving morphine (Fig 2). Meperidine was correlated with poorer performance in the trailmaking test and a higher rate of dry mouth. There were no between-drug differences in severity of nausea, mood, and incidence of unusual dreams.

Conclusion.—Morphine is the drug of choice for postoperative pain relief in patients with major abdominal operations. It is associated with a lower incidence of dry mouth and less impairment of ability to concentrate. Meperidine should still be considered in patients for whom morphine is judged inappropriate.

▶ The superiority of morphine over meperidine in this study was probably not related to differences in administration paradigms, as three different doses were used for each drug. Studies of analgesic efficacy in animals have demonstrated that meperidine is less efficacious as well as less potent than morphine. This has been demonstrated in studies assessing the ability of opiates to provide analgesia at high stimulus intensities and following the development of tolerance. The relatively low efficacy of meperidine plus the accumulation of a neurotoxic metabolite during prolonged administration, suggests that this drug should not be the first-line analgesic for most patients.

S.E. Abram, M.D.

Postoperative Epidural Infusion: A Randomized, Double-blind, Dose-finding Trial of Clonidine in Combination With Bupivacaine and Fentanyl

Paech MJ, Pavy TJG, Orlikowski CEP, et al (Women and Infants Research Found, Perth, Australia)

Anesth Analg 84:1323–1328, 1997 5–7

Introduction.—The clinical use of postoperative epidural clonidine is limited by insufficient analgesia, hemodynamic changes, and sedation. Epidural clonidine with bupivacaine and morphine substantially decreases movement pain scores but also decreases arterial blood pressure. A randomized, double-blind investigation was conducted to determine whether clonidine added to bupivacaine and fentanyl could provide an effective analgesia that would minimize sedative and hemodynamic effects in patients undergoing abdominal gynecologic surgery.

Methods.—Patients were randomized and stratified for gynecologic or gynecologic oncology surgery to receive 1 of 4 epidural combinations. The control group (group C0, 22 patients) received 0.125% plain bupivacaine with fentanyl 2 µg/mL. Clonidine was added in the amounts of 10, 15, or 20 µg/hr, respectively, in groups C10 (22 patients), C15 (24 patients), and C20 (24 patients). Patient-controlled epidural analgesia was available with fentanyl 20 µg in 4-mL demand bolus with 20-minute lockout.

Results.—A dose-dependent improvement in analgesia at rest was observed with the addition of clonidine. With the 20-µg/hr dose, clonidine significantly increased the percentage of patients who experienced no pain with coughing, decreased pain scores with coughing, and significantly diminished supplementary fentanyl requirements. A dose-dependent reduction in blood pressure and pulse rate and an increase in vasopressor requirement was observed with clonidine. There were no between-group differences in sedation, pruritus, nausea, time to ambulation, and satisfaction with analgesia.

Conclusion.—High-quality analgesia was achieved after abdominal gynecologic surgery with epidural bupivacaine-fentanyl and high doses of clonidine. This regimen is associated with hemodynamic changes and increased vasopressor requirement.

► Routine use of epidural clonidine does not seem justified, given the hemodynamic effect and modest dose-sparing effects when given with other agents. It may, however, be useful in patients previously on opioids and patients with difficult-to-control hypertension.

S.E. Abram, M.D.

Epidural and Intravenous Bolus Morphine for Postoperative Analgesia in Infants

Haberkern CM, Lynn AM, Geiduschek JM, et al (Univ of Washington, Seattle; Children's Hosp and Med Ctr, Seattle)
Can J Anaesth 43:1203–1210, 1996 5–8

Objective.—Epidural morphine is effective for relieving postoperative pain in infants; however, infants may be at increased risk for respiratory depression after its use. The effectiveness, use, side effects, respiratory effects, and pharmacology of bolus epidural morphine were compared with that of intravenous morphine administered to infants for the control of postoperative pain after abdominal or genitourinary surgery.

Methods.—After undergoing abdominal or genitourinary surgery, 18 infants aged 3–12 months were randomly assigned to receive epidural morphine, 0.025 mg/kg; epidural morphine, 0.050 mg/kg; or intravenous morphine, 0.050–0.150 mg/kg. Infants were monitored continuously with ECG, impedance pneumogram, pulse oximeter, and nasal thermistor pneumogram. Pain was measured by using a modified infant pain scale every 4 hours. Response to CO_2 was determined with the use of the rebreathing technique. Serum morphine concentrations were measured at 15, 30, 60, and 120 minutes. Group variables were compared statistically using 1-way analysis of variance.

Results.—Analgesia was effective within 5 minutes. Infants receiving intravenous morphine required a second dose after 4 hours, whereas infants receiving epidural morphine received a second dose after 7–8 hours. Doses had to be adjusted in all groups to achieve pain relief. Many infants in all groups had pruritus, apnea and bradycardia, major or minor hypoxemic events, and hemoglobin desaturation. Slopes of CO_2 response curves were shallower than baseline curve slopes in the high-dose epidural and intravenous groups.

Conclusions.—In infants who had undergone abdominal or genitourinary surgery, epidural groups required fewer morphine doses and less morphine than did the intravenous morphine group to achieve pain relief. Pruritus, apnea and bradycardia, major or minor hypoxemic events, and hemoglobin desaturation were common in all groups. These infants need continuous monitoring with pulse oximetry.

► There is evidence that, in adults, postoperative epidural analgesia provides more effective analgesia and, in certain patient populations, improved outcomes as compared with systemic analgesics. This study fails to show appreciable benefit from the epidural route of morphine administration in infants. Potentially serious side effects were seen with both routes of administration.

S.E. Abram, M.D.

Patient-maintained Propofol Sedation: Assessment of a Target-controlled Infusion System

Irwin MG, Thompson N, Kenny GNC (Univ of Hong Kong; Royal Infirmary, Glasgow, Scotland)

Anaesthesia 52:525–530, 1997 5–9

Background.—Regional anesthesia has various advantages over general anesthesia. Propofol has a rapid onset of action and recovery. It can be difficult to provide optimal sedation for each patient because of individual differences in sensitivity to sedative drugs, individual preferences in degree of sedation, and changes in stimulation and discomfort during long procedures. Patient-administered sedative medication may be a useful solution.

Methods.—The infusion system was used in 36 unpremeditated patients scheduled for local and regional anesthesia procedures lasting from 10 to 280 minutes. An IV propofol infusion was started at a target concentration of 1 $\mu g/mL^{-1}$. The target propofol concentration could be increased by 0.2

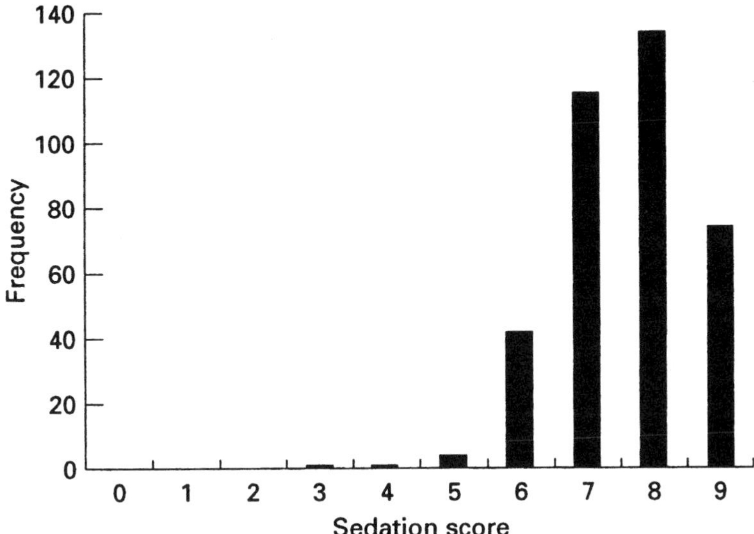

FIGURE 1.—Frequency of observed sedation scores. (Reprinted from Irwin MG, Thompson N, Kenny GNC: Patient-maintained propofol sedation: Assessment of a target-controlled infusion system. *Anaesthesia* 52[6]:525–530. Copyright 1997, by permission of the publisher, WB Saunders Company Limited, London.)

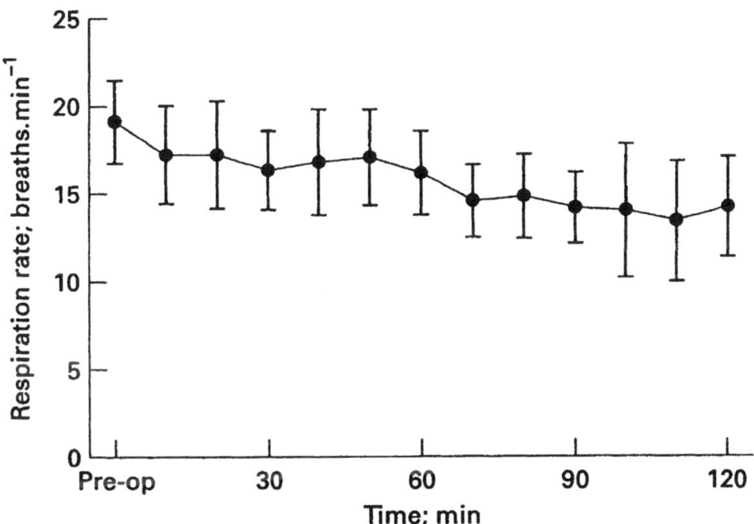

FIGURE 2.—Mean respiration rate before and during sedation. *Error bars* indicate ±2 SEM. (Reprinted from Irwin MG, Thompson N, Kenny GNC: Patient-maintained propofol sedation: Assessment of a target-controlled infusion system. *Anaesthesia* 52[6]:525–530. Copyright 1997, by permission of the publisher, WB Saunders Company Limited, London.)

μg/ml^{-1} increments by pressing a demand button. The lockout interval was 2 minutes and the maximum target concentration allowed was 3 μg/mL^{-1}.

Results.—The mean propofol consumption was 39.3 μg/kg^{-1}.min^{-1}; the range was 3–131 μg/kg^{-1}.min^{-1} (Fig 1). There was substantial variation in propofol consumption among individual patients, no cardiovascular instability, and little oversedation. A decrease in respiratory rate was noted with onset of sedation (Fig 2). Supplemental oxygen was needed in 8 patients. Median target concentrations of 0.8–0.9 μg/mL^{-1} provided optimal sedation. The target-controlled infusion system bias was −47% and inaccuracy was 48%. Patients were very satisfied with the system, and 89% reported they would definitely use it again.

Summary.—This infusion system combines the benefits of target-controlled infusion with a patient-controlled feedback loop. It offers a safe technique of administering intraoperative sedation during regional anesthesia with rapid recovery. Patients were very satisfied.

▶ Patient-controlled analgesia is well established, and we are now seeing an interest in extending this technique to patient-controlled sedation.

M. Wood, M.D.

Performance of Computer-assisted Continuous Infusion at Low Concentrations of Intravenous Sedatives

Veselis RA, Glass P, Dnistrian A, et al (Mem Sloan-Kettering Cancer Ctr, New York; Cornell Univ, New York; Duke Univ, Durham, NC)
Anesth Analg 84:1049–1057, 1997 5–10

Background.—Although still not routinely used clinically, computer-assisted continuous infusion (CACI) devices have been used in research settings for some time. Few studies have assessed the performance and usefulness of these devices when used to maintain constant serum concentrations during testing of pharmacodynamic effect, although studies have been performed to assess the accuracy of various target-controlled devices. The serum concentrations used in these studies have been in the range of general anesthesia purposes; few studies have addressed performance at the lower range, such as sedative concentrations, for clinical settings.

Methods.—The performance and temporal characteristics for 4 sedative drugs were assessed. Forty-one healthy volunteers were randomly assigned to receive midazolam, propofol, thiopental, or fentanyl with ondansetron pretreatment to prevent nausea. All drugs were given by CACI to achieve various constant target concentrations that would not result in loss of consciousness. An initial bolus was infused rapidly, followed by 3 increasing concentrations and 2 decreasing concentrations, each maintained at 45–70 minutes to allow time for data collection (Fig 1). A battery of psychomotor tests was administered at each target concentration. Twenty-

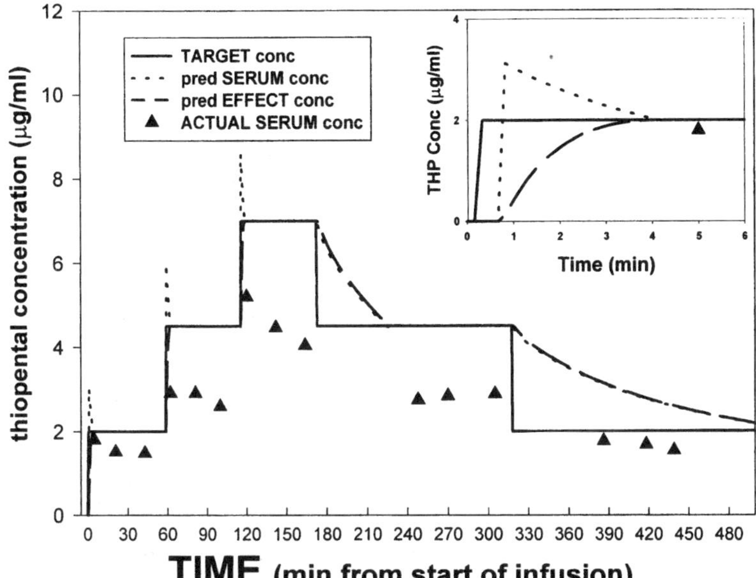

FIGURE 1.—Time course of various concentrations in 1 volunteer who received thiopental. Subjects were studied at 5 sequential constant target concentrations, 3 increasing followed by 2 decreasing. Note that in this subject, actual serum concentrations were substantially less than predicted. The *inset* shows the relationship between predicted serum (*dotted line*), predicted effect site (*long dashed line*), and desired target (*solid line*) concentrations over the initial few minutes at a given target concentration. The *triangle* indicates the first blood sample, which was taken for each drug after predicted equilibration between serum concentration and effect site concentration. An initial bolus was infused by computer-assisted continuous infusion to rapidly achieve the desired effect site concentration. Three blood samples were obtained at the beginning, middle, and end of each constant target level (triangle). Although not true in this volunteer, actual serum concentrations during the step-down phase were not necessarily the same as during the step-up phase. (Courtesy of Veselis RA, Glass P, Dnistrian A, et al: Performance of computer-assisted continuous infusion at low concentrations of intravenous sedatives. *Anesth Analg* 84[5]:1049–1057, 1997.)

six subjects had arterial sampling and 15 had venous sampling to determine drug concentrations. Median prediction error, median absolute prediction error, median absolute constancy error, and divergence were calculated as standard performance parameters (Fig 5).

Results.—Significant performance errors which were different among drugs, were demonstrated with CACI. Computer-assisted continuous infusion was able to maintain a constant serum concentration over time successfully, although performance errors could be large. The median absolute constancy error ranged from 5.6% (3.9% to 17.3%) for fentanyl to 11.2% (8.9% to 20.4%) for propofol. Differences between arterial and venous samples were few, but when they occurred, the largest errors were in the arterial sampling group.

Conclusion.—Computer-assisted continuous infusion is successful at monitoring constant serum concentrations of sedative drugs. Arterial sampling is preferred over venous sampling when testing performance of an infusion device. Venous sampling is adequate in determining serum con-

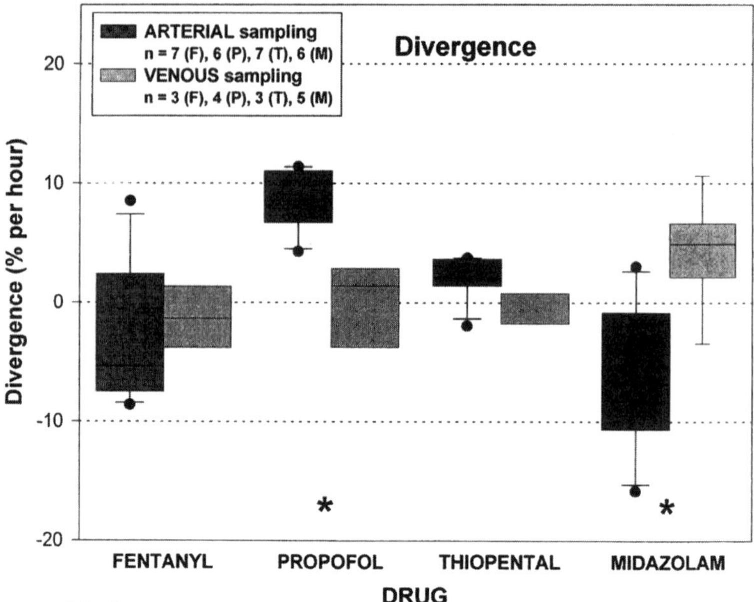

FIGURE 5.—Box and whisker plots indicating median, 25th and 75th percentile (*box*), 5th and 95th percentile (*whiskers*), and outlier values for divergence of computer-assisted continuous infusion when blood sampling was obtained using arterial (*left bar*) or venous (*right bar*) sampling for each drug. The number of subjects in each group are indicated. *Abbreviations: F*, fentanyl; *P*, propofol; *T*, thiopental; *M*, midazolam. Divergence was significantly different among drugs ($P < 0.05$ by one-way nonparametric analysis of variance). A significant difference between arterial and venous sampling (*) occurred for propofol and midazolam ($P < 0.05$). (Courtesy of Veselis RA, Glass P, Dnistrian A, et al: Performance of computer-assisted continuous infusion at low concentrations of intravenous sedatives. *Anesth Analg* 84[5]:1049–1057, 1997.)

centrations when a pseudosteady state has been achieved. Computer-assisted continuous infusion maintains stable serum concentrations for 45–70 minutes at low concentrations for sedative drugs. Future studies should use a device similar to CACI when drugs with rapid redistribution properties are being studied to examine the effects of sedative-hypnotic drugs.

▶ Although CACI devices have been a research tool for a number of years, they are still not used routinely in clinical practice. There is no doubt, however, that their availability has markedly dominated and changed pharmacokinetic and pharmacodynamic clinical studies, as plateau plasma concentrations and concentrations at the "effect site" can be more readily attained with this methodology.

M. Wood, M.D.

Magnetic Resonance Imaging and Spinal Cord Stimulation Systems
Liem LA, van Dongen VCPC (St Antonius Ziekenhuis, Nieuwegein, The Netherlands; Maasland Ziekenhuis, Sittard, The Netherlands)
Pain 70:95–97, 1997 5–11

Background.—The effects of MRI on neurostimulators used for spinal cord stimulation in pain treatment are debated. Three patients with a neurostimulation system implant who underwent MRI are presented.

Case Reports.—The first patient was a 50-year-old woman implanted with a pulse generator for stump and phantom limb pain in the amputated second digit of the right hand. The subcutaneous pocket containing the pulse generator was in the right infraclavicular region. This treatment adequately suppressed the pain. However, progressive sensory disturbances necessitated MRI of T7-T11. The presence of the neurostimulator, located out of the region of interest, did not affect the recordings. No pulse generator heating or electrode dislodgement occurred. Scanning had one permanent effect: erasure of the electronically coded serial number in the pulse generator memory. Several other changes occurred in the pulse generator's parameter settings but could be corrected. The patient experienced no effects from these changes.

The second patient, a 46-year-old man undergoing lumbar laminectomy procedures, was implanted with a pulse generator in the subfascial layer of the right lower abdominal quadrant. Subsequent development of cervicobrachialgia radiating into the arms prompted an MRI of the cervical spine, with C4–C7 included. During imaging, the patient reported a slight increase in temperature of the pulse generator. After imaging was completed successfully, the occurrence of 2 magnet activations of the pulse generator was discovered. In addition, the normal amplitude, set to zero before scanning, changed to 3.1 V, and the pulse width changes from 65 µs to 270 µs. These changes were easily corrected.

The third patient was a 48-year-old woman implanted with a neurostimulation system because of failed back treatment syndrome. Magnetic resonance imaging of the area including the radiofrequency receiver and epidural electrode was required subsequently. The images were intensely disturbed. Scattered images of the whole area were obtained. There was no heating in the area of the receiver system, and the patient reported no unusual sensations or adverse effects.

Conclusions.—Under certain circumstances, MRI can be performed safely in patients with neurostimulators. Caution is recommended when the neurostimulator is in the area to be scanned. Images are likely to be affected by the electrode, pulse generator, or receiver system.

▶ The fact that none of these patients suffered injury or substantial damage to the expensive pulse generators does not guarantee that such adverse events will not occur in other patients. In view of the generally poor images that result from the presence of metallic implants, it would seem prudent to use other imaging technologies, such as CT, in these patients.

S.E. Abram, M.D.

Oximetry/Capnography/Blood Pressure Monitoring

Measurement of Percent Oxyhemoglobin by Optical Densitometry in Perfluorocarbon Supplemented Blood

Murrah CP, Agnihotri AK, Spruell RD, et al (Univ of Alabama at Birmingham; Alliance Pharmaceutical Corp, San Diego, Calif)

ASAIO J 42:M769–M773, 1996 5–12

Background.—Clinical studies are currently being performed to evaluate some new perfluorocarbon emulsions for use as erythrocyte substitutes. However, there are still unanswered questions about how perfluorocarbon emulsions affect measurements of percent oxyhemoglobin ($\%O_2Hb$) by optical densitometry. The effects of perfluorochemical concentration in blood and hematocrit (Hct) in $\%O_2Hb$ measurements were studied in vitro.

Methods.—The experiments used stored porcine blood with an Hct of 18% or 9%. The blood was mixed with a perfluorocarbon emulsion (Oxygent) in concentrations of 0, 0.73, 1.45, and 2.90 g of perfluorochemical per deciliter of blood. Values for pH and PCO_2 were maintained at physiologic levels; tonometry was performed to determine the range of oxygen tensions within each Hct/perfluorocarbon concentration group.

Results.—As perfluorochemical concentration increased and Hct decreased, error in $\%O_2Hb$ measurements increased. These errors were predictable and could be used to generate an equation to correct $\%O_2Hb$ measurements for perfluorocarbon supplementation in blood. The influence of perfluorocarbon supplementation became apparent at PO_2 values of 30 mm Hg or greater.

Conclusions.—Perfluorocarbon concentration and Hct affect the error in $\%O_2Hb$ measurement in blood. This study proposes an equation for use in correcting for such aberrant oxyhemoglobin measurements. However, more research will be needed before such a correction equation can be used in clinical practice.

▶ This study provides a technique to make corrections to percent oxyhemoglobin when perfluorocarbon-supplemented blood is used, such as during cardiopulmonary bypass. I would estimate that each new substitute would require you to know its content. The problem, of course, is in the dynamic situation of the ongoing blood loss and perfluorocarbon loss. It will be hard to estimate the percent perfluorocarbon that remains in the circulating solution.

M.F. Roizen, M.D.

Use of a Neonatal Noninvasive Blood Pressure Module on Adult Patients

Green DW (King's College Hosp, London)

Anaesthesia 51:1129–1132, 1996 5–13

Purpose.—Automatic digital monitors, based on the principle of oscillometry, are now routinely used for noninvasive blood pressure measurement in anesthetized patients. These monitors can measure blood pressure in tiny newborns. As such, they should be able to measure blood pressure in the finger or thumb of adults, which would have some important advantages. The use of a neonatal automatic noninvasive oscillometric blood pressure monitor to measure blood pressure in adults was evaluated.

Methods.—The study included 18 adult patients undergoing general anesthesia for an elective major surgical procedure. Each patient had a neonatal oscillometric blood pressure monitor, with a size 2 Dinamap cuff, attached to the proximal phalanx of the thumb. In the other extremity, a radial artery catheter was placed for intra-arterial pressure monitoring. Measurements of systolic, mean, and diastolic arterial blood pressures made by the 2 devices were compared.

Results.—A total of 1,258 readings were analyzed. Mean differences between the invasive and noninvasive pressures recorded were +9.1 mm Hg for systolic pressure, −7.9 mm Hg for diastolic pressure, and −0.7 mm Hg for mean pressure. The standard deviations of the pressure differences were 14.4, 11.7, and 11.9 mm Hg, respectively.

Conclusion.—An oscillometric neonatal noninvasive blood pressure device attached to the thumb of an adult patient provides a reasonably accurate measurement of blood pressures, compared with invasive pressure recordings from a radial artery catheter. This technique offers some advantages over conventional arm cuff placement. The thumb pressure monitoring technique does tend to underestimate systolic pressures, particularly at pressures of less than 90 mm Hg.

► The author concludes that the thumb pressure monitoring technique via oscillometry is acceptable. Yet, if one looks at the data, pressure differences of as much as 50 mm Hg occur when blood pressure readings are around 100. I do not consider these differences acceptable. Similarly, differences of over 25 mm Hg are not uncommon when the diastolic pressure is around 50 mm Hg. I think this author does an excellent job of showing that this technique, rather than being acceptable, is unacceptable for perioperative care.

M.F. Roizen, M.D.

Airway Protection, Evaluation, and Monitoring

Cricoid Cartilage Pressure Decreases Lower Esophageal Sphincter Tone

Tournadre J-P, Chassard D, Berrada KR, et al (Hôpital de l'Hôtel Dieu, Lyon, France)

Anesthesiology 86:7–9, 1997 5–14

Introduction.—Cricoid cartilage pressure (Sellick's maneuver) has historically been used to occlude the esophagus and prevent pulmonary aspiration of gastric contents because of decreased upper esophageal sphincter pressure during induction of anesthetic agents. The effect of Sellick's maneuver on lower esophageal sphincter pressure (LESP) was evaluated in 8 unanesthetized volunteers.

Methods.—Four men and 4 women fasted for 12–16 hours before cricoid cartilage pressure was applied through a water-filled polyvinyl chloride balloon (25 mL) connected to a pressure transducer that displayed the applied force in newtons. Perfused polyethylene catheters were used to record lower esophageal sphincter, esophageal, and gastric pressure. The force applied to the cricoid was measured throughout and LESP was recorded during cricoid force of 20 and 40 newtons.

Results.—There was a significant decrease in LESP with cricoid pressure. The decrease in lower esophageal sphincter pressure was 15 mm Hg at a pressure of 20 newtons and 12 mm Hg at a pressure of 40 newtons. There was a significant difference in LESP between 20 and 40 newtons. The LESP returned to baseline values after release of cricoid pressure. Gastric pressure and heart rate were similar throughout (Table 1). Cricoid pressure was well tolerated and no volunteers reported difficulty in breathing.

Conclusion.—Cricoid pressure with 20 newtons decreased LESP and barrier pressure in conscious humans but did not occlude the esophagus. At least 40 newtons is needed to occlude the esophagus, although at this pressure, LESP is also reduced. These findings may help explain why gastric content aspiration may occur during induction of anesthesia de-

TABLE 1.—Manometric Data During Cricoid Pressure of 20 Newtons and 40 Newtons

	Before Cricoid Pressure	Cricoid Pressure 20 N	Cricoid Pressure 40 N	After Release
LESP (mmHg)	24 ± 3	15 ± 4*	12 ± 4†	24 ± 6
GP (mmHg)	5 ± 2	5 ± 1	5 ± 2	5 ± 0
BrP (mmHg)	18 ± 2	10 ± 3*	7 ± 3†	19 ± 4

Note: Data are means ± SD.
*$P < 0.05$ vs. control.
†$P < 0.01$ vs. control.
Abbreviations: LESP, lower esophageal sphincter pressure; *GP*, gastric pressure, *BrP*, esophageal barrier pressure (LESP − GP).
(Courtesy of Tournadre J-P, Chassard D, Berrada KR, et al: Cricoid cartilage pressure decreases lower esophageal sphincter tone. *Anesthesiology* 86:7–9, 1997.

spite the use of cricoid pressure. These are important data, particularly when anesthesia is used in patients with increased gastric pressure.

▶ This study challenges accepted dogma regarding the use of cricoid pressure, suggesting that the risk of gastric aspiration may actually be increased with this maneuver. Indeed, if poor technique is used, as is often the case when inexperienced personnel are involved, not only will there be inadequate pressure occluding the esophagus, but LESP may be decreased as well. Future studies corroborating these data, and deciphering the neural mechanism by which this phenomenon occurs, may change our standard methods of preventing gastric acid aspiration.

D.M. Rothenberg, M.D.

Ease of Insertion of the Laryngeal Mask Airway by Inexperienced Personnel When Using an Introducer

Dingley J, Baynham P, Swart M, et al (Univ Hosp of Wales, Cardiff)

Anaesthesia 52:756–760, 1997 5–15

Introduction.—To aid insertion of the laryngeal mask airway, the Portex introducer was designed. It overcomes one of the most common reasons for insertion failure—the folding back of the laryngeal mask airway. As a means of initial airway management during emergency in-hospital resuscitation, the laryngeal mask airway may be of use. During initial resuscitation, it was hypothesized that it could be inserted by the ward nurse who would have less experience than most anesthetists in inserting the laryngeal mask airway. The first-time success rate for laryngeal mask airway insertion in unskilled hands was explored and was compared with the first-time success rate using the Portex introducer.

Methods.—Made of soft plastic, the introducer is lubricated and placed in the mouth after induction of anesthesia. The deflated edges of the laryngeal mask airway cuff lie over the introducer, which is split into 2 bars at its proximal end (Fig 1). The introducer acts as an artificial hard palate to guide the tip of the laryngeal mask into the correct position (Fig 2). There were 89 adults scheduled to receive an anesthetic for a short day-case surgical procedure using the laryngeal mask airway. Doctors who were inexperienced in the insertion of the laryngeal mask airway inserted a maximum number of 4 laryngeal mask airways. Patients were randomly assigned to receive the laryngeal mask airway with or without the introducer.

Results.—There was a 68% success rate in the 44 patients with the laryngeal mask airway being inserted according to the manufacturer's instructions, with 14 failures. Eight of these resulted from the tip of the mask folding back, 2 were caused by an inability to pass the mask past the teeth, 2 were caused by obstruction in the pharynx, and 2 resulted from incorrect final positioning. There was a 96% success rate in the 45 patients

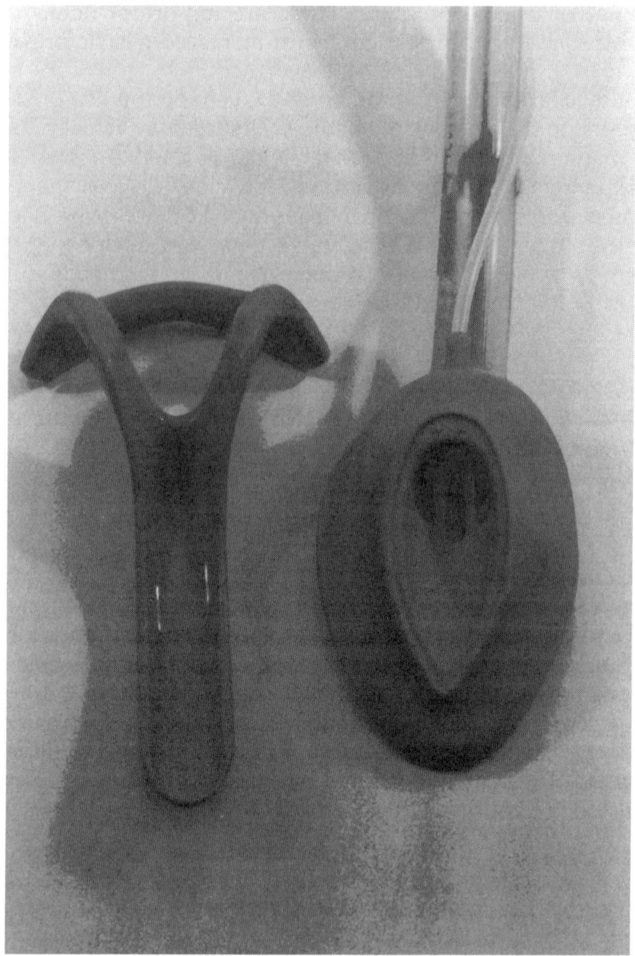

FIGURE 1.—View of introducer alongside a size 3 laryngeal mask airway. (Reprinted from Dingley J, Baynham P, Swart M, et al: Ease of insertion of the laryngeal mask airway by inexperienced personnel when using an introducer. *Anaesthesia* 52:756–760. Copyright 1997, by permission of WB Saunders Company Limited, London.)

with the laryngeal mask airway being inserted with the Portex introducer, with 2 failures.

Conclusions.—In the hands of inexperienced personnel, the success rate for laryngeal mask airway insertion at the first attempt was found to be significantly better when the Portex introducer was used. If difficulty has been encountered initially, this device can be used as an aide for a second insertion attempt and trainees may find the device helpful. Where restriction of head and neck movement is a problem, the device may also prove to be useful.

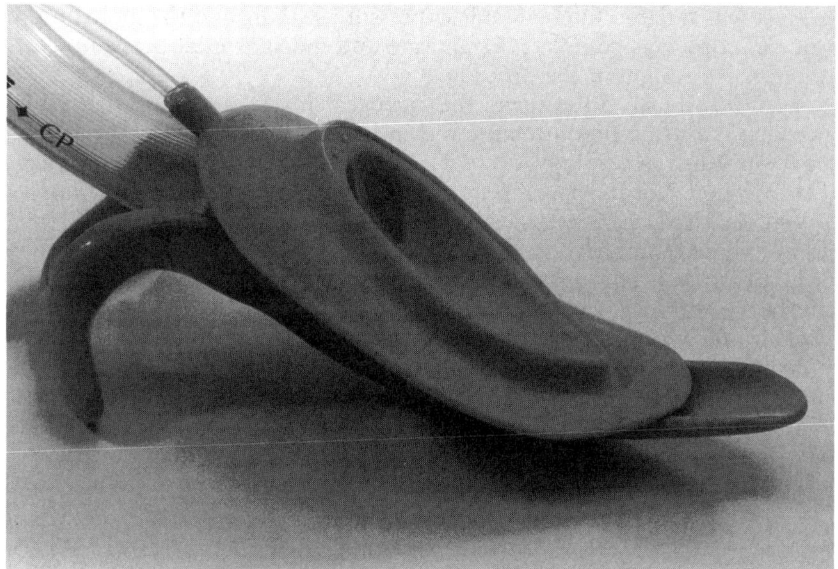

FIGURE 2.—The introducer acts as an artificial palate and is shaped to guide the tip of the laryngeal mask airway in the correct direction as it is inserted. (Reprinted from Dingley J, Baynham P, Swart M, et al: Ease of insertion of the laryngeal mask airway by inexperienced personnel when using an introducer. *Anaesthesia* 52:756–760. Copyright 1997, by permission of WB Saunders Company Limited, London.)

► This article nicely demonstrates the use of an introducer to facilitate a laryngeal mask airway placement. This may be especially useful in the emergency situation when novices are attempting to place the laryngeal mask airway. One word of caution in evaluating this article, however, is that this device was designed by one of the authors, and therefore the results of this study may be somewhat biased.

D.M. Rothenberg, M.D.

The Laryngeal Mask Airway: A New Standard for Airway Evaluation in Thoracic Surgery

Ferson DZ, Nesbitt JC, Nesbitt KK, et al (Univ of Texas, Houston)

Ann Thorac Surg 63:768–772, 1997 5–16

Background.—Fiberoptic bronchoscopy is typically performed before thoracotomy, after inserting a single-lumen endotracheal tube and before inserting a double-lumen endotracheal tube. Thus, this approach requires two intubations. The authors evaluated the use of a laryngeal mask airway, which requires no intubation, for fiberoptic bronchoscopy.

Methods.—Fifty patients undergoing elective thoracic surgical procedures received a laryngeal mask airway before fiberoptic bronchoscopy. The deflated cuff of the laryngeal mask airway was inserted into the hypopharynx until it encountered the upper esophageal sphincter. Then the cuff was inflated to create a low-pressure seal around the glottis until bronchoscopy was complete. Heart rate and mean arterial pressure were monitored throughout the procedure.

Findings.—In all 50 patients the laryngeal mask airway was inserted successfully on the first attempt, and in less than 10 seconds. Bronchoscopy confirmed accurate placement of the cuff against the upper esophageal sphincter. Vocal cord leukoplakia was seen in 2 patients. No complications occurred as a result of the procedure. Blood pressure and pulse rate did not change significantly from baseline.

Conclusions.—The laryngeal mask airway is a quick, easy-to-insert, and safe means of surveying the larynx and trachea. It is inexpensive and reusable and avoids the need for multiple insertions of endotracheal tubes. In fact, because this method involves no endotracheal tube, the clinician can easily inspect the supraglottic, aryepiglottic, glottic, and infraglottic areas for malignancies. Its effects on hemodynamic responses are minimal, and the authors recommend that use of the laryngeal mask airway should become the standard in airway evaluation before thoracic surgery.

▶ I include this paper to condemn a current practice. The practice that seems to be becoming widespread, performing a fiberoptic bronchoscopy immediately prior to routine thoracic surgery, and then routinely demanding a double-lumen tube, again prior to what used to be routine thoracic surgery, seems to be extraordinarily time consuming and wasteful. Having performed and supervised literally thousands of anesthetics for thoracotomies, I do not believe that a double-lumen tube is necessary or really beneficial for many routine thoracotomies that involve less than major pulmonary resections. I do not believe that a bronchoscopy prior to making a skin incision adds anything but a separate billing opportunity. I am cynical enough to wonder if perhaps someone is getting extra pay for that bronchoscopy! If that bronchoscopy prior to intubation with a double-lumen tube (which requires its own separate bronchoscope) wasn't done, then the laryngeal mask airway (LMA) step wouldn't be necessary at all. The idea that an LMA for performance of this perhaps unnecessary prior bronchoscopy is somehow better than the insertion of a single lumen tube fort is nonsense. The single lumen tube costs about $2.00. Although it may add some hemodynamic perturbation in an inadequately anesthetized patient, it certainly does not constitute hemodynamic jeopardy. For these authors to call the prior use of an LMA a "new standard" is the kind of hype I condemn. Maybe I'm simply turning into an old curmudgeon, but I do not understand the necessity of a prior bronchoscopy for routine thoracotomies. I do not understand the necessity for routine use of the double-lumen tube in those same circumstances, nor do I know of any compelling reasons why the LMA should become a "standard" here.

J.H. Tinker, M.D.

Hypothermia/Temperature Monitoring

Clinical Experience With Epidural Cooling for Spinal Cord Protection During Thoracic and Thoracoabdominal Aneurysm Repair

Cambria RP, Davison JK, Zannetti S, et al (Massachusetts Gen Hosp, Boston; Harvard Med School, Boston)

J Vasc Surg 25:234–243, 1997 5–17

Objective.—The incidence of spinal cord ischemic injury is 16% during thoracic aneurysm (TA) or thoracoabdominal aneurysm (TAA) repair. Regional hypothermia may prevent spinal cord injury. Results of 2½ years of experience with epidural cooling (EC) in 70 patients is reported.

Methods.—Between July 1993 and January 1996, 70 consecutive patients, aged 30 to 85, with type I (n = 24), type II (n = 11), type III (n = 26), and descending (n = 9) thoracic aneurysms (TAs) were treated with intraoperative EC. Iced (4°C) normal saline was infused through a 4F 40 cm catheter placed into the T_{11-12} epidural space an average of 74 minutes before aortic cross clamping. CSF temperature (CSFT) and pressure (CSFP) were continuously monitored via a second 4F thermistor catheter placed 4 cm into the subarachnoid space at the L_{3-4} interspace. The clamp-and-sew technique was used in all patients except for 1 with Marfan's syndrome who received an atriofemoral bypass. Neurological outcome was compared with data gathered retrospectively from control patients operated on before adoption of EC.

Results.—Epidural infusion values ranged from 200 to 3,500 mL and averaged 1,409 mL. CSFT changed from 28°C before cross-clamp to 25°C during cross-clamp to 32°C 1 hour after clamp removal. CSFP changed from 13 mm Hg at baseline to 40 mm Hg before cross-clamp to 31 mm Hg during cross-clamp to 11 mm Hg 1 hour after clamp removal. Within 60 days of surgery, 7 (10%) patients died, 18 had pneumonia, 4 had cardiac complications, 10 had renal complications, and 3 had a stroke. Lower extremity neurologic deficits developed in 2 (2.9%) EC patients and 13 (23%) deficits in control patients. Predicted deficits were 20% and 17.8%, respectively. Logical regression analysis showed that prolonged visceral aortic cross-clamp time (more than 60 minutes) (RR 4.4) and lack of epidural cooling (RR 9.8) were significantly associated with development of postoperative neurologic deficits.

Conclusion.—EC reduces the risk of ischemic cord injury and of lower extremity neurologic deficits during TA or TAA repair.

► This is a fascinating study that in a case-controlled fashion looked at the neurologic outcome after thoracoabdominal and thoracic aneurysm repair. I am often reminded of the experiments we did with the rabbit model a while ago, where we accidentally left the heating blanket on. We used heating blankets to initially maintain temperature in the animals and found that when the spinal cord was close to the heating blanket, neurologic damage increased.

This experiment tested the logical hypothesis that cooling would decrease neurologic damage, and it did. One worries whether it was just experience of the surgeons, as this was a case control trial with the more recent cases receiving this epidural cooling, rather than the epidural cooling, per say, that made a difference. Obviously, surgical techniques make a major difference in this operation. It is hard to find neurologic damage when the repair is done in an under 10-minute period of time, or at least the neurologic damage is reduced compared to what it would be if a 40-minute time frame or repair is done. Thus, as the authors state, it appears that epidural cooling can be a safe and effective technique to increase ischemic tolerance of the spinal cord and can help when the surgeons take longer than 10 minutes to complete repair.

M.F. Roizen, M.D.

The Use of Countercurrent Heat Exchangers Diminishes Accidental Hypothermia During Abdominal Aortic Aneurysm Surgery

Muth CM, Mainzer B, Peters J (Heinrich-Heine-Universität, Düsseldorf, Germany)

Acta Anaesthesiol Scand 40:1197–1202, 1996 5–18

Objective.—Accidental hypothermia during surgery can significantly increase the risk of cardiac morbidity. The effectiveness of fluid/blood warmers after surgery has not been tested. The use of an in-line fluid/blood warmer based on the principle of countercurrent heat exchange to reduce the incidence and severity of hypothermia was evaluated in patients undergoing elective abdominal aortic surgery.

Methods.—Fifty patients (ASA classification grade III) were prospectively randomized to receive an infusion via a countercurrent heat exchanger (Hotline, Level 1 Technologies Inc., Boston) (n = 25) or to receive infusion solutions stored at 21°C and blood products warmed to 37°C. Patients were classified based on esophageal temperature as mildly hypothermic (greater than 35.5°C), moderately hypothermic (34.5°C to 35.5°C), or severely hypothermic (less than 34.5°C). Groups were compared statistically.

Results.—Whereas the use of heat exchangers did not eliminate hypothermia, the mean temperature decrease in the group managed with heat exchangers was significantly less than that of the control group (−0.35°C vs. −1.5°C). The temperature decrease in patients managed with heat exchangers was less dependent on duration of surgery than was the temperature decrease in the control group. The postoperative temperature was significantly lower in the control group than in the heat-exchanger managed group (34.2°C vs. 35.1°C), and the incidence of severe hypothermia was significantly greater in the control group than in the heat-exchanger managed group (64% vs. 8%).

Conclusion.—Whereas countercurrent heat exchangers do not prevent hypothermia, they are an effective means for significantly reducing the degree and the incidence of hypothermia in patients undergoing abdominal aortic aneurysm repair.

▶ This study looks only at fluid warming and not forced air warming. Forced air warming or even greenhouse-type warming, in which a blanket is placed underneath the patient in a greenhouse effect and in which warm air in the covering gowns of the patient is used to keep the patient warm, are both effective at restoring normal thermia even after hypothermia has occurred. That is, as opposed to this type of warming of fluid where you only can maintain, or help maintain temperature. Thus, I believe that the forced air warming systems have been a substantial improvement over the fluid warming systems.

M.F. Roizen, M.D.

Regional Anesthesia Techniques

Comparison of Single, End-holed and Multi-orifice Extradural Catheters When Used for Continuous Infusion of Local Anaesthetic During Labour

Dickson MAS, Moores C, McClure JH (Royal Infirmary of Edinburgh, Scotland)

Br J Anaesth 79:297–300, 1997 5–19

Background.—Previous studies have compared the efficacies of the single, end-holed extradural catheter and the multi-orifice extradural catheter during bolus infusion of local anesthetic. The efficacies of these 2 extradural catheters during a continuous infusion were evaluated.

Methods.—Patients were randomly assigned to receive either a single, end-holed extradural catheter (n = 163) or a multi-orifice extradural catheter (n = 153) for the administration of local anesthetic. The proximal orifices of the multi-orifice catheter were positioned to lie similarly within the extradural space as the orifice of the single, end-holed catheter. A single dose of 0.25% or 0.5% bupivacaine was used to establish extradural block, and block height was measured after 20 minutes. Then, a continuous infusion of 0.1% bupivacaine was started, with dose increases as needed.

Findings.—Good pain relief was reported by 86% of patients in each group. At the 20-minute measurement, the frequency of unilateral block did not differ between the single, end-holed catheter and the multi-orifice catheter groups (18, or 12% vs. 16, or 11%, respectively). Similarly, unilateral block recurred at similar frequencies in both groups (between 4% and 5%). However, during continuous anesthetic infusion, new unilateral block developed significantly more often in the group with a single, end-holed catheter (29, or 16%) compared to the group with a multi-orifice catheter (14, or 8%).

Conclusions.—The frequency of unilateral block was similar with both types of epidural catheters during a bolus infusion of local anesthetic. However, with a continuous infusion, significantly more new unilateral blocks developed with the single, end-holed catheter. Thus, when a continuous infusion of local anesthetic is needed, the multi-orifice epidural catheter would seem to be the better choice.

► When multi-orifice epidural catheters were first introduced, some anesthesiologists expressed concern about the risk of unrecognized multi-compartment block, which might result in systemic local anesthetic toxicity or high spinal anesthesia. Nonetheless, these multi-orifice catheters have become increasingly popular, in part because many anesthesiologists perceive that they provide better analgesia—with a low incidence of complications—in clinical practice. In the present study, the authors noted no difference between groups in the initial incidence of unilateral block. However, they observed a twofold increase in the incidence of unilateral block in the single-orifice group during the continuous epidural infusion of 0.1% bupivacaine.

D.H. Chestnut, M.D.

Prevention of Hypotension During Spinal Anesthesia: A Comparison of Intravascular Administration of Hetastarch Versus Lactated Ringer's Solution

Sharma SK, Gajraj NM, Sidawi JE (Univ of Texas, Dallas)

Anesth Analg 84:111–114, 1997 5–20

Background.—The efficacy of preloading with colloid solutions in decreasing the incidence of hypotension after spinal anesthesia in patients undergoing tubal ligation has not been assessed. Six percent hetastarch was compared with crystalloid administration in a study.

Methods.—Forty women with ASA grade I scheduled for postpartum tubal ligations under spinal anesthesia were assigned randomly to 500 mL of hetastarch solution or 1,000 mL of lactated Ringer's solution before spinal anesthesia. Spinal anesthesia was identical in both groups.

Findings.—Hypotension occurred in 52% of the lactated Ringer's solution group and in 16% of the hetastarch group. This difference was significant. The need for 5-mg bolus doses of ephedrine to maintain systolic arterial blood pressure of more than 75% of baseline was significantly greater in the lactated Ringer's solution group than in the hetastarch group.

Conclusions.—An IV infusion of 500 mL of 6% hetastarch solution appears to be more effective than 1,000 mL lactated Ringer's solution in attenuating spinal anesthesia–induced hypotension in women undergoing postpartum tubal ligation. In both groups, however, hypotension was mild and quickly corrected with prompt treatment.

► It is pretty hard for me to get excited about the use of an expensive colloid solution to reduce the incidence of a nonproblem (i.e., hypotension during spinal anesthesia for postpartum tubal ligation). Indeed, the authors concluded that the "routine administration of expensive hetastarch . . . might not be justifiable."

D.H. Chestnut, M.D.

Postoperative Analgesia and Antiemetic Efficacy After Subarachnoid Neostigmine in Orthopedic Surgery
Lauretti GR, Reis MP (Univ of São Paulo, Brazil)
Reg Anesth 22:337–342, 1997 5–21

Introduction.—Subarachnoid neostigmine provides analgesia by inhibiting the breakdown of acetylcholine in the spinal cord. Side effects of nausea and vomiting, however, may limit its use in postoperative patients. Various antiemetics were evaluated for their ability to prevent neostigmine-related side effects in patients undergoing tibial or ankle reconstruction.

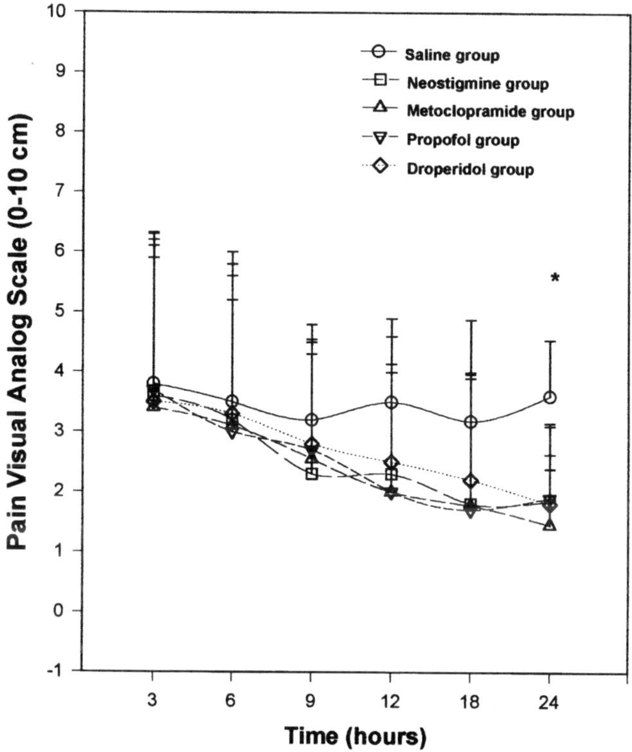

FIGURE 1.—Visual analog scores for postoperative pain at fixed intervals. Data expressed as mean ± SD. *Neostigmine, metoclopramide, propofol, and droperidol groups compared with the saline group, $P < 0.001$. (Courtesy of Lauretti GR, Reis MP: Postoperative analgesia and antiemetic efficacy after subarachnoid neostigmine in orthopedic surgery. *Reg Anesth* 22:337–342, 1997.)

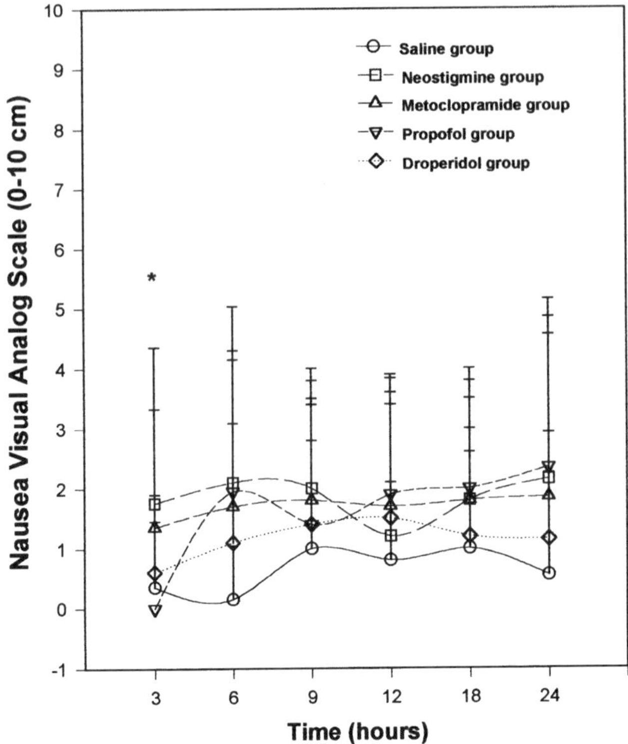

FIGURE 2.—Postoperative visual analog scores for nausea at fixed intervals. Data expressed as mean ± SD. *At 3 hours, neostigmine, metoclopramide, and propofol groups compared with the saline group, $P < 0.05$. (Courtesy of Lauretti GR, Reis MP: Post-operative analgesia and antiemetic efficacy after subarachnoid neostigmine in orthopedic surgery. *Reg Anesth* 22:337–342, 1997.)

Methods.—The prospective study enrolled 100 patients who were randomized to 1 of 5 groups of 20 each: saline, neostigmine, metoclopramide, droperidol, and propofol. A single-blind design was used in the propofol group and a double-blind design in the remaining 4 groups. The IV antiemetic test drug (except propofol) was given as premedication after IV midazolam (0.05 mg/kg). Subarachnoid drugs administered were 20 mg bupivacaine (0.5 mg) in conjunction with 100 µg neostigmine, except for the saline group which received bupivacaine and saline. The IV test drug was saline in the saline, neostigmine, and propofol groups. The droperidol and metoclopramide groups received these agents IV (0.5 mg and 10 mg, respectively). The propofol group received this agent as a continuous IV infusion (2–4 mg/kg/hr), started 10 minutes after the spinal injection. Patients were monitored in the first 24 hours after surgery for nausea, emetic episodes, and the need for analgesic or antiemetic medication. A visual analog scale (VAS) was also completed for pain and emesis.

Results.—The 5 groups were comparable in American Society of Anesthesiologists physical status, sex and age distribution, mean weight and height, type of surgery performed, surgical time, and duration of anesthesia. Although subarachnoid neostigmine (100 μg) had no overall effect on subarachnoid bupivacaine analgesia, it did decrease the 24-hour VAS scores and the need for postoperative analgesics during this period. Twenty-four hour VAS pain scores (Fig 1) were similar for the 4 active treatment groups and significantly lower than that of the saline group. Compared with the saline group, the neostigmine, droperidol, and metoclopramide groups had a higher incidence of intraoperative nausea and vomiting. The 3-hour VAS assessment for emesis (Fig 2) was higher for the neostigmine, propofol, and metoclopramide groups than for the saline group.

Conclusion.—Subarachnoid neostigmine reduced postoperative pain scores and analgesic requirement in these patients undergoing minor orthopedic procedures, but nausea and vomiting were common. It could not be determined whether neostigmine enhanced the mechanisms involved in spinal analgesia.

▶ Here is another study that confirms that neostigmine has some potentially useful analgesic properties but that nausea may limit the clinical utility of the technique.

S.E. Abram, M.D.

A Comparison of Catheter vs Needle Injection of Local Anesthetic for Induction of Epidural Anesthesia for Cesarean Section

Husain FJ, Herman NL, Karuparthy VR, et al (Univ of Texas Health Science Ctr, San Antonio; Cornell Univ, New York; Vanderbilt Univ, Nashville, Tenn)

Int J Obstet Anesth 6:101–106, 1997 5–22

Purpose.—In women undergoing epidural anesthesia for cesarean section, the local anesthetic can be administered either directly through the epidural needle or after placement of an epidural catheter. Bolus injections through the epidural needle are generally thought to produce a more rapid onset of blockade, but a higher incidence and severity of hypotension. Intermittent injections via catheter do not achieve anesthesia as quickly, but the risk of hypotension is lower. These 2 techniques of local anesthetic administration were compared for speed of anesthesia and occurrence of systemic hypotension in a randomized trial.

Methods.—The study included 100 healthy ASA class I or III patients scheduled to undergo elective cesarean section with epidural anesthesia. They were randomly assigned to receive anesthetic injected intermittently through the epidural needle or through a previously placed catheter. The time to full surgical anesthesia and quality of anesthesia were compared for the 2 groups. The incidence and severity of hypotension were compared as well. The study protocol was successfully carried out in 88 patients.

Results.—The needle group required a larger total volume of anesthetic (lidocaine 2% with 1:200,000 epinephrine) to achieve surgical anesthesia.

They were also more likely to require supplemental doses of anesthetic, which were given through the epidural catheter placed after injection. There was no difference in time to anesthesia. Thirty-one percent of the needle group and 36% of the catheter group had hypotension, a nonsignificant difference. Neither were there any significant differences in quality of anesthesia or degree of motor blockade.

Conclusions.—In women undergoing cesarean section, needle induction of epidural anesthesia produces no faster onset of surgical anesthesia than catheter induction. Neither is there any difference in the incidence or severity of maternal hypotension. Thus, given the safety advantages of the incremental catheter technique, it is preferred for induction of epidural anesthesia.

▶ This study refutes my long-held bias that the "through-the-needle" technique results in a faster onset of epidural anesthesia for cesarean section. The authors convincingly argue that the through-the-needle injection technique offers no advantages over the catheter technique. One disadvantage of the through-the-needle technique is that the anesthesiologist may be tempted to give a large bolus of local anesthetic rapidly, which may result in an increased risk of systemic toxicity or high spinal anesthesia. The therapeutic dose of epidural local anesthetic should be given slowly and incrementally, regardless of the technique.

D.H. Chestnut, M.D.

Changes in the Position of Epidural Catheters Associated With Patient Movement

Hamilton CL, Rilely ET, Cohen SE (Stanford Univ, Calif)
Anesthesiology 86:778–784, 1997 5–23

Introduction.—Unsatisfactory analgesia has been reported in 1.5% to 23% of obstetric patients receiving epidural anesthesia. In morbidly obese women, this failure may be as high as 42%. Properly placed catheters can become displaced, as a result of patient movement, after being secured. Two hundred fifty-five women undergoing epidural anesthesia for labor or cesarean section were evaluated to determine whether the displacement phenomenon occurred with patient movement and whether it is of clinical significance. A technique was developed to minimize epidural displacement.

Methods.—A multiorifaced lumbar epidural catheter was inserted with patients sitting in the flexed position. As patients moved from sitting flexed to sitting upright, then to the lateral decubitus position, the distance to the epidural space, length of catheter inserted, and amount of catheter position change were measured before securing the catheter to the skin. Adequacy of analgesia, need for catheter manipulation, and presence or absence of obesity were recorded. Data were grouped by body mass index (BMI) of less than 25, 25–30, and more than 30 kg/m^2.

Results.—There were no between-group differences in length of catheter initially inserted or changes in catheter position between initial taping and removal. With increasing BMI, there were significant differences between distances to the epidural space. Catheters seemed to be drawn inward with position change from the sitting flexed to lateral decubitus position, especially in patients with a BMI higher than 30. There were no analgesic failures in the group with BMI more than 30 kg/m^2. In that group, patients had a greater distance to the epidural space and more catheter movement with position change than nonobese women.

Conclusion.—There was a clinically significant amount of catheter movement with position change in all BMI groups. Many catheters would have been pulled partially out of the epidural space if secured to the skin before position change. It is suggested that multiorifaced catheters be inserted at least 4 cm into the epidural space and that patients (especially obese ones) be placed in the sitting upright or lateral position before the catheter is secured.

▶ This study does not prove that the authors' technique is better than other techniques. The authors did not compare outcomes with this technique vs. outcomes in a control group of women whose catheters were secured to the skin before the patient assumed the lateral decubitus position. However, the authors' methods and observations seem logical and credible. This study has changed my practice in obstetric anesthesia. I now follow their recommendations, and the results have been positive.

D.H. Chestnut, M.D.

Infection Issues

Prevention of Central Venous Catheter–related Bloodstream Infection by Use of an Antiseptic-impregnated Catheter

Maki DG, Stolz SM, Wheeler S, et al (Univ of Wisconsin, Madison)

Ann Intern Med 127:257–266, 1997 5–24

Introduction.—Nearly all vascular catheter–related bloodstream infections are related to the use of noncuffed central venous catheters. Preventive strategies include potent cutaneous antiseptic agents, topical application of antimicrobial agents, and attachment of a subcutaneous silver-impregnated cuff. A new antiseptic venous catheter was evaluated in a randomized, controlled clinical trial.

Methods.—The study was conducted in a medical-surgical ICU. Patients scheduled to have a catheter placed were randomly assigned to receive a control catheter or an antiseptic catheter. Test and control catheters were identical (noncuffed, triple-lumen, 30.5-cm, 16-G catheters) except that the test catheter's external surface was impregnated with minute quantities of chlorhexidine gluconate (0.75 mg) and silver sulfadiazine (0.70 mg). All catheters were examined for colonization and catheter-related bloodstream infection at removal, and patient tolerance of the catheter was

TABLE 3.—Outcomes of Catheter-related Infection

Variable	Control Catheters (n = 195)	Antiseptic Catheters (n = 208)	Relative Risk (95% CI)	*P* Value
Colonized catheters, *n* (*n per 100 catheters*)	47 (24.1)	28 (13.5)	0.56 (0.36–0.89)	0.005
Catheters leading to catheter-related bloodstream infection, *n* (*n* per 100 catheters)	9 (4.6)	2 (1.0)	0.21 (0.03–0.95)	0.03
Bloodstream infection with gram-negative bacilli, *Staphylococcus aureus*, enterococci, or *Candida* species, *n* (*n per 100 catheters*)	8 (4.1)	0 (−)	− (0.02–0.65)	0.003
Colonization, *n* (*n causing bloodstream infection*)*				
Coagulase-negative staphylococci	34 (1)	24 (2)		>0.05
Enterococci	4 (1)	3		>0.05
S. aureus	1 (1)	1		
Gram-negative bacilli	7 (2)	3		>0.05
Candida species	8 (4)	1		0.05
Other	6	4		>0.05

*Eleven control catheters and 8 antiseptic catheters were infected by more than 1 species.

Abbreviation: CI, confidence interval.

(Courtesy of Maki DG, Stolz SM, Wheeler S, et al: Prevention of central venous catheter–related blood stream infection by use of an antiseptic-impregnated catheter: A randomized, controlled trial. *Ann Intern Med* 127:257–266, 1997.)

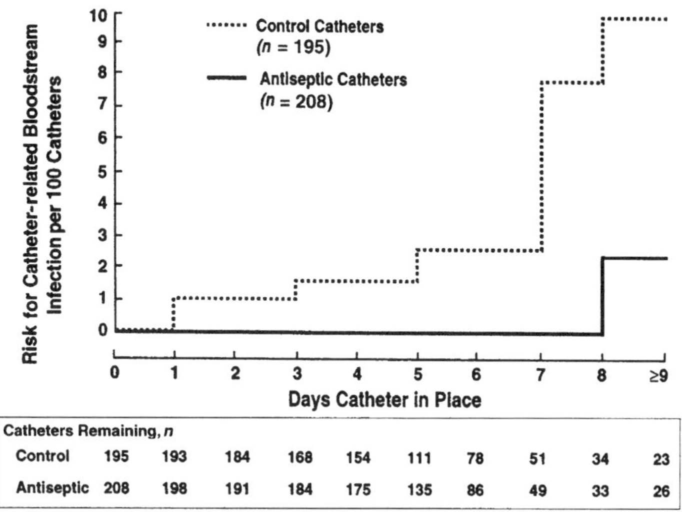

Catheters Remaining, *n*										
Control	195	193	184	168	154	111	78	51	34	23
Antiseptic	208	198	191	184	175	135	86	49	33	26

FIGURE 1.—Kaplan-Meier estimate of the cumulative risk for catheter-related bloodstream infection. The differences between groups are highly significant ($P = 0.01$, log-rank test). (Courtesy of Maki DG, Stolz SM, Wheeler S, et al: Prevention of central venous catheter–related bloodstream infection by use of an antiseptic-impregnated catheter: A randomized, controlled trial. *Ann Intern Med* 127:257–266, 1997.)

recorded. In the case of infection, all potential sources were cultured and findings confirmed by restriction-fragment DNA subtyping.

Results.—Complete data were obtained for 403 catheters (195 control and 208 antiseptic) in 158 patients. Most patients in each group were highly vulnerable to nosocomial infection because of their medical condition and multiple invasive medical devices. Catheters remained in place for an average of 6 days in each group. Compared with control catheters, antiseptic catheters were less likely to be colonized at removal (relative risk 0.56) and 5-fold less likely to produce bloodstream infection (relative risk 0.21). Eight patients in the control group, but none in the antiseptic group, had bloodstream infection caused by *Staphylococcus aureus,* gram-negative bacilli, enterococci, or *Candida* species (Table 3). There was a highly significant difference in the cumulative risk for catheter-related bloodstream infection in the 2 groups (Fig 1). The antiseptic catheter was not associated with any adverse effects.

Conclusions.—The antiseptic catheter was well tolerated, prevented catheter colonization, and reduced the incidence of bloodstream infection. Because nosocomial bloodstream infections are associated with high mortality, prolonged hospitalization, and additional cost (approximately $29,000), the antiseptic catheter should also prove cost-effective.

Central Venous Catheters Coated With Minocycline and Rifampin for the Prevention of Catheter-related Colonization and Bloodstream Infections: A Randomized, Double-blind Trial

Raad I, Darouiche R, Dupuis J, et al (Univ of Texas MD Anderson Cancer Ctr, Houston; Baylor College of Medicine, Houston; Ben Taub Gen Hosp, Houston; et al)

Ann Intern Med 127:267–274, 1997 5–25

Introduction.—Central venous catheters are the leading cause of primary nosocomial bloodstream infection. Topical application of antiseptic and antibiotic agents at the insertion site can lower the risk for catheter colonization and infection, but a more effective strategy might be the coating of venous catheters with these agents. The incidence of catheter-related colonization and bloodstream infections with coated and non-coated central venous catheters were compared.

Methods.—Study participants were 281 hospitalized patients at 5 university-based medical centers. The coated catheters were pretreated with tridodecylmethyl–ammonium chloride, then coated 18 hours later with minocycline and rifampin. Both coated and uncoated catheters were triple-lumen, polyurethane, 7 French, and 20 cm long. All were inserted into the subclavian, internal jugular, or femoral vein and were not exchanged over guidewires. Insertion sites were cleaned with an antiseptic agent at the time

TABLE 3.—Frequency and Microbiological Cause of Catheter Colonization and Bloodstream Infections

Variable	Uncoated Cultured Catheters (n = 136)	Coated Cultured Catheters (n = 130)	P Value
Catheter colonization, n (%)*	36 (26)	11 (8)	<0.001
Staphylococcus epidermidis	16 (12)	2 (2)	<0.001
Other coagulase-negative staphylococci	3 (2)	0	0.01
S. aureus	1 (1)	0	>0.2
Gram-negative bacilli	3 (2)	2 (2)	>0.2
Candida albicans	1 (1)	3 (2)	>0.2
C. tropicalis	0	1 (1)	>0.2
Polymicrobial	12 (9)	3 (2)	>0.02
Catheter-related bloodstream infections, n (%)†	7 (5)	0	<0.01
Infections confirmed by DNA typing, n (%)†	5 (4)	0	0.02
Infections/1000 catheter-days, n‡	7.34	0	<0.01
Infections confirmed by DNA typing/ 1000 catheter-days, n‡	5.16	0	0.03

*Catheter colonization was defined as the isolation of at least 15 colony-forming units of any organism by the roll-plate method or at least 10^3 colony-forming units by the sonication method. The Fisher exact test was used to compare the 2 groups. Relative risk for colonization for uncoated catheters was 3.13 (95% confidence interval, 1.66–5.88).

†Exact log-rank test was used; relative risks were undefined.

‡Binomial exact test was used.

(Courtesy of Raad I, Darouiche R, Dupuis J, et al: Central venous catheters coated with minocycline and rifampin for the prevention of catheter-related colonization and bloodstream infections: A randomized, double-blind trial. *Ann Intern Med* 127:267–274, 1997.)

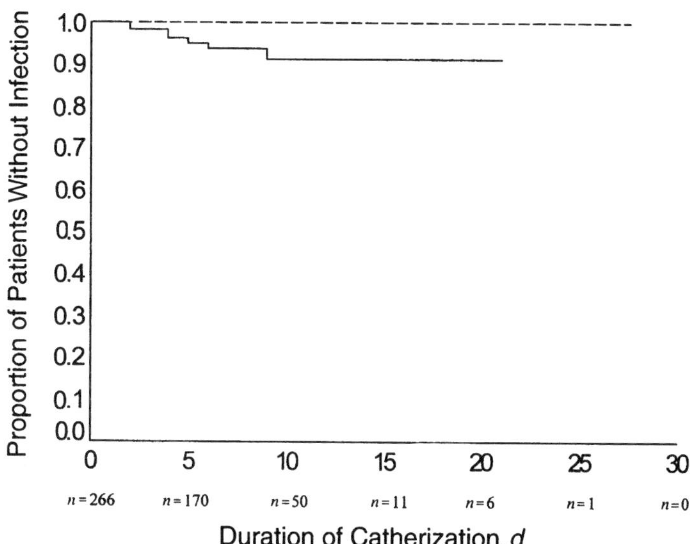

FIGURE 2.—Time to occurrence of catheter-related bloodstream infection according to study group. The difference between coated (*dashed line*) and uncoated catheters (*solid line*) was significant ($P < 0.01$, exact log-rank test). The numbers of catheters at risk in each group at various time points are indicated on the abscissa. (Courtesy of Raad I, Darouiche R, Dupuis J, et al: Central venous catheters coated with minocycline and rifampin for the prevention of catheter-related colonization and bloodstream infections: A randomized, double-blind trial. *Ann Intern Med* 127:267–274, 1997.)

of insertion and at each dressing change. Sites were inspected every 72 hours. Catheter segments were cultured at the time of removal; skin samples from the insertion site were cultured at insertion and within 24 hours after catheter removal.

Results.—Patients in the 2 catheter groups were similar in age, sex, underlying diseases, degree of immunosuppression, therapeutic interventions, and risk factors for catheter infections. The incidence of colonization was significantly lower in coated catheters (8%) than in uncoated catheters (26%). Seven patients in the uncoated catheter group, but none in the coated catheter group, had catheter-related bloodstream infections (Table 3). Rates of these infections (Fig 2) were 7.34 for uncoated vs. 0 for coated catheters (per 1,000 catheter-days). Coating central venous catheters with minocycline and rifampin was an independent risk factor against catheter-related colonization. These catheters caused no adverse effects, nor were they associated with antimicrobial resistance. Because of the high cost of treating colonization and bloodstream infections, the coated catheters could lead to significant savings.

Conclusions.—The venous catheters coated with minocycline and rifampin decreased the risk for colonization and infection without causing any adverse effects or promoting the development of bacterial resistance to the antimicrobial agents.

Central Venous Catheter Replacement Strategies: A Systematic Review of the Literature

Cook D, Randolph A, Kernerman P, et al (McMaster Univ, Hamilton, Ont; Harvard Univ, Boston; Univ of Toronto; et al)

Crit Care Med 25:1417–1424, 1997 5–26

Introduction.—Central venous catheters are associated with nosocomial morbidity and mortality. Replacement of the catheters can be achieved with new-site replacement or by guidewire exchange using the Seldinger technique. Compared with new-site venipuncture, exchanging catheters over a guidewire is reported to be associated with fewer serious mechanical complications and no increased risk of infection. The 2 strategies were assessed for frequency of catheter colonization and infection, catheter-related bacteremia, and mechanical complications.

Methods.—Published and unpublished research was reviewed for clinical trials evaluating the effect of guidewire exchange and new-site replacement in seriously ill patients and to compare outcome using scheduled catheter management vs. as-needed catheter management. Sources of data included MEDLINE, the Science Citation Index, a manual search of Index Medicus, citation review of primary and review articles, and contact with primary investigators. A pool of 151 randomized, controlled trials yielded 12 that were relevant to the review. These trials were examined for methodologic quality, study design, and outcomes.

Results.—The 12 trials were published between 1981 and 1995. Guidewire exchange was associated with a trend toward an increased frequency of catheter colonization (relative risk 1.26) and more frequent catheter exit-site infection (relative risk 1.52). There was also a trend toward an increased frequency of catheter-related bacteremia with guidewire exchange, both when all trials were pooled and when only the 4 trials meeting strict criteria for catheter-related bacteremia or sepsis were pooled (relative risk 1.68). Patients undergoing guidewire exchange did show a trend toward decreased mechanical complications (relative risk 0.48). Prophylactic catheter replacement at 3 days did not reduce catheter colonization in comparison with a protocol of replacement every 7 days or as needed.

Conclusions.—Guidewire exchange of central venous catheters is associated with fewer mechanical complications than new-site replacement, but the risk of catheter-related infection appears to be increased. Thus meticulous aseptic technique is required if guidewire exchange is used. The appropriate interval for scheduled catheter exchange has yet to be determined.

► Multiple studies have concluded that 90% of all nosocomial bloodstream infections are associated with the use of central venous catheters. These catheters often become colonized with microbacteria from the skin surrounding the insertion site. A number of factors are noted to increase the risk for infection and include the site of insertion (internal jugular greater than subclavian), lack of barrier precautions, the use of a multi-lumen catheter, and user inexperience. The 3 articles reviewed above (Abstracts 5–24, 5–25, and 5–26) would suggest that aseptic technique coupled with catheters impregnated with either antimicrobial or antibacterial agents could minimize bloodstream infections associated with triple-lumen central venous catheters. Guidewire exchange of central venous catheters appears to be associated with an increased risk of catheter-related infections, which again may be mitigated, as was shown in the study by Maki et al., by the use of antiseptic-impregnated catheters. Future studies need to address whether coating catheters for such procedures as femoral arterial monitoring, intra-aortic balloon counterpulsation, or pulmonary artery pressure monitoring could further decrease nosocomial infection from intravascular catheters.

D.M. Rothenberg, M.D.

Neurologic Monitoring

Continuous Intraoperative Monitoring of Middle Cerebral Artery Blood Flow Velocities and Electroencephalography During Carotid Endarterectomy: A Comparision of the Two Methods to Detect Cerebral Ischemia

Arnold M, Sturzenegger M, Schäffler L, et al (Univ of Berne, Switzerland)
Stroke 28:1345–1350, 1997 5–27

Objective.—Although carotid endarterectomy for high-grade internal carotid artery stenosis reduces the risk of death and stroke by 9.6% at 3 years and of ipsilateral stroke by 17% at 2 years, the overall benefit is lost if perioperative morbidity and mortality rate exceeds 9%. Velocities of middle cerebral artery blood flow (VMCAs) can be monitored by using transcranial Doppler (TCD) or electroencephalogram (EEG). The few studies that have compared the methods have yielded conflicting results. Results of a retrospective study comparing the results of both methods examined the degrees of changes in both methods and the ability to predict complications are presented.

Methods.—Over a 3-year period, 82 carotid endarterectomies were performed in 77 patients (16 women), aged 56–80 years, using 8-channel EEG and continuous TCD monitoring techniques. Thiopental administration interfered with EEG monitoring in 11 patients. VMCA decrease and frequency of intraoperative EEG changes, mean VMCA decrease and intraoperative EEG changes, and VMCA decrease and degree of contralateral carotid stenosis and shunt rates and degree of contralateral carotid stenosis were compared.

Results.—After cross clamping there was a significant correlation between percent decrease of VMCA and the incidence of EEG changes. Mean VMCA changes in patients with and without EEG changes were 53% and 20%, respectively (Fig 2). Although VMCA decreased significantly in contralateral stenosed or occluded carotid arteries compared with normal contralateral carotid arteries, only TCD findings were significant. Patients

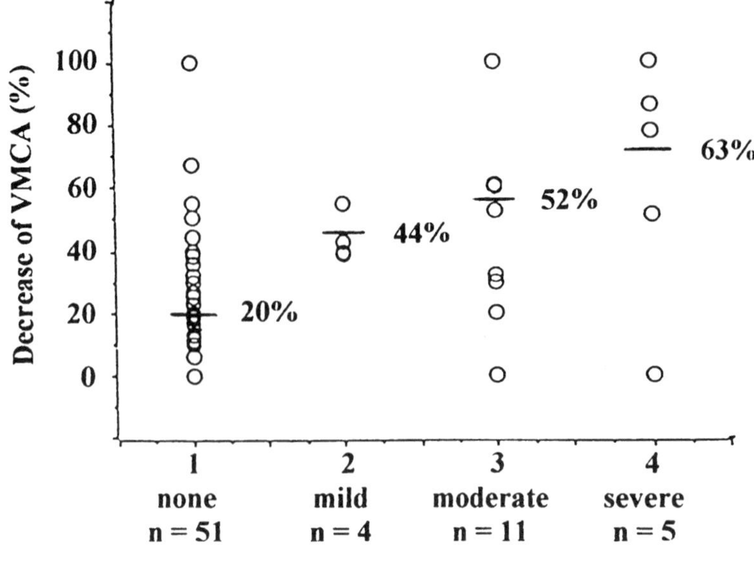

FIGURE 2.—Variation of TCD findings and EEG changes during cross clamping in the individual patients. Horizontal bars indicate the mean percentage decrease of VMCA in the 4 categories of EEG changes. (Courtesy of Arnold M, Sturzenegger M, Schäffler L, et al: Continuous intraoperative monitoring of middle cerebral artery blood flow velocities and electroencephalography during carotid endarterectomy: a comparison of the two methods to detect cerebral ischemia. *Stroke* 28:1345–1350, 1997.)

with a contralateral stenosed or occluded carotid artery required a shunt significantly more often than patients with a normal contralateral carotid artery. Cerebral complications included an intraoperative ipsilateral transient ischemic attack in 4 patients, a postoperative stroke in 2, and a postoperative transient ischemic attack in 1. The death and stroke rate was 3.6%.

Conclusion.—There was a significant correlation between EEG and TCD findings, although EEG findings did not add significantly to the information provided by TCD. Temporary shunting was provided in several patients on the basis of TCD findings.

▶ Within the literature, there is controversy between conclusions related to these two monitoring techniques. Although "EEG permits noninvasive continuous monitoring of bioelectrical activity of the superficial hemispheric cortex" and "TCD allows continuous noninvasive measurement of VMCA," to what extent do these different monitors predict cerebral injury, which, after all, is their purpose? As the authors correctly point out with EEG, there are a number of important considerations such as "...the influence of anesthesia, definition and grading of EEG changes, numbers of EEG channels recorded, and the method of analysis (computerized versus visual analysis by an experienced neurologist)." The authors appropriately define the per-

Subscribe to the Advances in your specialty

Yes! I would like my own copy of ***Advances in Anesthesia®*** at the price of **$81.00** plus sales tax, postage, and handling. Please begin my subscription with the current edition according to the terms described below.* I understand that I will have 30 days to examine each annual edition.

Name ______________________________

Address ______________________________

City ______________________ State __________ ZIP __________

Method of Payment

Check (in U.S. dollars, drawn on a U.S. bank, payable to ***Advances in Anesthesia®***)

❑ VISA ❑ MasterCard ❑ Discover ❑ AmEx ❑ Bill me

Card number ______________________ Exp. date: __________

Signature ______________________________

Prices are subject to change without notice. PMC-044

Reservation Card for the Year Book

Yes! I would like my own copy of ***Year Book of Anesthesiology and Pain Management®*** at the price of **$79.00** plus sales tax, postage, and handling. Please begin my subscription with the current edition according to the terms described below.* I understand that I will have 30 days to examine each annual edition.

Name ______________________________

Address ______________________________

City ______________________ State __________ ZIP __________

Method of Payment

Check (in U.S. dollars, drawn on a U.S. bank, payable to ***Year Book of Anesthesiology and Pain Management®***)

❑ VISA ❑ MasterCard ❑ Discover ❑ AmEx ❑ Bill me

Card number ______________________ Exp. date: __________

Signature ______________________________

Prices are subject to change without notice. PMC-006

*Your Year Book or Advances service guarantee:

When you subscribe to the *Year Book* or *Advances*, you will receive advance notice of future annual volumes about two months before publication. To receive the new edition, you need do nothing—we'll send you the new volume as soon as it is available. If you want to discontinue, the advance notice allows you time to notify us of your decision. If you are not completely satisfied, you have 30 days to return any *Year Book* or *Advances*.

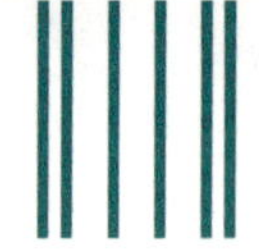

NO POSTAGE NECESSARY IF MAILED IN THE UNITED STATES

BUSINESS REPLY MAIL

FIRST-CLASS MAIL PERMIT NO 135 ST LOUIS MO

POSTAGE WILL BE PAID BY ADDRESSEE

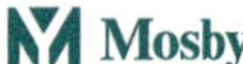

PAT NEWMAN
11830 WESTLINE INDUSTRIAL DRIVE
PO BOX 46908
ST. LOUIS MO 63146-9934

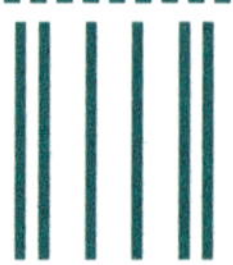

NO POSTAGE NECESSARY IF MAILED IN THE UNITED STATES

BUSINESS REPLY MAIL

FIRST-CLASS MAIL PERMIT NO 135 ST LOUIS MO

POSTAGE WILL BE PAID BY ADDRESSEE

Mosby

PAT NEWMAN
11830 WESTLINE INDUSTRIAL DRIVE
PO BOX 46908
ST. LOUIS MO 63146-9934

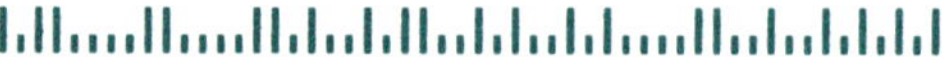

Want to speed up the process?

To order, you also may call 1-800-426-4545.

Mosby, Inc.
11830 Westline Industrial Drive
St. Louis, MO 63146 U.S.A.

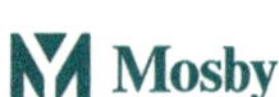

centage change in VMCA from baseline values and the definition of processed EEG changes that they considered mild, moderate, and severe. From Figure 2 they demonstrate a statistical correlation between VMCA and EEG changes ($P < 0.001$). However, the variability between the 2 was marked. There were patients who had a 100% reduction of VMCA (100 on they-axis) or no reduction of VMCA (0 on the y-axis) in all categories of EEG changes. In 1 of 4 patients with intraoperative neurologic injury, the event was predicted by both TCD and EEG monitoring.

Important points to consider are: (1) Three quarters of cerebral injury associated with carotid endarterectomies are due to emboli, presumably from the surgical field, and the remainder from inadequate blood flow over large areas (hemodynamic). (2) Emboli produce ischemia or infarction in small cerebral areas and therefore would not be expected to change the EEG, be seen easily on computed tomographic scan, or alter cerebral blood flow velocity. (3) EEG looks at the functional electrical integrity of large areas of cerebral cortex and, as such, reflects hemispheric blood flow. (4) The middle cerebral artery is a major vessel supplying blood to the cerebral cortex but is not the only vessel to do so. (5) The purpose of monitoring is to assess the adequacy of the hemodynamic component by determining the adequacy of collateral circulation to the brain based on cerebral functioning in the cortex (EEG) or cerebral blood flow in a major vessel (MCA) (TCD). To expect that either monitor will predict injury from emboli, which what most intraoperative injury is caused by, is a major misunderstanding of the pathogenesis of morbidity associated with CEA and the limitations of both monitors.

E.J. Heyer, M.D., Ph.D.

Intraoperative Identification of Spinal Cord Blood Supply During Repairs of Descending Aorta and Thoracoabdominal Aorta

Svensson LG (Lahey Hitchcock Clinic, Burlington, Mass)

J Thorac Cardiovasc Surg 112:1455–1461, 1996 5–28

Background.—Although repairs of the descending thoracic aorta and thoracoabdominal aorta have become much safer, paraplegia remains a problem, especially if the aortic crossclamp time is too long. Intraoperative identification of the spinal cord blood supply and shortening of the aortic crossclamp time were described in a current study.

Methods.—Five patients had descending aortic repairs; 3, type I thoracoabdominal aneurysm repairs; and 6, type II repairs. The surgeon placed a platinum electrode intrathecally by lumbar puncture alongside the spinal cord. The aorta was then crossclamped, and hydrogen in a saline solution was injected into the aorta. If the segment was seen to supply the spinal cord and there were multiple arteries, then individual injections were performed. The surgeon then performed the repair using a sequential segmental method.

Findings.—Highly selective angiography after surgery confirmed that reattached intercostal arteries supplied the spinal cord. In all patients, the technique was accurate. The spinal cord perfusion patterns observed were classified as direct, collateral, no direct supply from segment tested, from atriofemoral bypass, and occluded reattached intercostals. No response was obtained or further assessment required in 8 patients. This group had a testing time of 4.2 minutes and a crossclamp time of 41.9 minutes. When multiple segmental arteries necessitated further assessment, the mean testing time was 10.4 minutes, and the crossclamp time was 58.5 minutes, including reattachment of intercostal vessels.

Conclusions.—This research technique appears to be safe and effective in enabling radicular artery detection. It may also reduce the time for aortic crossclamping if no vessels are identified as supplying the spinal cord.

▶ The author describes an experimental technique that appears to have great value in identifying the segments supplying blood to the spinal cord. Early paraplegia after thoracoabdominal aortic repair is one of the major and most feared complications. Luckily, it doesn't happen in many patients. The extra time taken to do this testing was approximately 10½ minutes. Further, the discussion of the article by experts centers around whether there is danger with recurrent clamping of the aneursymal segment, and dislodgment of clot, causing more problems than this technique would solve. The author, a polished surgeon from the Lahey-Hitchcock Clinic in Burlington, Massachusetts, assures those questioning him that this is not a problem.

M.F. Roizen, M.D.

Other Techniques, Monitoring

Penile Intracorporeal Infusion—Possible Access to the Systemic Circulation: Pressure Flow Studies in Dogs and Humans

Gofrit ON, Leibovici D, Shapira SC, et al (Hadassah Univ, Jerusalem; Rambam Med Ctr, Haifa, Israel)

Eur J Surg 163:457–461, 1997 5–29

Introduction.—In patients with advanced shock or those who have sustained extensive limb injuries, achieving emergency peripheral intravenous access is difficult, time-consuming, and occasionally impossible. Even in severe shock, the penile corpora cavernosa are paired vascular spaces that do not collapse. There has been the possibility of infusing fluids into the corpora cavernosa of patients in shock, but this has not been heretofore attempted. Patients can tolerate the insertion of the needle into the corpora, which is safe and easy. The flaccid corpora cavernosa was used as access to the systemic circulation because large quantities of fluids can often be infused during cavernosometry when the venous occlusion mechanism of the corpora cavernosa is impaired.

Methods.—In 5 dogs and 10 humans, pressure-flow studies were conducted, and then were repeated in dogs during an episode of hypovolemic shock. As part of their evaluation for impotence, 10 men were referred for cavernosometry. A corpus cavernosum of the mid-shaft of the flaccid penis had 2 19-gauge scalp vein needles inserted obliquely. Using a pressure cuff inflated to 300 mm Hg, Ringer's lactate solution was infused through 1 of the needles. A sudden loss of resistance and backflow of blood is seen in the intravenous tubing as the needle pierces the tunica albuginea, indicating the needle is in the right place. A circular adhesive bandage was used to secure the needle to the shaft of the penis. Measurements were taken from the time from skin penetration to fixation of the needle.

Results.—For the Ringer's lactate solution, the mean infusion rate through the canine corpora was 110 mL/min and for autologous blood, it was 109 mL/min. Into the human corpora, the mean infusion was 89.7 mL/min in the psychogenic impotent patients, and in the organic impotent patients, it was 88.2 mL/min. To insert the needle, the mean time taken was 15 seconds.

Conclusions.—In a short period, an intracorporeal infusion line can be established. Through the human and canine corpora cavernosa, adequate quantities of fluids can be infused. The catheter's caliber dictates the flow rate because the resistance to flow through the flaccid corpora cavernosa is low. Using a wider catheter, a higher flow rate can be attained.

▶ This article redefines the concept of intraosseous infusion!

D.M. Rothenberg, M.D.

Sevoflurane Inhalation Induction for Emergency Cesarean Section in a Parturient With No Intravenous Access

Schaut DJ, Khona R, Gross JB (Univ of Connecticut, Farmington)

Anesthesiology 86:1392–1394, 1997 5–30

Background.—Patients who require emergency cesarean section because of fetal distress undergo rapid sequence induction of IV general anesthesia and paralysis. These patients are treated as if they are at risk of aspiration of gastric contents, with its attendant maternal morbidity. However, it is possible that the severity of fetal distress may mandate delivery before IV is available. Inhalation induction of anesthesia with a volatile, nonirritating anesthetic, sevoflurane, was used in 1 patient for emergency cesarean section, with a successful outcome.

Case Report.—Woman, 29, uniparous, gravida 2, at 38 weeks' gestation was admitted with labor pain. During the initial examination, her membranes ruptured and revealed a double footling breech fetus with 15–20 cm of prolapsed umbilical cord. The obstetrician manually attempted to retain the fetus in the uterus as the patient was wheeled to the delivery room. When the anesthesia call team was emergently summoned, the fetal heart rate was 50 beats/min, preparations were underway for an emergency cesarean section, and the obstetrician insisted that the infant be delivered immediately, because of worsening fetal distress. There was no IV access nor maternal monitors. No veins were apparent. An anesthesia mask was applied and 10 L/min of oxygen with 8% sevoflurane was administered. Within 30 seconds, the patient was no longer responsive to verbal commands and eyelash reflex was absent, but spontaneous ventilation continued. After incision, there was no change in respiratory pattern or increase in heart rate. The infant was delivered by cesarean section less than 5 minutes after the patient's arrival in the operating room, less than 3 minutes after initiation of anesthesia, and within 1 minute of incision. The 1-minute Apgar score was 2, the 5-minute score was 6, and the 10-minute score was 8. The neonate was intubated to assist oxygenation. Within 2 hours, he was extubated and spent time in his mother's room. After an uneventful night in neonatal intensive care, he was transferred to the nursery and was discharged home with his mother after 2 days.

Discussion.—For the anesthesiologist, the primary concern during an emergency cesarean section is the safety of the mother. However, when any delay in delivery may lead to the death of the fetus, there may not be sufficient time available to obtain the IV access necessary for rapid sequence induction. This case report describes the use of inhalation induction with sevoflurane for emergency cesarean section in a patient with a prolapsed umbilical cord and no IV access, which resulted in a favorable outcome for both mother and infant. A rapid-acting nonirritating anesthetic such as sevoflurane may prove useful in the treatment of patients requiring emergency cesarean section under difficult circumstances.

▶ This is a provocative case report. The authors acknowledged that "for the anesthesiologist, the first concern in an emergency cesarean section is to ensure the safety of the mother." Yet many would argue that it is inappropriate to anesthetize a parturient for an emergency cesarean section without IV access.

D.H. Chestnut, M.D.

New Agents, the Circle System and Short Procedures

Nel MR, Ooi R, Lee DJH, et al (Chelsea and Westminster Hosp, London)
Anaesthesia 52:364–381, 1997 5–31

Background.—Compared with other anesthetic breathing systems, the circle system has the advantage of permitting anesthesia with low fresh gas flows. This has physiologic, economic, and environmental benefits. Sevoflurane, desflurane, and isoflurane were compared in the circle system during short surgeries.

Methods.—Ninety-seven patients undergoing short surgical procedures were included in the study. The intervals to equilibration between inspired and end-expired agent concentrations were determined using initial high flows. Equilibration was defined as $F_E/F_I = 0.8$.

Findings.—Mean time to equilibration for sevoflurane was 8.2 minutes; for desflurane, 3.8 minutes; and for isoflurane, 19.7 minutes. The differences between these times were significant. Total flows were decreased to 500 ml/min^{-1} after equilibration. At these flows, the initial decline in end-expired agent concentration was minimal with desflurane, intermediate with sevoflurane, and greatest with isoflurane.

Conclusions.—Desflurane and sevoflurane are both suitable for the efficient use of the circle system during short anesthetic administration. Desflurane equilibrates more rapidly than sevoflurane and is almost ideal for circle system use in short cases. However, sevoflurane can also be used effectively.

► This paper contains some interesting data. The times required to achieve an expired to inspired ratio of at least 0.8 were 8.2 minutes for sevoflurane, 3.8 minutes for desflurane, and 19.7 minutes for isoflurane. Why was the time for sevoflurane so much longer than for desflurane? Sevoflurane's blood gas coefficient is only a little higher than that of desflurane. These patients were already anesthetized, so the pungency issues with respect to desflurane did not come into play here. Apparently the tachycardia seen with rapid changes in desflurane concentration was also avoided in this protocol. I think the answer to the disparate times to achieve equilibration has to do with the inspired concentrations administered. The authors gave sevoflurane at 2.5%, but they gave desflurane at 8.0%. Because of the concentration effect, the rate of rise to a high expired to inspired ratio was faster owing to the greater concentration of desflurane. I included the paper because it's an interesting commentary on uptake and distribution. Actual times for satisfactory clinical induction of anesthesia will be nowhere near that disparate between sevoflurane and desflurane because of the pungency issues; sevoflurane is generally considered to be a smoother agent with which to induce anesthesia.

J.H. Tinker, M.D.

Glucose Level and Myocardial Recovery After Warm Arrest

Ning X-H, Childs KF, Bolling SF (Univ of Michigan, Ann Arbor)

Ann Thorac Surg 62:1825–1829, 1996 5–32

Objective.—Warm cardioplegia confers superior cardioprotection during cardiac operations. Whether the addition of glucose facilitates cardiac functional recovery during reperfusion is controversial. The myocardial metabolic and functional recovery after global ischemia and reperfusion was investigated in rabbits using warm cardioplegia with increasing glucose concentrations.

Methods.—Rapidly excised rabbits hearts were retrograde-perfused. Cardioplegia solution was injected every 30 minutes with glucose concentration increasing from 0 to 88 mmol/L during the 2-hour warm ischemia period. Osmolarity was adjusted. Lactate, pH, and carbon dioxide content of coronary effluent were measured at baseline and during reflow. Nucleoside and nucleotide content of heart biopsy specimens were determined.

Results.—The addition of 5.5–88 mmol/L glucose significantly improved functional recovery. There were no significant differences between glucose increments in functional recovery, which peaked at 22 mmol/L glucose. Recovery of postischemic myocardial oxygen consumption and oxygen extraction and high-energy phosphate levels were significantly enhanced at 22 mmol/L glucose.

Conclusion.—During warm cardioplegia, moderately increasing glucose levels enhances functional recovery by increasing high-energy phosphate levels. Elevating glucose levels to extreme hyperglycemia does not improve functional recovery.

▶ As I started to read this article, I remembered how much I hate the systeme international for research reports. It turns out that the authors use a glucose value between 0 and 88 mmol/L to get the glucose in milligrams percent, so that one has to divide by 0.055 or multiply by 18. Thus, they find a value at which maximum benefit is 22 mmol/L, the equivalent of roughly 400 mg/dL. Clearly, their interpretation of "functional" means only what happens in the short term. That is, in fact, the major deficit of this study in rabbit hearts. The better immediate recovery of myocardial ennergetics as reflected by contractility does not indicate long-term well-being or survival based on what might happen 2 or 3 hours later after the effect of edema in the arteries, caused by the loss of auto-regulation that the high glucose results in, has its effects.

Thus, while this study does point out an important recovery of myocardial ennergetics with high glucose, or with a glucose level that is higher than we might conceive of using, this benefit may be only a short-term in vitro benefit and not a long-term in vivo benefit. Other authors have shown that a level this high may, in fact, be bad for both the heart and brain, and that a U-shaped response curve for glucose might show that a value between 100 and 200 mg (5–11 mmol/L) might be optimal in both warm and cold situations.

M.F. Roizen, M.D.

Environmental Monitoring During Gaseous Induction With Sevoflurane

Hall JE, Henderson KA, Oldham TA, et al (Univ of Wales, Cardiff)

Br J Anaesth 79:342–345, 1997 5–33

Objective.—Gaseous induction with sevoflurane has been shown to be safe. Triple vital capacity induction in adults was used to study whether pollution levels in the anesthetic room met the 20-ppm exposure level set by the manufacturer.

Methods.—Environmental monitoring of sevoflurane was carried out during 23 consecutive triple vital capacity sevoflurane inductions in 8% oxygen. Environmental monitoring of nitrous oxide was also performed during 12 inductions using 8% sevoflurane in nitrous oxide and oxygen (2:1). Time-weighted averages were calculated.

Results.—The time-weighted average for sevoflurane with sevoflurane monitoring was 1.1 ppm. The time-weighted average for sevoflurane when nitrous oxide was monitored was 17.3 ppm. The high concentration excursion rate for sevoflurane was 8.3 ppm, and for nitrous oxide monitoring, it was 172.4 ppm. Personal reservoir sampling concentrations were 1.2 ppm for sevoflurane monitoring and 45.9 ppm for nitrous oxide monitoring.

Conclusion.—Anesthetists receive low exposures to sevoflurane during gaseous induction.

► It appears that our British colleagues may be a bit ahead of (or behind?) us in determining permissible occupational exposures to various anesthetics, in this case, sevoflurane. The authors stated that the manufacturer (Abbott Laboratories) set an arbitrary target level of 20 ppm. This apparently was in response to the fact that the British Health and Safety Executive previously set the Occupational Exposure Standard for halothane at 10 ppm. The 20 ppm limit was chosen arbitrarily at 100 times less than the level at which there would be any clinical effect. The authors used peak levels and time-weighted exposures to study this issue. It is of special concern because sevoflurane is so useful for mask induction of pediatric and other kinds of patients.

What interests me about this study, primarily is the obvious "bias" and its apparent lack of attention. Although the authors carried out this sampling during entire operating room days, the anesthetists could not possibly help but understand that this sampling was going on. The question is whether or not they "tightened" their practices during the previous sampling. I don't know how to control for this either. Nonetheless, this elegant study may portend things to come in the United States.

J.H. Tinker, M.D.

Relationship of the Train-of-four Fade Ratio to Clinical Signs and Symptoms of Residual Paralysis in Awake Volunteers

Kopman AF, Yee PS, Neuman GG (New York Med College, Valhalla; St Vincent's Hosp, New York)

Anesthesiology 86:765–771, 1997 5–34

Background.—When train-of-four (TOF) ratio had spontaneously recovered to more than 0.70, acceptable neuromuscular function returned. Little information exists regarding subjective experience accompanying residual neuromuscular block when TOF ratio is 0.70–0.90. Because of the ambulatory surgery being done, where rapid return of cognitive function is normal, examination of standards of neuromuscular recovery seems necessary.

Methods and Materials.—Ten volunteers of American Society of Anestheseologists' physical status 1 were studied. Grip strenth in kilograms, ability to perform 5-sec head- and leg-lift, and ability to hold a wooden tongue depressor between the incisors against resistance were measured. Neuromuscular function was monitored with an electromyographic monitor, and TOF stimulation was done every 20 seconds and the measured TOF fade ratio recorded. Mivacurium (5 mg/kg) was administered as a bolus and an infusion at 2 mg/kg^{-1}/min^{-1} was started and continued until the TOF ratio decreased to less than 0.70. The infusion was adjusted to keep the range between 0.65 and 0.75. Weakness was recorded when the TOF ratio was stable for 10 minutes (± 0.03) when the infusion was not adjusted. All tests were repeated and the TOF allowed to recover to 0.85–0.90, and when stable, all tests were repeated again and the infusion was discontinued. The TOF was measured until a ratio of 1.0 was reached and a final set of observations was recorded.

Results.—No intervention was required to maintain a patent airway and hemoglobin oxygen saturation was always 96% or higher. Diploplia and difficulty tracking moving objects was noted in all subjects when TOF ratio was 0.90 or less; the subjects were not able to strongly appose the incisors until the TOF ratio was greater than 0.85; a 5-sec head-lift was not attained until the TOF averaged 0.60 (range, 0.45–0.75); and grip strength averaged 59% of control (range, 50% to 70%) at a TOF ratio of 0.70. Generally, symptomatology between patients varied widely for any given TOF ratio. Reliable break points for signs and symptoms to be present or absent are not possible.

Conclusions.—Significant signs and symptoms of residual block occur at a TOF of 0.70. Train-of-four fade is slow in developing. In a time when patients may be discharged 2–3 hours after sugery, lingering paresis is an important consideration. Ability to perform a 5-sec head-lift may not be sufficient to protect the airway from regurgitation and aspiration. An area of further interest is the masseter sensitivity to nondepolarizing neuromuscular blocking agents. Satisfactory recovery of neuromuscular function after mivacurium-induced neuromuscular block requires return of TOF ratio to greater than 0.90 and preferably to 1.00.

► Mivacurium is commonly administered to patients undergoing ambulatory surgery, and therefore recovery of neuromuscular function and avoidance of residual neuromuscular weakness is very important for patient safety. I selected this article because Kopman et al. describe in this elegant clinical study the relationship between TOF ratio and clinical signs and symptoms of residual paralysis in awake volunteers who received a mivacurium infusion, and make new recommendations for adequate return of neuromuscular function. An editorial that accompanies the article[1] discusses measurement of neuromuscular function and asks if we should change our practice, because the investigators suggest that recovery of neuromuscular function in an ambulatory setting requires return of the TOF ratio to 0.9 and ideally to unity.

M. Wood, M.D.

Reference

1. Brull SJ: Indicators of recovery of neuromuscular function: Time for change? (editorial) *Anesthesiology* 86:755–757, 1997.

Ethanol Monitoring of the Transurethral Resection Syndrome

Hahn RG, Olsson J (South Hosp, Stockholm; Sundsvall Central Hosp, Sweden)

J Clin Anesth 8:652–655, 1996 5–35

Objective.—The risk of transurethral resection (TUR) syndrome increases significantly when glycine-containing irrigating fluid absorption exceeds 1,000 mL. Addition of 1% to 2% ethanol to the fluid permits quantitative monitoring of absorption by measuring the patient's end-expiratory ethanol concentration with a breathalyzer either with an expired-breath test every 10 minutes in awake patients or with the breathalyzer connected to the ventilation system close to the tracheal tube in anesthetized patients. A case is reported.

Case.—A man, 67, undergoing transurethral resection of the prostate (TURP), received bladder irrigation with prewarmed fluid containing 2% ethanol at an intravesical pressure less than 10 cm of water. The surgeon noticed a small perforation in the prostatic capsule. The breath test indicated an increase in blood ethanol concentration to 30 mg/dL. Forty to 50 minutes into surgery the blood ethanol concentration had reached 95 mg/dL at which point the surgery was terminated. Total blood loss was 1.1 liters. The patient's systolic blood pressure decreased from 130 mm Hg to 80 mm Hg, and he was transferred to intensive care. He became hypothermic and had bradycardia and frequent supraventricular arrhythmias. The patient was warmed and given oxygen, and his electrolyte balance was restored. He recovered and was returned to the urology unit the next afternoon.

Conclusion.—A trace amount of ethanol in irrigating fluid provides an effective and quantitative indicator of fluid absorption during TURP and is a valuable technique for preventing TUR syndrome. Urologists should discontinue surgery immediately when fluid absorption exceeds 2 L. A lower threshold should be selected in high-risk patients.

▶ The authors describe a case report using the breath test from alcohol absorption in transurethral resection. We wonder if there might be an easier method to use, such as the skin patch described years ago. Nevertheless, this is a very effective use of the breathalyzer for an alcohol detection device in the operating room during transurethral resection to provide early detection of the typical fluid absorption syndrome.

M.F. Roizen, M.D.

6 Complications, Mishaps, and Other Perioperative Troubles

Incidence/Severity

Detection of Intraoperative Incidents by Electronic Scanning of Computerized Anesthesia Records: Comparison With Voluntary Reporting
Sanborn KV, Castro J, Kuroda M, et al (Columbia Univ, New York)
Anesthesiology 85:977–987, 1996 6–1

Objective.—Performance measurement requires collecting and analyzing data related to the process and outcome of medical care. Automated anesthesia records (AAR) were investigated to detect intraoperative incidents, to determine if anesthesiologists underreport intraoperative incidents, and to study the occurrence of intraoperative incidents associated with intraoperative and postoperative mortality.

Methods.—Between September 1, 1993, and June 30, 1994, records from 5,454 patients undergoing noncardiothoracic surgery collected using the AAR system were analyzed for deviations from procedure. Physiologic data (recorded every 15 seconds) and blood pressure, heart rate, arterial oxygen saturation, and temperature measurements were reviewed as were computer records of voluntary reports by anesthesiologists of intraoperative deviations. Reports identified as intraoperative incidents were reviewed by 2 independent investigators to eliminate artifacts.

Results.—There were 494 intraoperative incidents reported in 473 anesthesia records. Of these records, 16 reported 2 incidents, and 4 reported 3 incidents. When artifacts and irrelevant incidents were eliminated, there were 434 incidents left. Risk of intraoperative incidents was higher for patients undergoing emergency surgery than for patients undergoing elective surgery (OR 1.4), higher for men than for women (OR 1.4), significantly higher for children and adolescents than for adults, significantly higher for patients age 70 or more than for younger adults, and increased significantly as patient's ASA status increased. Eighteen voluntary reports were found that matched the 434 intraoperative incidents. The sensitivity and specificity of electronic scanning were 97.2% and 98.4%, respectively. Significantly more electronically detected incidents were voluntarily reported for inpatients than for outpatients, for emergency than for elective surgery, and for male than for female patients. There were 29 (7.0%) deaths among the 413 electronically detected incidents and 79 (1.6%) among the 5,041 non-electronically detected incidents.

Conclusion.—The sensitivity and specificity of the anesthesia information management system for detecting intraoperative incidents were 97.2% and 98.4%, respectively. There was a significant association between inpatient mortality and voluntarily reported incidents.

▶ This article is an extremely important one because it gives a value to the intraoperative record, and further it indicates areas where voluntary compliance does not work. One is constantly concerned about voluntary compliance that does not work and puzzled by why it does not work. Did it not work because the physicians did not think things were serious? What happened to the patients whose voluntary compliance did not record a quality assurance indicator, yet the quality assurance check of the automated record did? Did these patients have the same incidence of postoperative problems, or not? Thus, one wants to know if the reason for the low level of compliance with voluntary reporting is due to the fact that these are trivial incidences, or due to lack of understanding that they are important, or due to lack of belief that there is a relationship between the intraoperative incidences and in-hospital morbidity or mortality? Because there was, on the overall set, a strong association between intraoperative incidences and in-hospital mortality, one wonders if that was especially true or not true where no voluntary reports were submitted. Thus, once again, one wonders whether the editors of this journal were simply remiss in not asking for this obvious piece of data, or whether this, like many other good studies, just brings up more questions than it answers.

M.F. Roizen, M.D.

Visual Loss as a Complication of Spine Surgery: A Review of 37 Cases

Myers MA, Hamilton SR, Bogosian AJ, et al (Orthopedic Physician Associates, Seattle; Eye Associates Northwest, Seattle; Physicians Anesthesia Service, Seattle)

Spine 22:1325–1329, 1997 6–2

Background.—Visual loss after spinal surgery is a rare complication, although several cases have been reported in the last few years. The cause of this devastating complication is unknown. Possible risk factors include chronic hypertension, diabetes, smoking, vascular disease, and disorders causing increased blood viscosity.

Methods.—Twenty-seven patients who had visual loss after spinal surgery were identified through a survey of members of the Scoliosis Research

TABLE 1.—Matched Group Comparison

	Blindness Group	Controls
N	28	28
Age (yr)	45.4	45.6
Surgery		
No. of fusions	28	28
No. of revisions	11	11
Mean no. of levels	3.4	3.3
Operative time (min)	430	250*
Intraoperative blood loss (mL)	3600	880*
Hematocrit (%)		
Preoperative	41	40
Lowest recorded	28	29
Systolic blood pressure (mm Hg)		
Preoperative	129	124
Lowest recorded	77	79
Lowest (ION only)	78	80

*$P \leq 0.05$.

Abbreviation: ION, ischemic optic neuropathy.

(Courtesy of Myers MA, Hamilton SR, Bogosian AJ, et al: Visual loss as a complication of spine surgery: A review of 37 cases. *Spine* 22:1325–1329, 1997.)

Society. Another 10 patients were identified from the literature. Medical records were reviewed and risk factors were evaluated.

Results.—The mean patient age was 46.5 years. In 92% of cases, surgery included instrumented posterior fusion. The average operative time was 410 minutes and the average blood loss was 3,500 mL. Significant intraoperative hypotension occurred in most patients. The mean decrease in systolic blood pressure was 130 mm Hg to 77 mm Hg. There were no differences in hematocrit or blood pressure values in these patients compared to a matched group of patients who had no visual loss (Table 1). Visual loss resulted from ischemic optic neuropathy, retinal artery occlusion, or cerebral ischemia. Eleven patients had bilateral visual loss, and 15 patients had complete blindness in at least 1 eye (Table 5). Most cases of visual loss were permanent.

TABLE 5.—Visual Symptoms

Unilateral [no. (%)]	26	(70)
Bilateral [no. (%)]	11	(30)
Partial deficits [patients (eyes)]		
Visual field loss	18	(22)
Acuity loss only	5	(8)
Complete blindness [patients (eyes)]	15	(18)
Diagnoses (cases)		
Central retinal artery occlusion	9	
Ischemic optic neuropathy		
Posterior	14	
Anterior	8	
Cortical ischemia	3	
Other or unspecified	3	

(Courtesy of Myers MA, Hamilton SR, Bogosian AJ, et al: Visual loss as a complication of spine surgery: A review of 37 cases. *Spine* 22:1325–1329, 1997.)

Discussion.—The incidence of visual loss after spinal surgery is estimated to be 1 patient per 100 spine surgeons per year. Many patients have no preoperative risk factors. Hypertension, smoking, diabetes, and vascular disease may increase the risk. Most cases of visual loss occur after instrumented posterior fusion, long operative times, and significant blood loss. Several recommendations were made for selected high-risk patients.

▶ I selected this article because I believe that visual problems after spinal surgery are more common than is recognized in the literature. It is a serious complication, because these deficits are often permanent. A review article on postoperative optic neuropathy suggested that this complication results from multiple factors, but is often associated with hypotension, blood loss, a low hematocrit, older age, and a variable such as venous obstruction.[1]

M. Wood, M.D.

Reference

1. Williams EL, Hart WM, Tempelhoff R: Postoperative ischemic optic neuropathy. *Anesth Analg* 80:1018–1029, 1995.

Residual Neuromuscular Block Is a Risk Factor for Postoperative Pulmonary Complications: A Prospective, Randomised, and Blinded Study of Postoperative Pulmonary Complications After Atracurium, Vecuronium and Pancuronium

Berg H, Viby-Mogensen J, Roed J, et al (Copenhagen Univ)

Acta Anaesthesiol Scand 41:1095–1103, 1997 6–3

Objective.—Patients receiving pancuronium anesthesia, particularly for lengthy operations, have high rates of residual neuromuscular block and postoperative pulmonary complications (POPC). No randomized, controlled studies have addressed the significance of postoperative residual neuromuscular block to the development of postoperative complications. The incidence of POPC was compared for patients receiving pancuronium, atracurium, and vecuronium. The impact of residual neuromuscular block on the rate of POPC was also evaluated.

Methods.—The study included 691 adult patients undergoing major abdominal, gynecologic, or orthopedic operations. They were randomly assigned to receive pancuronium, atracurium, or vecuronium. During the perioperative period, neuromuscular monitoring was carried out with a nerve stimulator. Supramaximal train-of-four (TOF) stimulation of the ulnar nerve was repeated every 12 seconds, with manual evaluation of the response. Postoperatively, mechanomyographic measurement of the TOF ratios was performed. The study definition of residual block was a TOF ratio of less than 0.7. For 6 days after surgery, clinical tests for residual neuromuscular blockade were performed, with clinical monitoring of patients for the development of pulmonary complications.

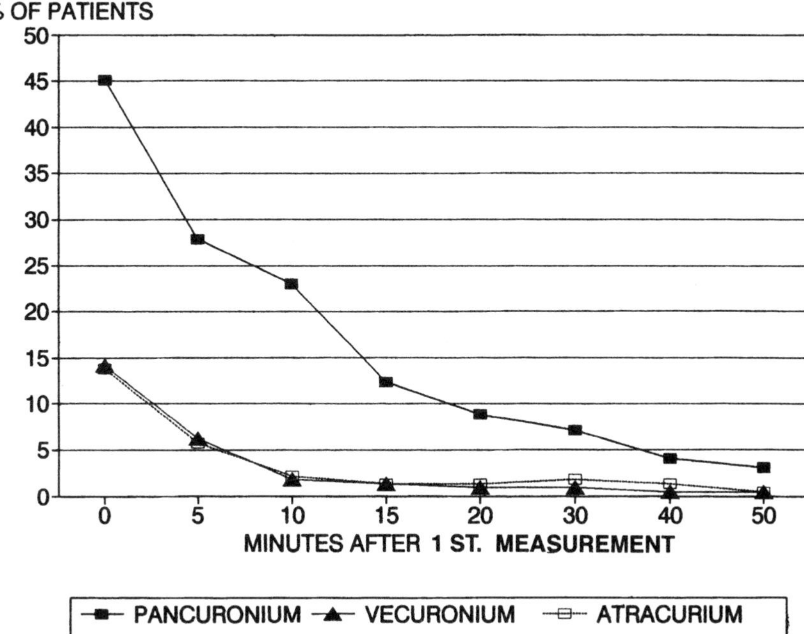

FIGURE 3.—Number of patients (in %) with a TOF ratio < 0.80 following pancuronium, vecuronium, and atracurium within 50 minutes of the first mechanomyographic recording. (Courtesy of Berg H, Viby-Mogensen J, Roed J, et al: Residual neuromuscular block is a risk factor for postoperative pulmonary complications: A prospective, randomised, and blinded study of postoperative pulmonary complications after atracurium, vecuronium and pancuronium. *Acta Anaesthesiol Scand* 41:1095–1103, 1997.)

Results.—The incidence of residual block was 26% in the pancuronium group vs. 5% in the atracurium and vecuronium groups combined. The time to reach a TOF ratio of 0.80 was significantly longer in the pancuronium group (Fig 3). Among patients in the pancuronium group, the rate of POPC was 17% for those with residual block vs. 5% for those without residual block. In the other 2 groups, the rate of POPC was only 4% for patients with residual block vs. 5% for those without (Table 4). Potential risk factors for POPC, identified by multiple regression analysis, were abdominal surgery, age, long-lasting surgery, and a TOF ratio of less than 0.7 after the use of pancuronium.

Conclusions.—In patients undergoing lengthy operations, residual block caused by the long-acting neuromuscular blocking agent pancuronium is a significant risk factor for the development of POPC. This relationship is particularly strong for elderly patients and those undergoing abdominal surgery. For patients receiving the intermediate-acting agents atracurium and vecuronium, residual block is unrelated to risk of POPC. If the use of pancuronium is to continue, more careful monitoring of neuromuscular block may be indicated.

TABLE 4.—Relationship Between TOF Ratio at First Postoperative Recording and Postoperative Pulmonary Complications (POPC)

	Pancuronium (n=226)			Atracurium or vecuronium (n=450)		
		Patients with POPC			Patients with POPC	
	No of patients	n	%	No of Patients	n	%
TOF ≥0.70	167	8	4.8	426	23	5.4
TOF <0.70	59	10	16.9*	24	1	4.2

Note: In 4 of the 46 patients with POPC (1 in the pancuronium group and 3 in the atracurium-vecuronium groups) the TOF ratio was not available. As there were no significant differences in the two groups of patients given the intermediate-acting muscle relaxants, the data from these groups are pooled.

*$P < 0.02$ as compared to patients in the same group with TOF ratio ≥0.7.

(Courtesy of Berg H, Viby-Mogensen J, Roed J, et al: Residual neuromuscular block is a risk factor for postoperative pulmonary complications: A prospective, randomised, and blinded study of postoperative pulmonary complications after atracurium, vecuronium and pancuronium. *Acta Anaesthesiol Scand* 41:1095–1103, 1997.)

► I have always believed that intermediate-duration muscle relaxant use was safer than long-acting muscle relaxant (e.g., pancuronium) administration; the low incidence of adverse effects after anesthesia makes safety issues difficult to prove. However, this study is a useful one to show to those individuals who advocate pancuronium use for economic reasons and not therapeutic grounds.

M. Wood, M.D.

Masseter Muscle Rigidity and Nondepolarizing Neuromuscular Blocking Agents

Albrecht A, Wedel DJ, Gronert GA (Mayo Clinic, Rochester, Minn; Univ of California, Davis)

Mayo Clin Proc 72:329–332, 1997 6–4

Background.—Masseter muscle rigidity is a possible risk factor for malignant hyperthermia; it is more common in children after induction with halothane and succinylcholine chloride. It is believed that nondepolarizing muscle relaxants are safe for individuals susceptible to malignant hyperthermia. A case of jaw rigidity in the absence of succinylcholine after administration of a nondepolarizing muscle relaxant was described. This case was reported to the Malignant Hyperthermia Association of the United States hot line.

Case 1.—Woman, 33, underwent diagnostic laparoscopy and hysteroscopy. Endotracheal entubation was attempted after loss of the train-of-four response, but the anesthetist was unable to open the patient's mouth. A second dose of vecuronium, 4 mg, and atracurium besylate, 30 mg, was administered, but the degree of mouth opening did not improve. An atypical reaction to vecuronium or a malignant hyperthermia episode was then considered.

The procedure was canceled, with no malignant hyperthermia triggering in the postoperative period. Five days later, the patient returned for surgery. A trial dose of mivacurium chloride, 4 mg, was given and masseter muscle rigidity again developed. The patient was given mivacurium, 6 mg, and full loss of the train-of-four response to the peripheral nerve stimulator was observed, but with no effect on the degree of masseter muscle spasm. The masseter muscle rigidity resolved during recovery. The patient was discharged with no further complications.

Discussion.—This case involved masseter muscle rigidity associated with nondepolarizing muscle relaxants, which was reproducible during later anesthesia. Masseter muscle rigidity has also been reported during administration of pancuronium. It is a rare response that probably does not predict susceptibility to malignant hyperthermia. In this case, the masseter muscle rigidity did not resolve until reversal of neuromuscular blockade. Adequate mask ventilation is necessary before these agents are administered because direct laryngoscopy may be difficult to perform after development of masseter muscle rigidity.

► Masseter muscle rigidity formerly was sufficient to cancel the procedure and to ask that the patient be worked up for malignant hyperthermia. More recently, dogma has it that one can go ahead with reasonable assurance that malignant hyperthermia will not develop just because masseter muscle rigidity occurred with succinylcholine. This report concerns 3 cases wherein such rigidity occurred after administration of nondepolarizers, as opposed to succinylcholine. One third of these patients—i.e., 1 patient—, did test positive for malignant hyperthermia. I read this paper several times and, in all honesty, do not understand what the authors would like us to do when we get a patient with masseter muscle rigidity after nondepolarizing muscle relaxants. I am also not sure what they want us to do after administration of succinylcholine to such a patient, either! I included this paper so that the reader could at least consider the problem, but I do not think these authors have helped us in our understanding of what to do in this situation.

J.H. Tinker, M.D.

Laryngeal Mask Airway and the Incidence of Regurgitation During Gynecological Laparoscopies

Bapat PP, Verghese C (Royal Berkshire Hosp, Reading, England)

Anesth Analg 85:139–143, 1997 6–5

Background.—The laryngeal mask airway is an alternative to the face mask and endotracheal tube for providing a secure airway during general anesthesia. The laryngeal mask airway does not always provide an airtight seal around the larynx and may not protect against aspiration of gastric contents that may be regurgitated into the pharynx. Regurgitation of gastric contents is more common during laparoscopic surgery in gynecologic patients. In a survey from this institution, there were no reports of regurgitation or aspiration of gastric contents associated with the laryngeal mask airway with positive pressure ventilation in 1,469 gynecologic laparoscopic procedures. It is possible that some regurgitated fluid may not be detectable clinically.

Methods.—The rate of regurgitation was examined in 100 patients under general anesthesia during gynecologic laparoscopic procedures using intermittent positive pressure ventilation and a laryngeal mask airway. Methylene blue capsules were given to patients before anesthesia. A fiberoptic laryngoscope was used to detect traces of dye.

Results.—Insertion of a laryngeal mask airway was successful in 95 patients at the first attempt and in all patients within 2 attempts. In 96 patients, fiberoptic examination revealed the vocal cords, vocal cords and posterior epiglottis, or vocal cords and anterior epiglottis. There was no trace of dye in 99 patients. Immediately after induction of anesthesia, 1 patient regurgitated dye, and the stain was later seen on the laryngeal mask airway. The other 99 laryngeal mask airways had no stain. Regurgitation did not occur in 91 patients with complete pH data. There was no stain in 30 patients randomly selected for fiberoptic examination of the laryngopharynx before neuromuscular block was antagonized. The 95% confidence limit for a true probability of regurgitation was 0.041.

Discussion.—The general view that intermittent positive pressure ventilation during general anesthesia is safe with a laryngeal mask airway in patients having gynecological laparoscopic surgery is supported, provided that the patient is carefully monitored and there is great attention to detail.

▶ Using methylene blue as a marker—and some sophisticated statistical legerdemain—the authors came to the conclusion that there is a "true rate of regurgitation" of about 4% using the laryngeal mask. Because that rate is obviously unacceptably high, the authors somehow managed to conclude that a larger study would be required to possibly demonstrate a lower incidence of regurgitation. I think there is a reasonable likelihood that a larger study would indicate the same, or a larger, incidence of regurgitation! The truth is that regurgitation does occur with the laryngeal mask airway. It is more likely there than it is with an endothracheal tube, at least to the point of producing symptoms. The endothracheal tube is not a guarantee either, of course. There are those who would like the laryngeal mask airway to be all things to all people, but it is not. That's the way most things turn out.

J.H. Tinker, M.D.

The Claims of Compensation for Awareness With Recall During General Anaesthesia in Finland

Ranta S, Ranta V, Aromaa U (Helsinki Univ)

Acta Anaesthesiol Scand 41:356–359, 1997 6–6

Background.—An estimated 0.2%–0.4% of patients undergoing general surgery remain aware during anesthesia. In the current study, claims for compensation involving awareness under anesthesia filed in Finland were analyzed.

Methods.—Claims filed between May 1987 and December 1993 were reviewed. Hospital notes, expert advisor's comments, and the comments of the anesthesiologist in charge of the anesthesia were also reviewed. The decisions of the Patient Injury Association (PIA), which determines whether compensation is to be paid for injury caused by medical treatment, were noted.

Findings.—Of 23,363 patient injury claims filed during the study period, 391 claims were related to anesthetic treatment. Only 4 were cases of awareness with recall during anesthesia. All 4 patients were granted compensation.

Conclusions.—Given the number of general anesthesias administered in Finland during the study period, the number of awareness cases reported to the PIA were remarkably few. The compensations awarded to the 4 patients filing claims were low compared with compensations given in other countries.

▶ This paper goes against one of my (many) long-held biases. I have long believed that the inclusion of a volatile anesthetic in the "mixture" we call anesthesia will go a long way toward preventing episodes of awareness. In the 4 cases included here, volatile agents were used in 3, though only in low concentration (isoflurane) in case 4. In cases 1 and 2, reasonable doses of isoflurane and enflurane were used, yet recall occurred anyway. I have one other comment to make about the issue of recall. As medicolegal concern increases for such cases, will anesthetists respond to their own increased "awareness" of this threat by routinely deepening anesthesia in their patients? I hope not. We already err on the heavy side much of the time, don't we?

J.H. Tinker, M.D.

Serious Complications Related to Regional Anesthesia: Results of a Prospective Survey in France

Auroy Y, Narchi P, Messiah A, et al (Begin Military Hosp, Saint-Mande, France; Hotel Dieu de France Hosp, Beirut, Lebanon; Bicetre Hosp, Le Kremlin-Bicetre, France; et al)

Anesthesiology 87:479–486, 1997 6–7

Objective.—The literature reporting serious cardiac and neurologic complications resulting from regional anesthesia consists mainly of retrospective or case studies. A large number of anesthesiologists were surveyed to determine the incidence of serious cardiac and neurologic complications associated with regional anesthesia occurring with current drugs, equipment, and techniques.

Methods.—A survey was mailed to 4,927 anesthesiologists in France asking for reports of cardiac arrest, seizures, radiculopathy, cauda equina syndrome, paraplegia, or death associated with regional anesthesia between January 1, 1994 and May 31, 1994. Surveys were reviewed by 3 anesthesiologists. Follow-up information was requested via a second questionnaire.

Results.—The 736 (14.9%) surveys returned reported 103,730 regional anesthetics including 40,640 spinal, 30,413 epidural, 21,278 peripheral nerve blocks, and 11,229 IV regional anesthetics. There were 98 serious complications. Follow-up information was received on 97. The number and incidence of severe complications were tabulated (Table 3). Age and American Society of Anesthesiologists' physical status class were significant risk factors for death after cardiac arrest. Pain during injection or paresthesia during puncture was common in patients who experienced neurologic complications during administration of spinal anesthesia. Nine of 12 patients who had radiculopathy or cauda equina received 5% hyperbaric lidocaine.

Conclusion.—Whereas the incidence of severe complications related to regional anesthesia was less than 0.1%, the 5% cardiac arrest and neurologic injury rate for spinal anesthesia needs to be investigated further.

▶ Quite some time ago, I remember a well-known speaker who flatly stated, at a national meeting, something to the effect that "although regional anesthesia is fun to do, and it is our dogmatic belief that we should be teaching it, doing it, and vigorously selling it to our patients, in truth it is associated with lots of complications." I think that is possibly a valid interpretation of this article, perhaps not. Of greater interest to me is the clear evidence presented that indeed spinal anesthesia maybe is more dangerous than other kinds of regional anesthesia. Robert Kaplan pointed this out in his controversial article several years ago. I believe this is elegant confirmation of his early warning. In fact, rapidly taking away most if not all of the sympathetic nervous system would not necessarily be something you would want to do in many patients. In this study, cardiac arrest and neurologic

TABLE 3.—Number and Incidence of Severe Complications Related to Regional Anesthesia

Critical Serious Event	Spinal (40,640)	Epidural (30,413)	Type of Anesthesia Peripheral Nerve Blocks (21,278)	Intravenous Regional (11,229)	Total (103,730)
Cardiac arrest	26	3	3	0	32
	(6.4)	(1.0)*	(1.4)†		(3.1)
	(3.9–8.9)	(0.2–2.9)	(0.3–4.1)	(0–3.3)	(2.0–4.1)
Death	6	0	1	0	7
	(1.5)		(0.5)		(0.9)
	(0.3–2.7)	(0–1.2)	(0–2.6)	(0–3.3)	(0.2–1.2)
Seizures	0	4	16	3	23
		(1.3)	(7.5)‡	(2.7)	(2.2)
	(0–0.9)	(0.4–3.4)	(3.9–11.2)	(0.5–7.8)	(1.3–3.1)
Neurological injury	24	6	4	0	34
	(5.9)	(2.0)*	(1.9)‡	(2.7)§	(3.3)
	(3.5–8.3)	(0.4–3.6)	(0.5–4.8)	(0.5–7.8)	(2.2–4.4)
Radiculopathy	19	5	4	0	28
	(4.7)	(1.6)*	(1.9)		(2.7)
	(2.6–6.8)	(0.5–3.8)	(0.5–4.8)	(0–3.3)	(1.7–3.7)
Cauda equina syndrome	5	0	0	0	5
	(1.2)				(0.5)
	(0.1–2.3)	(0–1.2)	(0–1.7)	(0–3.3)	(0.2–1.1)
Paraplegia	0	1	0	0	3
		(0.3)			(0.1)
	(0–0.9)	(0–1.8)	(0–1.7)	(0–3.3)	(0–0.5)

Note: Values are, in order, the number, the incidence/10,000, and the 95% confidence interval.
*Epidural vs. spinal ($P < 0.05$).
†Peripheral nerve blocks vs. spinal ($P < 0.05$).
‡Peripheral nerve blocks vs. epidural ($P < 0.05$).
§Intravenous regional vs. epidural and spinal ($P < 0.05$).
(Courtesy of Auroy Y, Narchi P, Messiah A, et al: Serious complications related to regional anesthesia: Results of a prospective survey in France. *Anesthesiology* 87:479–486, 1997. Copyright American Society of Anesthesiologists, Inc. Used with permission of Lippincott-Raven Publishers.)

injury were more than 3 standard deviations greater after spinal anesthesia than with other kinds of regional anesthesia procedures.

J.H. Tinker, M.D.

Coagulation Alterations in Patients Undergoing Elective Craniotomy

Heesen M, Kemkes-Matthes B, Deinsberger W, et al (Justus-Liebig Univ Giessen, Germany)

Surg Neurol 47:35–38, 1997 6–8

Objective.—Because they do not receive standard anticoagulation therapy, patients scheduled for craniotomy are at risk of thromboembolism. Immobilization during long operations may also contribute to the problem of thrombosis. Coagulation and fibrinolysis parameters were studied in 15 patients undergoing elective craniotomy.

Methods.—The patients were 10 men and 5 women, mean age 49 years. Parameters measured included plasma thrombin antithrombin III complex (TAT), a marker of coagulation activation; prothrombin fragment 1 + 2 (F1 + 2), another marker of activation; and D-dimer, a marker of fibrinolysis. Measurements were made before and after induction of anesthesia, 1 and 3 hours after the start of surgery, and on the day after surgery.

Results.—There was a significant increase in TAT from the preoperative period to 1 hour after the start of surgery. The TAT level peaked 3 hours after the start of surgery. The course of F1 + 2 was similar, again peaking during the intraoperative period. A slight increase in D-dimer was noted 3 hours after the start of surgery; this value peaked the day after surgery. The only significant increase was that for TAT.

Conclusions.—Patients undergoing elective craniotomy show a transient activation of coagulation, peaking during the intraoperative period. This change could reflect thromboplastin liberated from the brain parenchyma, because TAT levels are lower in patients undergoing procedures with less extensive brain tissue damage.

▶ This is an interesting article because of the danger in patients undergoing elective craniotomy of using prophylactic anticoagulants to reduce deep venous thrombosis and subsequent pulmonary embolism and its consequences. For obvious reasons, including the fear of bleeding at the operative site or rebleeding, standard anticoagulation therapy is not used. This article does document that in these patients, there is a significant activation of coagulation. Thus, this article highlights the importance of the problem but does not provide any more information about how to solve it.

M.F. Roizen, M.D.

Grading of Severity of Postdural Puncture Headache After 27-gauge Quincke and Whitacre Needles

Corbey MP, Bach AB, Lech K, et al (Grindsted Sygehus, Denmark)

Acta Anaesthesiol Scand 41:779–784, 1997 6–9

Introduction.—It has been suggested that the use of small-gauge needles for spinal anesthesia carries a low complication rate. In research, postdural puncture headache (PDPH) can be graded as I (mild), II (moderate), or III (severe), based on the results of a visual analog scale and functional rating. This grading system was used to compare the severity of PDPH after spinal anesthesia with 27-gauge Quincke or Whitacre needles.

Methods.—The study included 200 day-care surgery patients undergoing spinal anesthesia. All were younger than 45 years. The patients were randomly assigned to have anesthesia performed with a 27-gauge Quincke or Whitacre spinal needle. The previously described PDPH grading system was applied to compare the severity of PDPH in the 2 groups.

Results.—Postdural spinal puncture headache occurred in 6% of patients in whom the Quincke needle was used vs. none of those in whom the Whitacre needle was used. In the Quincke needle group, the severity of headache was grade II in 3 patients and grade III in 2 patients. In all of these patients, the bevel of the Quincke needle was withdrawn perpendicular to the dural fibers after having been inserted in parallel fashion. As long as the bevel was inserted and removed parallel to the dural fibers, there were no cases of PDPH. The rate of postdural headache was similar for patients with and without a history of recurrent headaches or migraine, and for male and female patients.

Conclusions.—For patients of normal body stature, the 27-gauge Whitacre needle is the preferred needle for use in spinal anesthesia. For patients in whom Quincke needles are used, the risk of PDPH is affected by the direction of the bevel during both insertion and removal. The Quincke needle is preferred for patients in whom difficulties are expected, because of obesity or other reasons. Patients with a history of recurrent or migraine headaches are not at increased risk of PDPH.

▶ To my knowledge, this is the first report describing the importance of how the Quincke needle is withdrawn, as well as the manner in which it was placed, in the incidence of postdural PDPH. It is not long ago that I remember being instructed to rotate the needle in all four quadrants after inserting a spinal needle, to make sure that there was CSF. I guess we need to test that maneuver as well to determine if it is still applicable, and that it is more than the way it is inserted and withdrawn, but actually the number of positions the needle is in during the insertion that may determine whether PDPH occur. I am continuously amazed by the science that develops on this important clinical problem and how the results are relatively unpredictable.

M.F. Roizen, M.D.

Neurologic Complications of 603 Consecutive Continuous Spinal Anesthetics Using Macrocatheter and Microcatheter Techniques

Horlocker TT, and the Perioperative Outcomes Group (Mayo Clinic, Rochester, Minn)

Anesth Analg 84:1063–1070, 1997 6–10

Background.—The occurrence of cauda equina syndrome after continuous spinal anesthesia has been reported recently, prompting a reassessment of the indications for and applications of this anesthetic technique. However, the frequency of neurologic complications using macrocatheter and microcatheter methods has not been thoroughly investigated in large studies.

Methods.—Six hundred three continuous spinal anesthetics performed between 1987 and 1992 were reviewed retrospectively. One hundred twenty-seven were administered through a 28-gauge microcatheter. Orthopedic procedures were done in 83.4% of the 476 patients with macrocatheters. All patients with microcatheters were parturients.

Findings.—Three patients reported pain after surgery. The symptoms resolved in 4 days in 2 patients, and the third was discharged on postoperative day 8 with residual foot pain. In addition, 1 patient had aseptic meningitis, and 1 had a sensory cauda equina syndrome, which persists after 15 months. Postdural puncture headache (PDPH) occurred in 9.6% of the patients, including 33.1% of those with microcatheters. In 6.8% of the patients, an epidural blood patch was performed (Table 3).

Conclusion.—In this series, the frequency of neurologic complications, excluding PDPH, is comparable to that in previously published reviews. The frequency of PDPH in patients with microcatheters was greater than previously reported.

▶ This article describes the complications of continuous spinal anesthesia—a technique recently in vogue because of the introduction of a micro-

TABLE 3.—Neurologic Complications

Complication	Macrocatheter (N = 476) *n* (%)	Microcatheter (N = 127) *n* %
Inadequate anesthesia	15 (3.2)	5 (3.9)
Sacral anesthesia only	0 (0)	0 (0)
Postdural puncture headache*		
Overall	16 (3.4)	42 (33.1)
No treatment	6 (1.3)	7 (5.5)
Caffeine	0 (0)	6 (4.7)
Epidural blood patch	10 (2.1)	31 (24.4)
Persistent paresthesia/numbness	2 (0.4)	1 (0.8)
Aseptic meningitis	1 (0.2)	0 (0)
Sensory cauda equina syndrome	1 (0.2)	0 (0)

*Two patients with postdural puncture headaches received IV caffeine and an epidural blood patch.

(Courtesy of Horlocker TT, and the Perioperative Outcomes Group: Neurologic complications of 603 consecutive continuous spinal anesthetics using macrocatheter and microcatheter techniques. *Anesth Analg* 84[5]:1063–1070, 1997.)

catheter. This is a retrospective survey, but a large number of patients were studied and the findings are of interest. In 1992, the United States Food and Drug Administration mandated removal of microcatheters smaller than 24 gauge because of reports of cauda equina syndrome after continuous spinal anesthesia.

M. Wood, M.D.

Incidence of Neurologic Complications Related to Thoracic Epidural Catheterization

Giebler RM, Scherer RU, Peters J (Klinikum der Universität, Essen, Germany)

Anesthesiology 86:55–63, 1997 6–11

Background.—Because of the perceived potential for neurologic sequelae, the risk-benefit ratio of thoracic epidural analgesia is debated. The incidence of neurologic complications after thoracic epidural catheterization was established in patients undergoing abdominal or abdominothoracic surgery.

Methods.—The prospective phase of the study included 1,059 patients, and the retrospective phase, 2,126. General anesthesia was provided to all patients after thoracic epidural catheterization.

Findings.—One hundred twenty-eight patients experienced complications after thoracic epidural catheterization, for an overall incidence of 3.1%. Dural perforation occurred in 0.7% overall; unsuccessful catheter placement, in 1.1%; postoperative radicular-type pain, in 0.2%; and peripheral nerve lesions, in 0.6%. Fourteen of these 24 peripheral nerve lesions were peroneal nerve palsies probably associated with surgical positioning or other transient peripheral nerve lesions. There was no evidence of epidural hematoma. No permanent sensory or motor defects were attributable to epidural catheterization. Unintentional dural perforation occurred significantly more often in the lower thoracic region than in the mid- or upper regions. Severe respiratory depression occurred after epidural buprenorphine in 1 patient, who recovered without complication.

Conclusions.—The incidence of serious neurologic complications associated with thoracic epidural catheterization in patients undergoing abdominal and thoracoabdominal surgery is not high. The maximum predicted risk for permanent neurologic sequelae is only 0.07%.

► I selected this article because it is a useful reference source to quote to physicians in other specialties who might require information on this procedure. Thoracic epidural catheterization for patients undergoing abdominal and thoracic surgery is increasing, and it is of interest that these authors report that this procedure may be as safe as lumbar epidural catheterization.

M. Wood, M.D.

Severe Respiratory Depression in the Obstetric Patient After Intrathecal Meperidine or Sufentanil

Jaffee JB, Drease GE, Kelly T, et al (Rush-Presbyterian-St Luke's Med Ctr, Chicago)

Int J Obstet Anesth 6:182–184, 1997 6–12

Introduction.—Opioids combined with spinal anesthetic are commonly used for pain relief during labor. Two patients were seen with respiratory depression after subarachnoid opioid administration.

Case 1.—Woman, 36, was seen at 8–10 weeks' gestation for incomplete spontaneous abortion. The pregnancy was complicated by hypertension and gestational diabetes. She was premedicated with IV metoclopramide 10 mg and famotidine 20 mg. In the operating room, meperidine 50 mg was administered intrathecally. Surgery lasted approximately 30 minutes. She was awake and alert when placed on a stretcher, but was apneic and responsive only to painful stimuli upon arrival to recovery room. Her blood pressure was 69/21 mm Hg, heart rate was 60–70 beats/min, and she required ventilation. Naloxone 0.2 mg was administered IV and she regained consciousness immediately. Her blood pressure rose to 90–100/50–60 mm Hg. She remained awake and alert with stable vital signs and was discharged later that day with no further respiratory depression.

Case 2.—Girl, 16, was admitted for induction of labor at 41 weeks' gestation of primigravida pregnancy. She was given oxytocin and asked for spinal analgesia for pain control. She received 50 μg IV fentanyl (total dose 200 μg in preceding 4 hours) 30 minutes before spinal-epidural placement and administration of sufentanil 10 μg. She experienced complete pain relief and mild pruritus within 2 minutes. At 5 minutes, she was apneic and unresponsive to verbal commands, but responded to mild sternal rub. Blood pressure was 135/78 mm Hg and fetal heart rate was 130 beats/min. She recovered rapidly after administration of 50 μg of naloxone. She remained stable and good analgesia was maintained throughout labor and delivery using epidural infusion of bupivacaine 0.08% and fentanyl 0.0002% at 8 mL/hr. Mother and baby were discharged with no further events after routine postpartum care.

Conclusion.—Administration of neuraxial opioids has many advantages, but serious side effects may occur, even with a modest dose of intrathecal meperidine. This approach to pain control must be practiced with vigilance when neuraxial opioids are used, since respiratory depression and arrest may occur, even in healthy patients.

Maternal Respiratory Arrests, Severe Hypotension, and Fetal Distress After Administration of Intrathecal, Sufentanil, and Bupivacaine After Intravenous Fentanyl

Lu JK, Manullang TR, Staples MH, et al (Univ of Utah, Salt Lake City)

Anesthesiology 87:170–172, 1997 6–13

Introduction.—There are several reports of respiratory depression in patients who receive combined spinal epidural analgesic techniques. Two patients were seen who had respiratory arrest after intrathecal sufentanil (ITS) and bupivacaine following IV fentanyl.

Case 1.—Woman, 19, was primigravida and at 40 weeks' gestation when admitted in labor. She received IV fentanyl, 100 μg, on admission and again at 0.75 and 2 hours after admission. Active labor was arrested, so a pitocin infusion was administered. She underwent a combined spinal epidural technique for complaints of extreme discomfort. Five minutes after injection, the patient was difficult to arouse. Pulse oximeter reading was 54%. In the next 2 minutes, apnea, cyanosis, and loss of consciousness developed. The patients' heart rate was 45 beats/min, blood pressure was 108/47 mm Hg, and fetal heart rate was 60 beats/min. Naloxone, 0.4 mg, was administered and she regained consciousness and spontaneous breathing within 2 minutes. The baby was delivered by vacuum extraction 9 hours after admission. Apgar scores were 10 at 1 minute and 10 at 5 minutes.

Case 2.—Woman, 22, was primigravida and at 40 weeks' gestation when admitted in labor. She was given 2 doses of fentanyl 50 μg 130 minutes apart. A combined spinal epidural was performed using sufentanil and bupivacaine. She became unresponsive, apneic, bradycardic, and cyanotic at 10 minutes after injection. The maternal and fetal heart rates were 40 and 60 beats/min, respectively. Cardiopulmonary resuscitation was given in conjunction with naloxone, 0.4 mg. Within 10 chest compressions, her pulse was palpable, Sa_{O2} rose from 50% to 95%, and she regained consciousness and spontaneous ventilation. Delivery was spontaneous 4 hours later. Apgar scores were 9 at 1 minute and 9 at 5 minutes.

Conclusion.—Significant respiratory depression may occur when intrathecal sufentanil is combined with small doses of bupivacaine or when it is preceded by IV fentanyl.

► Laboring women who receive systemic opioids, followed by epidural or spinal analgesia, are at risk for respiratory depression. These 2 case reports (Abstracts 6–12 and 6–13) suggest that laboring women who receive IV fentanyl, followed by intrathecal sufentanil, are at risk for clinically significant respiratory depression, including respiratory arrest. Both groups of authors suggested that when giving systemic opioid analgesia during labor, it may be preferable to give an IV opioid agonist-antagonist such as nalbuphine rather than IV fentanyl in parturients who may later receive an intrathecal opioid.

D.H. Chestnut, M.D.

Parenteral Ketorolac: The Risk for Acute Renal Failure

Feldman HI, Kinman JL, Berlin JA, et al (Univ of Pennsylvania, Philadelphia; Univ of Medicine and Dentistry of New Jersey, New Brunswick)

Ann Intern Med 126:193–199, 1997 6–14

Introduction.—Ketorolac tromethamine is a nonsteroidal anti-inflammatory drug (NSAID) approved for use as a parenteral analgesic. The adverse events are similar to those of other NSAIDs, including gastrointestinal effects, rare allergic reactions, and liver dysfunction. Acute renal failure has also been reported in association with ketorolac use. The risks of acute renal failure associated with ketorolac were compared with that associated with opioid administration.

Methods.—The retrospective study included 9,850 hospitalized patients who received ketorolac and 10,145 who received opioids. The total number of courses was 10,219 for ketorolac and 10,145 for opioids. All patients were treated in 35 Philadelphia-area hospitals during a 3-year period. The 2 groups were compared for their incidence of acute renal failure. The study definition of acute renal failure was an increase in serum creatinine concentration of 50% or greater, an absolute increase of 44.2 μmol/L or greater for patients with an initial concentration of less than 132.6 μmol/L, or an absolute increase of 88.4 μmol/L or greater for patients with an initial concentration of 132.6 μmol/L or greater. A secondary definition required diagnosis by a physician.

Results.—The incidence of acute renal failure in the entire study group was about 1.1% in each group. On multivariate analysis, the adjusted rate ratio for acute renal failure with ketorolac compared with opioids was 1.09 overall, 1.00 for patients receiving less than 5 days of therapy, and 2.08 for patients receiving more than 5 days of therapy. The results were comparable using the secondary definition of acute renal failure. Predisposing factors for acute renal failure included congestive heart failure, chronic renal disease, cirrhosis, and hypertension. No particular subgroup at increased clinical risk of acute renal failure could be identified, however.

Conclusions.—Acute renal failure is uncommon in hospitalized patients receiving parenteral analgesics. Patients receiving ketorolac for less than 5 days are at no greater risk for renal failure than those receiving opioids. However, risk may be doubled for patients receiving ketorolac for more than 5 days.

► This study failed to stratify patients by whether they had or had not undergone surgery; therefore, I am unsure how to apply these findings in the perioperative setting.

D.M. Rothenberg, M.D.

Infectious Complications

Conservative Management of Extradural Abscess Complicating Spinal-extradural Anaesthesia for Caesarean Section

Dysart RH, Balakrishnan V (Wellington Hosp, Wellington South, New Zealand)

Br J Anaesth 78:591–593, 1997 6–15

Introduction.—There are no reports of conservative treatment of an extradural abscess in an obstetric patient. In a patient with a lumbar extradural abscess treated 9 days after cesarean section was performed using spinal-extradural anesthesia, conservative treatment was followed by complete recovery. The clinical course included development and resolution of mild paraparesis.

Case Report.—Woman, 26, had an elective cesarean section at 39 weeks' gestation. Combined extradural-spinal anesthesia was used, and an extradural catheter was inserted for pain relief postoperatively. A routine aseptic procedure was followed. When it was noted that blood could be aspirated from the extradural catheter, it was removed and a new one inserted at a higher space. The patient had normal postoperative pain. Between 9 and 11 days later, the patient's symptoms progressed from increasing backache, pyrexia, tenderness over the extradural site, and shivers to pain radiation down both lower limbs, neck pain, headache, a numb feeling in the right leg, a mild weakness in the left leg, tachycardia occasionally approaching 150 beats/min^{-1}, variable sensation in the legs, patchy numbness to pinprick, photophobia, and a heavy feeling in the legs. Blood cultures showed gram-positive *Staphylococcus*. Conservative treatment was recommended for a suspected extradural infection because there were no focal neurologic signs. Treatment progressed from an opioid analgesia and patient-controlled analgesia with morphine to MRI scan, which showed a lesion 2.4 × 1.2 cm at L2 to L3. T1-weighted and T2-weighted images indicated space-occupying fluid collection, rather than old bleeding or fibrosis. A diagnosis of extradural abscess was supported by the clinical findings and extent and loculation of the lesion. Spinal surgery was not performed because the patient had mild neurologic signs and subjective improvement. Twelve days postoperatively, the patient improved and had no headache and less severe backache. *Staphylococcus aureus* was confirmed by blood cultures, and the patient's antibiotics were changed to floxacillin and rifampicin. The patient steadily improved during the next 2 weeks. On postoperative day 25, the patient was discharged. Floxacillin was continued for 6 weeks, and the patient continued physiotherapy. A month later, the patient was completely recovered.

Discussion.—There are an increasing number of reports of extradural infections associated with extradural anesthesia. It is unclear whether the rate of infections is on the rise because of increasing use of extradural anesthesia, or whether such infections are being reported more often. Most of the reported extradural abscesses have been associated with older age, immunocompromise, infection, IV drug abuse, and trauma. The preferred diagnostic tool is MRI with contrast enhancement. Treatment is often surgical drainage and treatment with antibiotics, though no one treatment course is recommended over another.

▶ The authors noted that "the variable rate of progression of neurological symptoms after presentation of an extradural abscess makes many neurosurgeons uneasy about conservative treatment." It makes me uneasy too! Bromage noted: "Occasionally, an epidural abscess will resolve with aggressive antibiotic therapy, but recovery is less certain than with surgical drainage."[1] The consequences of failed conservative therapy are grave. Timely surgical decompression remains the definitive treatment of epidural abscess.

D.H. Chestnut, M.D.

Reference

1. Bromage PR: Neurologic complications of labor, delivery, and regional anesthesia, in *Obstetric Anesthesia: Principles and Practice*. Chestnut DH (ed): St Louis, Mosby, 1994, p 621.

Transmission of *Mycobacterium tuberculosis* by a Fiberoptic Bronchoscope: Identification by DNA Fingerprinting

Michele TM, Cronin WA, Graham NMH, et al (Johns Hopkins Univ, Baltimore, Md; Baltimore City Health Dept, Md; Maryland Dept of Health and Mental Hygiene, Baltimore; et al)
JAMA 278:1093–1095, 1997 6–16

Introduction.—In recent outbreaks of drug-susceptible and drug-resistant tuberculosis, nosocomial transmission of *Mycobacterium tuberculosis* has been an important factor. Lack of adequate isolation of patients, poor ventilation, irrigation of tuberculous abscesses, performance of cough-inducing procedures without appropriate air filtering and exhaust, and congregation of susceptible individuals with tuberculosis patients are factors identified in tuberculosis epidemics in health care facilities. Because of the inherent difficulty of disinfection procedures for the bronchoscope, propagation of infection via the flexible fiberoptic bronchoscope has long been a concern. Bronchoscopic transmission of tuberculosis from a patient with active disease to a susceptible patient was described.

Methods.—Both patients' medical charts and bronchoscopic records were reviewed. The hospital locations that were visited by both patients were examined. The hospital ventilation systems were evaluated, and the cleaning and disinfection of bronchoscopes were observed to determine whether nosocomial transmission had occurred.

Results.—Bronchoscopy was performed on a patient with cough, hoarseness, and fever, leading to a diagnosis of tuberculosis. Another patient with a mediastinal mass also underwent bronchoscopy, and small-cell carcinoma was diagnosed. The second patient had fever and an infiltrate of the right upper lobe of the lung after 6 months of chemotherapy and radiation therapy. Acid-fast bacilli were revealed with bronchoscopic washings, which were culture positive for *M. tuberculosis.* The same instrument in the same operating room was used for both patients having bronchoscopy, with no intervening bronchoscopies having been performed. National guidelines were not followed in bronchoscope cleaning and disinfection procedures.

Conclusions.—Between these 2 patients, a contaminated bronchoscope was the most likely source of *M. tuberculosis.* This nosocomial source of transmission was detected by the restriction fragment length polymorphism analysis of *M. tuberculosis* isolates. To prevent further spread of infection and disease, public health measures were implemented. Continued vigilance in endoscope cleaning techniques is necessary.

Transmission of a Highly Drug-resistant Strain (Strain W1) of *Mycobacterium tuberculosis*: Community Outbreak and Nosocomial Transmission via a Contaminated Bronchoscope

Agerton T, Valway S, Gore B, et al (Ctrs for Disease Control and Prevention, Atlanta, Ga; South Carolina Dept of Health and Environmental Control, Columbia)

JAMA 278:1073–1077, 1997 6–17

Introduction.—There have been several outbreaks of multidrug-resistant tuberculosis (MDR TB) in New York prisons and hospitals in the 1990s. In 1996, the Centers for Disease Control and Prevention reported strain W1 MDR TB in 8 patients from South Carolina and investigated this community outbreak.

Methods.—All 8 patients were resistant to 7 drugs and had matching DNA fingerprints (strain W1). Community links were determined for 5 patients (patients 1–5). Other than being hospitalized in the same hospital, no links were identified for patients 6–8. The hospital staff was cross-matched with the state tuberculosis registry and patient family members were extensively interviewed. Laboratory reports were reviewed and infection control policies were reviewed with staff personnel in the infection control, laboratory, respiratory therapy, and endoscopy departments.

Results.—Four of the 5 community patients were from the same family and 1 was a close friend and neighbor of patient 1. Patient 1 was hospitalized in New York in 1991 in a hospital that was experiencing an outbreak of MDR TB. Patient 5, a family member of patient 1, was hospitalized while in an infectious period in May 1995 and was the source of the nosocomial outbreak in the hospital. The only common factor for patients 5–8 was that they all underwent bronchoscopies in May 1995. Patients 5 and 8 had clinical courses, smear-positive and culture-positive specimens, and chest radiographs with cavity lesions consistent with MDR TB. Both patients died of MDR TB within a month of diagnosis. Patients 6 and 7 had 1 positive culture for MDR TB on specimens collected during bronchoscopy. Patient 6 had a skin test conversion after undergoing bronchoscopy. Neither of these patients had a clinical course consistent with MDR TB, nor were they treated for MDR TB. They both remain alive and well. Patients 6, 7, and 8 underwent bronchoscopy at 1, 12, and 17 days, respectively, after patient 5. Bronchoscopy cleaning was inadequate and the bronchoscope was never immersed in disinfectant; both actions were contrary to hospital guidelines for cleaning and disinfecting endoscopic equipment.

Conclusion.—This is the first documented nosocomial transmission of MDR TB from a contaminated bronchoscope. The inadequate cleaning and disinfection of the bronchoscope used with patient 5 led to false positive cultures in patients 6 and 7, transmission of infection to patient 6, and active and subsequently fatal MDR TB to patient 8. Bronchoscopies should be avoided in patients with active TB, unless absolutely necessary.

▶ Many patients undergo fiberoptic bronchoscopy as part of an anesthetic procedure; infectious complications are rarely reported. I selected these 2 reports (Abstracts 6–16 and 6–17) to highlight the possibility of tuberculosis transmission from patient to patient with a bronchoscope that has been contaminated. Bronchoscope cleaning requires established protocols and guidelines, followed by proper quality assessment/quality improvement.

M. Wood, M.D.

An Epidural Abscess Due to Resistant *Staphylococcus aureus* Following Epidural Catheterisation

Yuste M, Canet J, Garcia M, et al (Hosp Universitari Germans Trias i Pujol, Barcelona)

Anaesthesia 52:163–165, 1997 6–18

Introduction.—Epidural abscess is difficult to diagnose, and delay in treatment can result in permanent neurologic damage. In the case presented, this rare complication of epidural cannulation led to paraplegia.

Case Report.—Man, 44, received emergency treatment after a traffic accident. Initial findings included rib fractures and a possible pulmonary contusion, but no pneumothorax was present. A thoracic epidural catheter for patient-controlled analgesia was inserted at the level of T5 before the patient was transferred to the ICU. The catheter was in place for 96 hours, with aseptic conditions maintained throughout the entire period. The patient made good progress in the ICU and was discharged after 3 days.

At a follow-up visit 5 days later, the patient complained of general discomfort in the upper back. He was readmitted the next day with fever, persistent thoracic back pain, and hyperreflexia of both legs. Eight hours after admission, the patient experienced paraplegia and loss of sphincter control. Methylprednisolone and ampicillin and gentamicin were administered and MRI was performed. Imaging studies showed a lesion with compression of the spinal cord from T1 to T6. An emergency decompressive laminectomy was performed within 12 hours of the first sign of neurologic symptoms. Bacterial culture of the drained abscess grew methicillin-resistant *Staphylococcus aureus* sensitive only to vancomycin and phosphomycin. Despite immediate treatment with these antibiotics, the patient was still paraplegic 6 months later.

Discussion.—The incidence of epidural abscess is estimated to be 15 per 1 million cases of extradural anesthesia. In the case presented here, the usual recommendations for asepsis were followed; nevertheless, contamination of the epidural space appears to have occurred after the catheter was inserted in the emergency room. The patient's condition deteriorated rapidly despite early diagnosis and treatment.

► I included this article to again emphasize what I have been saying for many years, namely, beware of dismissing the risk of complications that are devastating, even if the risk is very low. How many of these horrible staphylococcal abscesses or other infections of the neuraxis are we willing to accept per hundred, even per thousand, epidurals. When something becomes as routine as epidural cannulation has become, these complications bring us up short and should be constant reminders, despite the rarity of the complication, that this kind of complication is devastating. The *magnitude* of any complication should be taken into consideration as well as its *incidence*.

J.H. Tinker, M.D.

Compartment Syndrome

Compartment Syndrome Associated With Bupivacaine and Fentanyl Epidural Analgesia in Pediatric Orthopaedics

Dunwoody JM, Reichert CC, Brown KLB (Univ of British Columbia, Vancouver)

J Pediatr Orthop 17:285–288, 1997 6–19

Background.—Epidural analgesia is being used increasingly for pain relief after orthopedic extremity surgery. Two children are described in whom compartment syndromes developed in association with reduced skin and deep-tissue sensitivity in the presence of bupivacaine 0.1% and fentanyl epidural analgesics.

> *Case Reports.*—The patients were 2 boys, aged 14 and 7 years. The boys underwent orthopedic procedures under a continuous lumbar infusion of a mixture of narcotic (fentanyl) and local anesthetic (bupivacaine 0.1%). In both patients, excessive pressure had been applied inadvertently to the limb distally. Neither was able to perceive the pain in the presence of his analgesia. After the pressure was relieved, signs of a compartment syndrome were evident. The sensation of pathologic pain was not masked by the epidural infusion.

Conclusions.—After this experience, the authors changed their practice to limit the use of bupivacaine for extremity surgery to patients for whom the use of local anesthetics would be advantageous, such as sympathetic block for microvascular surgery or in amputation surgery to decrease the incidence of phantom limb pain. Additional research is needed to determine the best solution for epidural analgesia and assessment of the potential use of patient-controlled epidural analgesia to see if this type of complication can be reduced.

▶ Although this study confirms the notion that epidural analgesia with bupivacaine and fentanyl does not mask the perception of pain associated with compartment syndrome, the level of sensory blockade was sufficient to block the sensation of pain associated with tissue compression sufficient to cause damage. The authors advocate the use of epidural fentanyl alone rather than a combination of fentanyl and bupivacaine. It has been shown repeatedly that epidural infusions of fentanyl are no more effective than intravenous infusions. Perhaps IV PCA opioid analgesia is the most appropriate postoperative analgesic technique for patients at risk of compression or ischemia from a cast or splint. However, as the authors point out, for patients with conditions that may benefit from continuous sympathetic denervation the benefits may outweigh the additional risk.

S.E. Abram, M.D.

Prevention of Compartment Syndrome Associated With the Dorsal Lithotomy Position

Scott JR, Daneker G, Lumsden AB, et al (Emory Univ, Atlanta, Ga)

Am Surg 63:801–806, 1997 6–20

Objective.—The dorsal lithotomy position is thought to be a contributing factor to postoperative compartment syndrome. Diagnosis, particularly in young patients, may be difficult, resulting in delayed therapy. Four cases of compartment syndrome in young patients were seen and cause of the syndrome, contributing factors, and recommendations for prevention and early diagnosis were reviewed.

Discussion.—All patients spent 6–11 hours in the dorsal lithotomy position. All subsequently experienced a painful and sometimes swollen and tense right calf, and some had hypotension. Compartment pressures, when measured, were widely divergent, and emergency 4-compartment fasciotomies were performed. Protracted leg elevation, hypotension, hypoxemia, vasoconstricting drugs, hip and knee flexion, direct pressure, and compressive bandages contribute to the development of compartment syndrome. These intraoperative events result in a reduction of perfusion pressure, leading to ischemia, followed by reperfusion, capillary leakage from ischemic tissue, an increase in tissue edema leading to compounded perfusion and reperfusion problems and ultimately ending with neuromuscular compromise. Preventive measures included repositioning the patient when the lithotomy position is not required, eliminating areas of direct local pressure, and positioning the extremities at the level of the heart.

Conclusion.—Every patient in the lithotomy position should be considered at risk of compartment syndrome. Early diagnosis and intervention are critical to preventing long-term neuromuscular compromise.

▶ The dorsal lithotomy position is not a position into which patients can be placed for protracted time periods without risking big problems. In 1 of the present cases, the patient was in this position for 9 hours. Is there really any excuse for that? In addition to the authors' 4 cases, I have consulted on 2 in my own experience, and they are indeed as devastating as the authors discuss. In the past some "wags" have suggested, perhaps tongue in cheek, that for some of these very long cases, we should bring trained physical therapists into the operating room to go through range-of-motion and other preventive exercises. Perhaps this would not be a bad idea, but I think figuring out how to do these operations more quickly might be better.

J.H. Tinker, M.D.

Compartment Syndromes Associated With Postoperative Epidural Analgesia: A Case Report

Price C, Ribeiro J, Kinnebrew T (Orlando Regional Med Ctr, Fla)

J Bone Joint Surg Am 78–A:597–599, 1996 6–21

Objective.—Compartment syndrome of the thigh is a rare condition that can result from trauma, prolonged compression, or vascular injury. However, it has never been previously reported after elective femoral osteotomy. A patient with compartment syndromes of the thigh and leg developing after corrective osteotomies of the femur and tibia—and in association with postoperative epidural analgesia—was reported.

Case.—Boy, 16 years, with hypophosphatemic rickets was evaluated because of bilateral genu valgum. The valgum deformities had recurred after bilateral corrective osteotomies performed 10 years earlier. Osteotomies were performed on the distal part of the femur and proximal part of the tibia in the right leg, without complications. Postoperative pain was controlled with narcotic medications. A few months later, similar osteotomies were performed on the left leg. The operations were as before, except that epidural fentanyl was used for postoperative pain control. This provided excellent analgesia until discomfort and slight numbness developed after 18 hours. The thigh was swollen and the skin shiny and tense. Anterior and posterior compartment pressures were measured at 64 and 32 mm Hg, respectively, compared with a normal pressure of less than 30 mm Hg. Fasciotomies were performed to relieve the pressure. Surgery revealed consolidated hematomas at the osteotomy sites, with histologic findings consistent with ischemic myonecrosis. There were no neurologic sequelae of the compartment syndromes.

Discussion.—Compartment syndromes of the thigh and leg can develop after simultaneous osteotomies of the femur and tibia. Because of the rarity of this condition, it could be easily missed. The use of epidural analgesia is a potential contributing factor, as it may mask the classic symptoms of compartment syndrome. In this case, epidural analgesia may have played a role in the development of compartment syndrome through increased blood flow secondary to sympathetic blockade.

▶ In their discussion, the authors speculate regarding how the epidural might have contributed to the occurrence of compartment syndrome. Part of their speculation that the epidural was responsible for the problem was based on the fact that compartment syndrome of the thigh is rare and the fact that the same surgeons had successfully done the other leg previously without epidural analgesia and without this complication. They further speculate that epidural fentanyl may have produced vasodilation of the operated limb. They cite evidence that epidural meperidine can produce peripheral vasodilation and state that it may be that fentanyl can do so as well, ignoring the fact that meperidine has a local anesthetic effect at clinically relevant doses whereas fentanyl does not.

There is certainly a risk to using epidural analgesia in patients who are at risk of compartment syndrome, not because it contributes to the development of the condition but because it may mask the condition, delaying its recognition. This was certainly not the case here. It is now well known that epidural fentanyl is no more effective than systemic fentanyl, and because this case was recognized promptly, serious sequelae were avoided. Here is another case of "anesthesia" being unjustly blamed for a surgical complication.

S.E. Abram, M.D.

Individual Cases and Other Complications

Management of Malignant Hyperthermia Susceptible Parturients
Pollock NA, Langton EE (Palmerston North Hosp, New Zealand)
Anaesth Intensive Care 25:398–407, 1997 6–22

Introduction.—A woman who is malignant hyperthermia susceptible (MHS) has increased risks at the time of labor and delivery, and there are potential risks for the newborn as well. A prospective study identified MHS women and partners of MHS men who were delivering, and followed their course through labor, cesarean section, and the postpartum period.

Methods.—The area served by the study institution has 4 MHS families, and up to 10 deliveries per year are children of MHS individuals. A protocol for the management of the MHS parturient was introduced in 1990. Referral to a hospital with specialist obstetric and anesthetic services is recommended. Epidural analgesia is started early in labor and an operating room with a dedicated vapor-free anesthesia machine is prepared. Specific monitoring guidelines are followed during labor, regional anesthesia, general anesthesia, and the postpartum period. When the father is MHS, the newborn has a 50% chance of susceptibility, and appropriate precautions are observed.

Results.—Eleven MHS women had 20 deliveries at the study center. The age range of the group was 16–34 years; 7 were primiparous. There were 10 vaginal deliveries, 4 emergency cesarean sections, 4 elective cesarean sections, 1 Ventouse delivery, and 1 delivery using Kielland's forceps. All cesarean sections were managed with regional anesthesia. Only 3 deliveries (all cesarean sections) had abnormal indicators that achieved any score on the MHS grading scale. There were 2 cases each of elevated temperature and tachycardia and 1 case of acidosis. The most commonly used drugs were syntocinon (5–40 IU, IM or IV) and bupivacaine (14–195 mg). Only 1 infant had an Apgar score of less than 9 at 5 minutes, and her score had risen to 10 at 10 minutes. The 3 infants with temperatures of more than 37.5° C all were normal by 4 hours after delivery. Five women with MHS partners had 8 deliveries. These women had no extra monitoring, but their infants were closely monitored during labor and after delivery. None had signs or symptoms of malignant hyperthermia.

Conclusion.—The identification of MHS women and those whose partners are MHS allows appropriate monitoring and precautions to be taken at the time of childbirth. In the deliveries reported here, there was little evidence that the stress of labor can trigger an MH episode. Sympathomimetics were used without adverse effects, but inhalational anesthetic agents and Suxamethonium should be avoided.

▶ There are few published reports of malignant hyperthermia (MH) during parturition. Some have hypothesized that the rarity of MH in pregnant patients suggests that pregnancy may protect against the occurrence of MH.

However, Douglas[1] noted that "It also may reflect the widespread use of regional anesthesia for labor, vaginal delivery, and cesarean section."

D.H. Chestnut, M.D.

Reference

1. Douglas J: Malignant hyperthermia, in Chestnut DH (ed): *Obstetric Anesthesia: Principles and Practice.* St Louis, Mosby, 1994, p 896.

Magnetic Resonance Imaging of Cerebrospinal Fluid Leak and Tamponade Effect of Blood Patch in Postdural Puncture Headache

Vakharia SB, Thomas PS, Rosenbaum AE, et al (State Univ of New York, Syracuse)

Anesth Analg 84:585–590, 1997 6–23

Introduction.—The incidence of postdural puncture headache (PDPH) has decreased substantially with advances in needles and needle tips, but PDPH continues to occur in association with spinal anesthesia, myelography, and accidental dural puncture during epidural anesthesia. Epidural blood patch is the definitive treatment for PDPH that does not respond to conservative therapy. The ability of MRI to visualize CSF leak in patients with PDPH and to determine the spread of the blood patch in the epidural space and the extent of tamponade on the thecal sac was assessed prospectively.

Methods.—The 5 patients who took part in the study all had PDPH that had failed to respond to 3 days of conservative management. Three had undergone spinal anesthesia, 1 had myelography, and 1 had an accidental dural puncture with an 18-gauge Touhy needle during epidural anesthesia. In all cases, PDPH occurred within 72 hours of dural puncture. After the MRI studies, 20 mL of autologous blood was injected into the lumbar space with the patient in the lateral recumbent position. Patients remained supine for at least 45 minutes. Repeat proton density and T2-weighted imaging was done in sagittal and parasagittal planes. Patients were observed in the hospital for 24 hours and discharged when free of pain. Follow-up was scheduled for 1 week later.

Results.—The patients' severe headaches with nausea and vomiting resolved immediately after placement of the epidural blood patch. Before the patch was placed, MRI revealed extrathecal CSF and hemosiderosis in 4 patients, indicating the site of dural puncture. Postprocedure MRI showed the bloody patch as a large extradural collection with anterior displacement of the thecal sac; the mean spread was 4.6 intervertebral spaces. Both MRI and CSF flow images (performed in 1 case) demonstrated the tamponade effect of the blood patch.

Conclusion.—Development of PDPH is attributed to the effect of postdurally related decreases in CSF pressure caused by persistent leak of CSF from the dural hole. With MRI, the tamponade effect of the 20-mL epidural blood patch was clearly demonstrated; this effect is thought to be responsible for the immediate resolution of PDPH. Both the site of the CSF leak and the correct placement of the blood patch can be confirmed with MRI.

► For years, I have been impressed that an epidural blood patch provides immediate relief of PDPH. I experienced instantaneous relief of my PDPH when a colleague gave me an epidural blood patch several years ago. Others have observed that epidural administration of a local anesthetic may result in a transient increase in intracranial pressure. In the present study, the authors observed that epidural administration of 20 mL of blood resulted in anterior displacement of the thecal sac. They commented that the expansion of the epidural space results in relative contraction of the subarachnoid space, and thus increases the CSF pressure, which helps explain the immediate resolution of PDPH.

D.H. Chestnut, M.D.

Two Cases of Cauda Equina Syndrome Following Spinal–Epidural Anesthesia

Kubina P, Gupta A, Oscarsson A, et al (Örebro Hosp Med Ctr, Sweden; Univ Hosp, Linköping, Sweden)

Reg Anesth 22:447–450, 1997 6–24

Introduction.—Cauda equina syndrome is a recognized but rare complication of spinal or epidural anesthesia, caused by damage to the sacral roots of the neural canal. Lidocaine, chloroprocaine, and procaine have all been reported as causes of cauda equina syndrome, but bupivacaine has not. Two cases of cauda equina syndrome related to spinal-epidural anesthesia with bupivacaine were reported.

Patients.—The first patient was a 63-year-old man undergoing transurethral resection of the prostate. He received spinal anesthesia with intrathecal injection of 3.6 mL of bupivacaine with glucose, 5 mg/mL. The procedure was performed without complications. However, general anesthesia—induced with thiopentone and maintained with isoflurane in nitrous oxide—was needed because of inadequate cephalad spread of bupivacaine with glucose. On the day after surgery, the patient had urinary incontinence and difficulty in defecation. Damage to the sacral roots was confirmed by electromyography; MRI showed spinal stenosis at the L2–L3 level. The patient's condition was unchanged, with inability to control the sphincter muscles, over 2 years' follow-up.

The second patient was a 70-year-old woman undergoing hip replacement surgery. She received combined spinal-epidural anesthesia using bupivacaine without glucose. The epidural bupivacaine infusion was stopped 42 hours postoperatively. However, the patient was unable to micturate, causing urinary retention. Rectal incontinence developed later. No abnormal findings were apparent on MRI of the lumbar and spinal canals. Bladder function returned slowly, but the patient was left without significant rectal function.

Discussion.—Cauda equina syndrome developed in these patients after the use of bupivacaine for spinal-epidural anesthesia. One case (the first) was clearly associated with spinal stenosis, but the other is unexplained. The second case could involve needle or catheter trauma at the time of insertion, contamination of the bupivacaine, and the long use of bupivacaine for postoperative pain relief.

▶ Cauda equina syndrome is bad—really bad. Local anesthetics can sometimes, somehow be neurotoxic. When we inject local anesthetics in or near the neuraxis, we must be prepared for the possibility that a devastating complication such as this can occur. We need to ask ourselves, in each case, just how often we can tolerate such a devastating complication. It is nice to talk glibly of the "risk-benefit" ratio in these cases, but so often, a clear benefit of 1 type of anesthesia over another is not obvious. I think these cases call upon us to, once again, question our near-universal dogmatic belief that it is important to "sell" regional anesthesia as often as possible to our patients. I am just not sure the available evidence supports that sell job.

J.H. Tinker, M.D.

Markedly Prolonged Paralysis After Mivacurium in a Patient Apparently Heterozygous for the Atypical and Usual Pseudocholinesterase Alleles by Conventional Biochemical Testing

Rosenberg MK, Lebenbom-Mansour M (Sinai Hosp, Farmington Hills, Mich; Wayne State Univ, Detroit)
Anesth Analg 84:457–460, 1997 6–25

Introduction.—Because of rapid hydrolysis by pseudocholinesterase, the neuromuscular blocker mivacurium has a very short duration of effect. This characteristic may make it appropriate for use in the ambulatory setting. However, the duration of action may be increased in some people with variants of the pseudocholinesterase gene. A case of prolonged paralysis after mivacurium administration in a patient heterozygous for the atypical cholinesterase gene is reported.

Case.—Woman, 39, was undergoing laparoscopic tubal ligation under general anesthesia at a freestanding ambulatory surgical center. The procedure was performed using lidocaine, propofol, and fentanyl anesthesia, with mivacurium 12 mg given to facilitate endotracheal intubation. At the end of the procedure, 35 minutes after mivacurium administration, the patient had no response to train-of-four ulnar nerve stimulation. When neostigmine and glycopyrrolate were given 10 minutes later, there was no effect. The patient still had no spontaneous muscle activity or response to nerve stimulation 2 hours after mivacurium, so she was transferred to the hospital postanesthesia care unit for mechanical ventilation. Spontaneous muscle activity began to appear 3.5 hours after mivacurium. By 6.25 hours the patient could lift her head, and extubation was performed. Measurement of pseudocholinesterase activity and dibucaine number suggested that the patient was heterozygous for the atypical pseudocholinesterase gene, as was 1 of her daughters. Subsequent genotyping studies identified the patient as genotype AA and her husband as usual silent type.

Discussion.—A patient with a very long duration of paralysis after mivacurium administration is described. Although this patient appeared heterozygous for the atypical pseudocholinesterase gene on conventional biochemical tests, subsequent genetic testing clarified the reasons for her clinical course, and its implications for her children. Such sophisticated testing may sometimes be needed when conventional tests cannot adequately explain the clinical situation.

► The seemingly endless introduction of new neuromuscular blockers has been a source of consternation to me, because I cannot remember the dosage of the older ones, only to have people in my department talking about some new one. I am not sure why drug companies keep introducing these new blockers, but one reason might be that they are relatively straightforward drugs to get through the Food and Drug Administration (little off-label usage or usage by untrained personnel). This particular new "...curium" seems to be occasionally associated with prolonged paralysis. Back in the days when we used succinylcholine infusions regularly, and indeed succinylcholine for intubation much more often than we do now, we saw a substantial number of patients who had "atypical pseudocholinesterase." These days, with much less use of succinylcholine, the presence of various alleles for plasma cholinesterase is less clinically obvious, but seems to have reared its ugly head again with mivacurium. In other words, because nowadays we don't use succinylcholine anywhere near as much as in the past, we are perhaps lulled into a false sense of security with respect to atypical pseudocholinesterase. The incidence is unlikely to have diminished. With mivacurium, it may be that at least some of these prolonged paralysis episodes we are hearing about now may be simply the uncovering of various kinds of atypical genetics. It is also possible, though speculation, that mivacurium may "unmask" some forms of heterozygotes that might not be problematic with succinylcholine.

J.H. Tinker, M.D.

Cardiovascular Collapse During Anesthesia in a Patient With Preoperatively Discontinued Chronic MAO Inhibitor Therapy

Sprung J, Distel D, Grass J, et al (Cleveland Clinic Found, Ohio)

J Clin Anesth 8:662–665, 1996 6–26

Introduction.—Monoamine oxidase (MAO) inhibitor therapy is often discontinued 2 weeks before surgery, but recent studies suggest that this widely recommended practice may not be necessary even for patients treated long term with these agents. Severe reactions may occur, however, even when MAO inhibitor therapy has been discontinued for as long as 3 weeks before general anesthesia.

Case Report.—Woman, 79, was scheduled for partial colectomy for rectal cancer. Her medical history included chronic obstructive pulmonary disease, congestive heart failure, and severe depression. Preoperative medications were theophylline, verapamil, bumetanide, potassium supplements, 2% nitroglycerin topical ointment, prednisone, triamcinolone inhalation, albuterol and ipratropium nebulizers, and the MAO inhibitor tranylcypromine (10 mg 4 times daily for 25 years). Tranylcypromine was discontinued 20 days before surgery.

An epidural catheter was used to deliver local anesthetic during surgery. After administration of 10 mg of bupivacaine, severe hypotension developed with a precipitous decrease in blood pressure (from 90/40 mm Hg postintubation to 40/20 mm Hg 30 minutes later). Several bolus injections of phenylephrine failed to maintain hemodynamic stability, and an infusion of the drug (40 µg/min) was started. The phenylephrine infusion maintained systolic blood pressure between 100 and 120 mm Hg for the rest of surgery. After surgery, muscle relaxation was not reversed and maintenance of systolic blood pressure above 100 mm Hg required infusion of norepinephrine and epinephrine. The patient was able to be transferred out of the ICU on day 7.

Discussion.—Hemodynamic instability in this patient was attributed to attenuation of sympathetic tone. Three contributing mechanisms were identified: a decrease in the number of β-adrenergic receptors, the residual effect of long-term MAO inhibitor therapy; recovered MAO activity causing effective degradation of sympathetic amines; and the combined effects of general and epidural anesthesia on sympathetic tone. Some patients may need to stop MAO inhibitor therapy more than 3 weeks before surgery to allow recovery of depressed adrenergic receptor activity.

▶ Monoamine oxidase inhibitors have long been controversial. Older "dogma," namely, that MAO inhibitors should be discontinued 14 days or more before elective anesthesia and surgery, has more recently been challenged and ignored. The challenges came from anecdotes of patients receiving

MAO inhibitors who were guided successfully through complicated and difficult anesthetics by expert anesthesiologists. The challenges to the dogma also came from emergent patients who couldn't have had their MAO inhibitors discontinued. Further, MAO inhibitors these days are usually reserved for patients who are refractory to less "major" antidepressants, and, therefore, it might be possible to affect a seriously ill patient's course adversely by forcing discontinuation of this drug.

I included this report because it is important that we think hard about patients taking MAO inhibitors. The "old timers" who had trouble with anesthesia in such patients were not stupid, not by any means. In the current case, the drug was stopped 20 days before anesthesia and surgery, yet the patient underwent cardiovascular collapse. To be sure, the patient was anesthetized with techniques that were additively antisympathic. Nonetheless, this report can serve as a warning that in a patient who continues taking MAO inhibitors before elective remotely major anesthesia and surgery, anesthetic management will not necessarily be easy and straightforward.

J.H. Tinker, M.D.

Ocular Explosion After Peribulbar Anesthesia: Case Report and Experimental Study

Magnante DO, Bullock JD, Green WR (Wright State Univ, Dayton, Ohio; Johns Hopkins Univ, Baltimore, Md)

Ophthalmology 104:608–615, 1997 6–27

Introduction.—The incidence of ocular penetration during peribulbar and retrobulbar anesthesia is reported to be less than 0.1% for eyes of axial length less than 26 mm and less than 1% for eyes of axial length greater than 26 mm. Scleral laceration and lens extrusion occurred after intraocular fluid injection in a patient undergoing peribulbar anesthesia before cataract surgery. Eye bank eyes were used in an experimental study which sought to recreate the clinical situation.

Case Report.—A woman, 66, was scheduled for cataract surgery on the left eye (axial length 23.08 mm). Peribulbar anesthesia was injected first in the inferior orbit, then in the superior orbit. Details of needle size or exact volume of anesthetic solution were not known. Surgery was canceled when a hyphema, hypotony, and vitreous hemorrhage were noted after the second injection. Examination of the eye suggested a retinal tear, a posterior vitreous detachment, and moderate vitreous hemorrhage.

Surgical exploration 6 days later revealed a subconjunctival hemorrhage covering a 10.5-mm irregular, jagged, and shelved scleral rupture located 2 mm posterior to the limbus from the 11- to 2-o'clock meridians. Uveal and vitreous prolapse through the rupture was evident, together with a yellowish subjunctival mass that represented the extruded crystalline lens. Treatment interventions included anterior segment reconstruction, a pars plana vitrectomy, a scleral-buckling procedure, endolaser therapy, and a perfluoropropane gas-fluid exchange. Six months later, visual acuity in the eye was light perception, intraocular pressure was 12 mm Hg, and a retinal detachment with proliferative vitreoretinopathy was inoperable.

Experimental Study.—Twenty-one human eye bank eyes were ruptured by intraocular injection of saline with 23- and 25-gauge Atkinson needles. In 7 globes, the hydrostatic pressure at which rupture occurred was determined. Three different techniques were employed for measuring hydrostatic pressure. The pressure transducers in cardiac catheterization equipment were used to capture peak pressure at the point of globe rupture. Scleral lacerations were equatorial in 48% of eyes and perilimbal in 52%. The mean length of perilimbal ruptures was 8.5 mm; mean length of equatorial ruptures was 7.6 mm. Lens extrusion occurred with 3 of the perilimbal lacerations. Mean rupture pressures varied with the 3 techniques: 3,065, 4,972, and 5,648 mm Hg.

Conclusion.—Ocular explosion can occur as a result of peribulbar injection. The 1–injection site technique carries a lower risk of this complication, which is more likely to occur when a nonophthalmologist administers the anesthetic. Extremely high intraocular pressure is achieved before globe rupture, resulting in corneal whitening and resistance to advancement of the syringe's plunger.

▶ These authors destroyed 21 human eye bank eyes by rupturing them with intraocular injections of saline! I hope these eyes were not considered useful for anything else! They undertook this study because a nurse anesthetist had injected a patient's eye both inferiorly and superiorly, for the purpose of producing a retrobulbar block, which somehow resulted in a 10.5-mm rupture to the sclera. These authors found that to rupture an eye, one needed enormous pressures in the thousands of milimeters of mercury. Despite their own finding, they concluded that it is possible to rupture an eye from a peribulbar injection. I would have reached a different conclusion from their findings. I would have concluded that it was virtually impossible from a simple needle stick in the sclera to rupture the eye. The rupture in the case they reported must have occurred because the needle ran sufficiently tangential to the sclera to actually cause a laceration in the sclera, which was subsequently lengthened by increased periorbital and/or intraocular pressure during the injection (depending on where the needle tip was actually located during the injection). I'll bet the cutting edge of the needle passed tangential to the sclera, cutting a path through it.

I included this amazing article for numerous reasons, most importantly to raise the issue as to whether anesthesia personnel of any stripe should be performing periorbital anesthesia in the absence of ophthalmalogic training.

I know several medical malpractice cases in which periorbital block attempts resulted in permanent retinal detachments and legal blindness.

As you can tell, I'm not a big fan of anesthesia personnel doing this. I realize that it's done all the time, with excellent results, but again, how many of these kinds of devastating complications are you willing to tolerate?

J.H. Tinker, M.D.

Hyperkalemic Cardiac Arrest During Anesthesia in Infants and Children With Occult Myopathies

Larach MG, Rosenberg H, Gronert GA, et al (North American Malignant Hyperthermia Registry; Univ of California, Davis; Hahnemann School of Medicine; et al)

Clin Pediatr 36:9–16, 1997 6–28

Background.—The Malignant Hyperthermia Association of the United States and the North American Malignant Hyperthermia Registry received reports in 1992 of cardiac arrest in healthy children given succinylcholine. Patients with denervating injuries, direct muscle or thermal trauma, and disuse atrophy have a risk of fatal hyperkalemia after administration of succinylcholine resulting from upregulation of acetylcholine receptors. In individuals with progressive myopathies, hyperkalemia resulting from rhabdomyolysis from abnormal muscle membranes may develop. Cardiac arrest can be induced by hyperkalemia resulting from efflux of potassium from muscle.

Methods.—All reports of pediatric cardiac arrest within 24 hours of anesthesia during a 3-year period were reviewed. The cause of arrest and presence of myopathy were recorded.

Results.—Of 25 patients who had cardiac arrest, 92% were male and 23 were to undergo minor surgery. The patients were healthy and had no history of myopathy. An inhalational anesthetic and/or succinylcholine was used. In 18 patients, serum potassium was measured during arrest. In 13 of 18 patients, hyperkalemia was detected. Postarrest resuscitation lasted a median of 42 minutes. Of the 25 patients, 10 died, 1 is vegetative, and 14 returned to baseline neurologic function. In 12 patients, an unknown Duchenne dystrophy or unspecified myopathy was diagnosed. In 8 of these 12 patients, the arrest was associated with hyperkalemia. There was no association between patient or treatment variables and survival.

Discussion.—Pediatricians should screen their patients, especially if male and young, for occult myopathy and notify the anesthesiologist if a myopathy is detected. Outcome may be improved by suspicion of hyperkalemia and aggressive treatment after arrest. A risk-benefit and cost analysis is needed before population creatine kinase screening can be recommended.

► This paper comes from the growing database of the Malignant Hyperthermia Association of the United States. The authors' contention is that if cardiac arrest, in fact, does occur, it may mean that the child has an occult myopathy. I do not think that the authors are advocating extensive expensive preoperative testing for occult myopathy. I cannot even figure out whether the authors are advocating the performance of creatine kinase screening preoperatively. If they are, they haven't addressed the various risk-benefit ratios, what to do about false positives, incidences of false negatives, etc. The authors have introduced an interesting idea, namely, that if cardiac arrest occurs, perhaps there was an occult myopathy. If this is so, it should require considerable follow-up and careful study.

J.H. Tinker, M.D.

Treating Intraoperative Hypotension in a Patient on Long-term Tricyclic Antidepressants: A Case of Aborted Aortic Surgery

Sprung J, Schoenwald PK, Levy P, et al (Cleveland Clinic Found, Ohio)

Anesthesiology 86:990–992, 1997 6–29

Introduction.—Conflict exists as to which sympathomimetic drugs should be given to patients receiving tricyclic antidepressant (TCA) therapy. Little study has been done to differentiate managing hypotension in patients receiving acute TCA therapy vs. those receiving long-term therapy.

Case Report.—Man, 68, with a history of hypertension managed with nifedipine and a 6-year history of depression controlled with 75 mg of nortriptyline daily was scheduled for repair of a thoracic aortic pseudoaneurysm. Results of ECG and dobutamine stress test were normal. The patient took his usual dose of nortriptyline the morning of surgery; he became anxious and his preoperative blood pressure was 190/90 mm Hg. Bradycardia developed and blood pressure dropped. These changes resolved quickly and surgery was begun, with ephedrine and phenylephrine given to keep the systolic blood pressure greater than 100 mm Hg. The pressure again fell markedly and surgery was stopped. The patient was weaned from vasopressors and TCA was discontinued. Surgery was rescheduled. After a psychiatry consult, nortriptyline therapy was reinstituted; 4 hours afterward the patient collapsed with a blood pressure of 70/45 mm Hg and a heart rate of 100 beats/min. Hypotension was corrected, nortriptyline was not given the morning of subsequent surgery, and the pseudoaneurysm was repaired without complications. During surgery, blood pressure never exceeded 110/65 mm Hg and heart rate did not exceed 85 beats/min.

Discussion.—For managing TCA-induced hypotension, recommendations range from using only sympathomimetics that act directly to using those that act indirectly. Short-term TCA therapy may increase central and peripheral adrenergic tone; however, chronic treatment or acute TCA overdose may have the opposite effect on noradrenergic transmission and responsiveness. Short-term TCA therapy increases pressor responsiveness to direct-acting sympathomimetics, whereas long-term therapy does not. The period necessary to recover depressed adrenergic function may be longer than that required to eliminate TCA from the body. The less potent sympathomimetics may not effectively manage hypotension in patients receiving long-term TCA therapy because their adrenergic receptors are either desensitized or catecholamine stores are depleted. Potent, direct-acting sympathomimetics may be the only effective management for hypotension in these patients.

► I selected this case report to remind us that long-term treatment with tricyclic antidepressants may produce intractable hypotension, and that effects of acute and long-term administration of TCA therapy may differ.

M. Wood, M.D.

A Rapid Increase in Foot Tissue Temperature Predicts Cardiovascular Collapse During Anaphylactic and Anaphylactoid Reactions

Kotani N, Kushikata T, Matsukawa T, et al (Univ of Hirosaki, Japan; Yamanashi Med Univ, Japan; Univ of California, San Francisco; et al)

Anesthesiology 87:559–568, 1997 6–30

Objective.—Histamine, the most important mediator of anaphylactic and anaphylactoid reactions, alters core temperature and distribution of heat within the body. Intense vasodilation may be associated with the worst cardiovascular consequences. Whether an acute increase in foot temperature precedes cardiovascular collapse and whether the magnitude of the temperature increase correlates with hemodynamic severity were investigated.

Methods.—Between September 1983 and February 1996, 120,000 patients were screened for evidence of intraoperative anaphylactic and anaphylactoid reactions. Patients experiencing unexplained cardiovascular collapse were treated according to prospective guidelines. Foot tissue temperature was measured on the sole, and core temperature was measured in the distal esophagus. Of the 32 patients with unexplained cardiovascular collapse, 15 met the criteria for anaphylactic ($n = 9$) or anaphylactoid reactions ($n = 6$), and anaphylaxis was confirmed in 9 using the in vitro leukocyte histamine-release test or the Praunitz-Küstner test.

Results.—Anaphylactic or anaphylactoid reactions developed according to a pattern: The baseline foot temperature, an average of 3.3°C below core temperature, increased to within 0.3°C of core temperature an average of 3.2 minutes after drug administration, and end-tidal P_{CO_2} increased significantly from an average of 33 mm Hg to 38 mm Hg. Cardiovascular collapse followed an average of 1.8 minutes later, and angioedema occurred at an average of 5.1 minutes. End-tidal P_{CO_2} increased significantly to 44 mm Hg, and core temperature increased from 34.7°C to 37.1°C at an average of 13.5 minutes.

Conclusion.—During the development of anaphylactic and anaphylactoid reactions, foot temperature increased nearly to core temperature, and cardiovascular collapse occurred less than 2 minutes later. The faster the temperature increases, the more severe the reaction.

▶ I couldn't resist including this article because it amazed me that the authors measured both distal esophageal temperatures and "deep" foot tissue temperatures on the sole of the foot in each and every one of 120,000 patients! Why they actually did that, I can't imagine. I also can't imagine that the records from all 120,000 patients were accurate enough to really be able to conclude, as the authors did, that the obliteration of the normal core vs. foot temperature differential occurred "minutes" before other manifestations of toxic anaphylactic reactions to drugs occurred. They must have been measuring these foot temperatures for a reason. I cannot believe that they were measuring these foot temperatures to try to monitor for anaphylaxis. The authors had monitored all these foot temperatures and had this incredible amount of data. Why did somebody say "I wonder if this is an early warning sign of anaphylaxis?"! I found it interesting to think a little bit about a study that purports to have actually reviewed records from 120,000 patients! WOW!

J.H. Tinker, M.D.

Postoperative Nausea and Vomiting

Vomiting After Strabismus Surgery in Children: Ondansetron vs Propofol

Splinter WM, Rhine EJ, Roberts DJ (Univ of Ottawa, Ont)
Can J Anaesth 44:825–829, 1997 6–31

Objective.—As many as 85% of patients undergoing strabismus surgery experience vomiting. Although both ondansetron and propofol have been shown to be effective in reducing postoperative emesis, they have not been compared. The efficacy and cost of halothane, nitrous oxide, and ondansetron were compared with those of propofol and nitrous oxide in children undergoing strabismus surgery.

Methods.—After sedation with nitrous oxide, anesthesia was induced in 144 children, average age 6.1 years, with halothane/nitrous oxide/oxygen (group O) and in 156 children, average age 6.0 years, with propofol 2.5–3.5 mg/kg plus lidocaine IV 0.5 mg/kg (group P). Before surgery, group O children received ondansetron 0.15 mg/kg (maximum dose 8 mg) IV over 2 minutes. All patients were given atropine 20 μ/kg and midazolam 50 μ/kg IV. Anesthesia was maintained during surgery with 70% nitrous oxide and 0.75% to 2.0% halothane in group O and with 70% nitrous oxide and propofol 10 mg/kg/hr initially in group P. Patients were observed for 24 hours after surgery and monitored for emesis and medications taken. Variable and fixed costs per patient were determined for each method.

Results.—Postoperative vomiting incidences were similar between groups. Of the premedicated patients, 36% had vomiting. Of patients receiving neostigmine, 20% had vomiting. The incidence of in-house vomiting was 11% for both groups. The incidence of out-of-hospital vomiting on days 0 and 1 was 26% for both groups. Each incidence of in-hospital vomiting significantly delayed discharge by an average of 17 minutes. The number of muscles involved was related to the incidence of vomiting. The total costs associated with anesthesia averaged Canadian $17.15 in group O and Canadian $20.71 in group P ($P < 0.01$).

Conclusion.—The 2 methods had similar antiemetic effects with ondansetron therapy costing less than propofol therapy.

▶ This article is interesting because the authors found that ondansetron was effective (no surprise); that propofol was similarly effective in limiting this sometimes devastating complication in children; but that the propofol-based anesthesia was *more expensive*. We are constantly told that ondansetron is so very expensive. In this study, at least compared to propofol, it was not.

J.H. Tinker, M.D.

7 Critical Care Medicine

Mechanical Ventilation

Effect on the Duration of Mechanical Ventilation of Identifying Patients Capable of Breathing Spontaneously

Ely EW, Baker AM, Dunagan DP, et al (Wake Forest Univ, Winston Salem, NC; Lynchburg Pulmonary Associates, Va; Mayo Clinic, Jacksonville, Fla)

N Engl J Med 335:1864–1869, 1996 7–1

Introduction.—Clinical judgment alone does not accurately predict timing of successful discontinuation of mechanical ventilation. It is possible that if patients could be screened daily with a trial of spontaneous breathing, physician behavior could be altered to discontinue mechanical ventilation earlier in appropriate patients.

Methods.—Three hundred adult patients receiving mechanical ventilation in medical and coronary ICUs were randomly assigned to either an intervention or control group (149 and 151, respectively). Patients in the intervention group were screened daily by physicians, respiratory therapists, and nurses to identify those capable of breathing spontaneously. Physicians were notified by a preprinted message on the medical record when the patient had successfully completed a 2-hour trial of spontaneous breathing. Patients in the control group were screened daily, but did not undergo trials of spontaneous breathing. All decisions about patient care were made by the attending physician.

Results.—Patients in the intervention group had more severe disease, but received mechanical ventilation for a mean of 4.5 days, compared to 6 days for patients in the control group. The mean interval between when a patient met screening criteria for discontinuation of ventilation and actual discontinuation was 1 day for the intervention group and 3 days for the control group. Controls had significantly higher incidence of removal of the breathing tube by the patient, reintubation, tracheostomy, and mechanical ventilation for more than 21 days, compared to the intervention group (41% vs. 20%). There were no between-group differences in the number of days in the ICU and hospital, but costs for these services were significantly lower: $15,740 vs. $20,890 for intensive care and $26,229 vs. $29,048 for hospitalization.

Conclusion.—Notifying physicians regarding results of spontaneous breathing in mechanically ventilated medical patients resulted in earlier removal (about 2 days) of mechanical ventilation and a 25% reduction in intensive care costs.

▶ This article underscores the need for intensivist support in "open" ICUs. Experts in mechanical ventilation can facilitate "liberation from" the mechanical ventilator while minimizing complications and reducing ICU costs. Additionally, the results of this study support the need for systematic protocols designed to expedite discontinuation from mechanical ventilation.

D.M. Rothenberg, M.D.

Prolonged "Phantom" Square Wave Capnograph Tracing After Patient Disconnection or Extubation

Ginosar Y, Baranov D (Hebrew Univ, Jerusalem)

Anesthesiology 86:729–735, 1997 7–2

Introduction.—Accidental disconnection from mechanical ventilation occurs frequently in the operating room and critical care setting. In a series of experiments, a phenomenon in which the appearance of misleading square wave "phantom" capnograph tracings appear for about 3 minutes after disconnection from a Siemens Servo 900c ventilator was evaluated.

Methods.—The Siemens Servo 900c ventilator was used to ventilate patients with these settings: minute volume 5 L/min; respiratory rate, 8

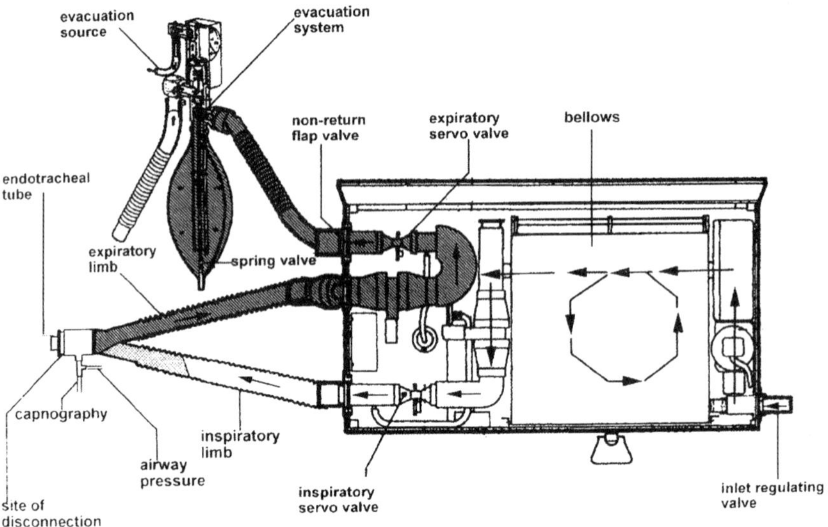

FIGURE 1.—The Siemens Servo Evac 180 evacuation system and the genesis of "phantom" capnography are shown. The *dark shaded area* is the carbon dioxide-containing gas within the expiratory limb and the evacuation system; the *light shaded area* is the carbon dioxide-containing gas within the portion of the inspiratory limb adjacent to the Y piece. The arrows show the flow of fresh and exhaled gas. (Courtesy of Ginosar Y, Baranov D: Prolonged "phantom" square wave capnograph tracing after patient disconnection or extubation. *Anesthesiology* 86: 729–735, 1997. Copyright American Society of Anesthesiologists, Inc. Used with permission of Lippincott-Raven Publishers.)

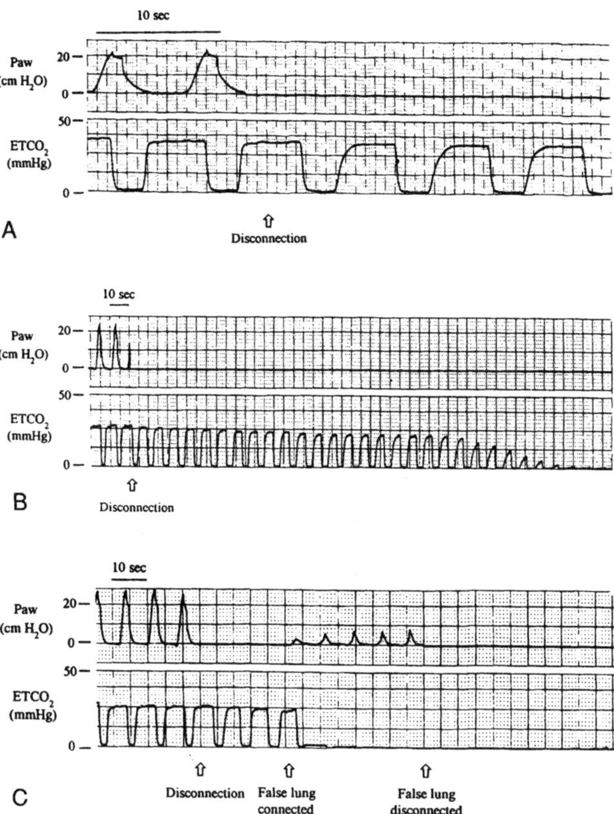

FIGURE 2.—A, the "phantom" capnograph. (*upper trace*): Airway pressure recording at the Y piece when ventilating a patient with the Siemens Servo 900c ventilator before and after disconnection. Minute volume was 5 L/min, respiratory rate was 8 breaths/min, positive end-expiratory pressure (PEEP) was 0 cm water, trigger sensitivity was −20 cm water, with a Siemens Servo Evac 180 evacuation system connected (25 L/min on evacuation flowmeter). (*lower trace*): Sidestream capnography recorded at the Y piece. "Phantom" capnograph tracings after disconnection closely resemble the square wave capnograph tracing before disconnection, both in amplitude and in shape. Note the slight blunting of the exhalation portion of the "phantom" capnograph B, decay of the "phantom" capnograph when ventilation is maintained under the conditions as outlined in Figure 2 (A). Note that, although the shape and amplitude of the tracings decline over time, a recognizable waveform persists for more than 3 minutes. C, connection of a false lung (1–L breathing bag) to the Y piece while maintaining ventilation after disconnection (note the positive deflections on the airway pressure trace when ventilating the false lung). Conditions otherwise as described earlier. The "phantom" capnograph trace disappeared immediately and did not reappear, even after the false lung was disconnected. Conclusion: The expiratory limb was washed out by fresh gas "exhaled" by the false lung. The expiratory limb is the source of carbon dioxide for the "phantom" capnograph (see also Fig 2C). D, disconnecting the evacuation system caused the "phantom" capnograph e to disappear immediately. If the evacuation system had been covered and not allowed to void to the atmosphere, then reconnection led to an immediate return of the "phantom" waveform. No interruption in the "phantom" capnograph tracing was observed if the evacuation system was left connected to the exhaust outlet but the suction source was disconnected. Conclusion: A weak positive pressure gradient between the evacuation bag and the atmosphere creates the force for reverse flow in the expiratory system; remove the bag, eliminate the reverse flow. (E, PEEP setting and the phantom capnograph are shown. Setting PEEP (note the baseline airway pressure trace) before disconnection prevented the phantom capnograph. In addition, if after an interval, the PEEP dial was then turned to 0 again, the phantom capnograph appeared. Conclusion: For reverse flow in the expiratory limb, the expiratory servo valve must be open at least intermittently. Setting PEEP will force this valve to close in the presence of disconnection

(*Continued*)

FIGURE 2 (cont.)

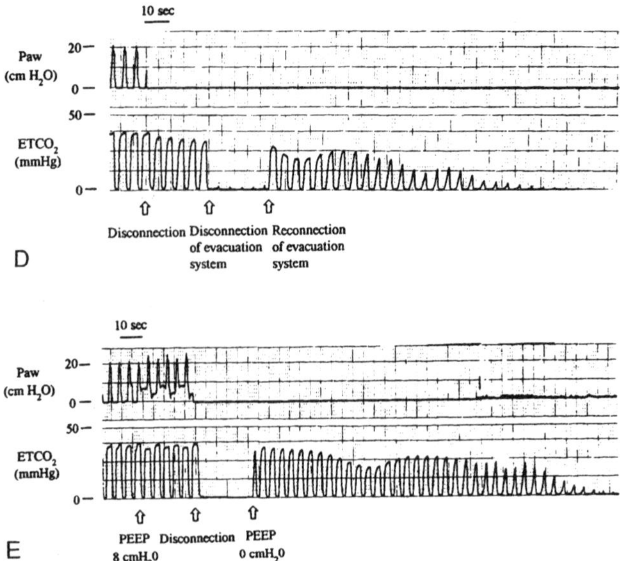

and, therefore, no phantom capnograph tracing will be seen. *Abbreviations*: *Paw*, mean airway pressure; *ETCO₂*, end-tidal carbon dioxide concentration; *PEEP*, positive end-expiratory pressure. (Courtesy of Ginosar Y, Baranov D: Prolonged "phantom" square wave capnograph tracing after patient disconnection or extubation. *Anesthesiology* 86:729–735, 1997. Copyright American Society of Anesthesiologists, Inc. Used with permission of Lippincott-Raven Publishers.)

breaths/min; positive end-expiratory pressure, 0 cm water; and trigger sensitivity, −20 cm water. The ventilator was linked to the Siemens Servo Evac 180 evacuation system at 25 L/min on evacuation flowmeter. During ventilation and after disconnection, airway pressure and capnography were recorded at the Y piece (Fig 1). The patient was supported by a back-up ventilator during disconnection of the ventilator being examined.

Results.—At first the "phantom" capnograph tracing was similar to the square wave capnograph tracing before disconnection, but with a gradual decay in the amplitude and shape of the waveform (Fig 2). The phantom capnograph was created by the establishment of a weak positive pressure gradient between the evacuation bag and the atmosphere, thus forcing a reversal of flow of exhaled gases trapped in the expiratory limb before disconnection.

Conclusion.—Several modifications could be made to eliminate phantom capnography. However reliable, monitoring techniques are no substitute for vigilant clinical observation, as evidenced by the phantom capnograph tracings described.

► In spite of the multitude of disconnect alarms commonly employed during mechanical ventilation, this article highlights how a clinician may be misled into believing that a patient disconnected from a Siemens Servo 900c is still being ventilated. This may be especially critical in patients in whom positive end-expiratory pressure is being avoided (e.g., after sleeve lobectomy or bronchopleural fistula repair).

D.M. Rothenberg, M.D.

Dramatic Effect on Oxygenation in Patients With Severe Acute Lung Insufficiency Treated in the Prone Position

Mure M, Martling C-R, Lindahl SGE (Karolinska Hosp, Stockholm)

Crit Care Med 25:1539–1544, 1997 7–3

Introduction.—A clinical follow-up study was conducted to confirm the positive effect on gas exchange that is achieved by treating patients with impaired respiratory function in the prone position. Although this finding was first presented in 1974, few reports since then have evaluated patients treated in the prone position.

Methods.—At the study institution the prone position has been the routine treatment of patients with severe lung insufficiency for several years. Thirteen patients treated in the ICU were the subjects of this study. Two had severe burns, 3 had experienced multiple trauma, 5 had septicemia, 2 were diagnosed with intoxication, and 1 had aspiration pneumonia. Severe hypoxia was present in 11 patients. Treatment in the prone position was performed without changing other ventilatory settings than FIO_2

TABLE 2.—Changes in the Ratio Between Hemoglobin Oxygen Saturation (SpO_2) and FIO_2 During the First 3 Hours Treated in the Prone Position

Patient	Supine before		Prone 1 hour		Prone 2 hours		Prone 3 hours	
nos.	SpO_2/FIO_2	Ratio	SpO_2/FIO_2	Ratio	SpO_2/FIO_2	Ratio	SpO_2/FIO_2	Ratio
1	90/0.60	150	94/0.60	157	97/0.60	162	95/0.60	158
2	90/1.00	90	95/0.90	106	97/0.80	121	97/0.70	138
3	73/1.00	73	77/1.00	77	81/1.00	81	86/1.00	86
4	93/0.65	143	97/0.60	162	95/0.50	190	95/0.50	190
5	89/1.00	89	99/0.60	165	98/0.55	178	–	–
6	97/0.80	121	97/0.70	139	97/0.60	162	–	–
7	47/1.00	47	92/1.00	92	95/0.80	119	96/0.80	120
8	72/1.00	72	91/0.75	121	86/0.75	115	90/0.75	120
9	87/0.75	116	97/0.50	194	98/0.50	196	96/0.45	213
10	91/0.60	152	97/0.60	162	96/0.55	175	94/0.55	171
11	91/0.75	121	96/0.75	128	95/0.65	146	97/0.60	162
12	91/0.75	121	94/0.55	171	93/0.50	186	94/0.50	188
13	83/1.00	83	95/0.75	127	93/0.75	124	95/0.75	127
Mean		106		139		150		152
SD		33		34		36		38
p			ns		< 0,0083		< 0,0083	

(Courtesy of Mure M, Martling C-R, Lindahl SGE: Dramatic effect on oxygenation in patients with severe acute lung insufficiency treated in the prone position. *Crit Care Med* 25[9]:1539–1544, 1997.)

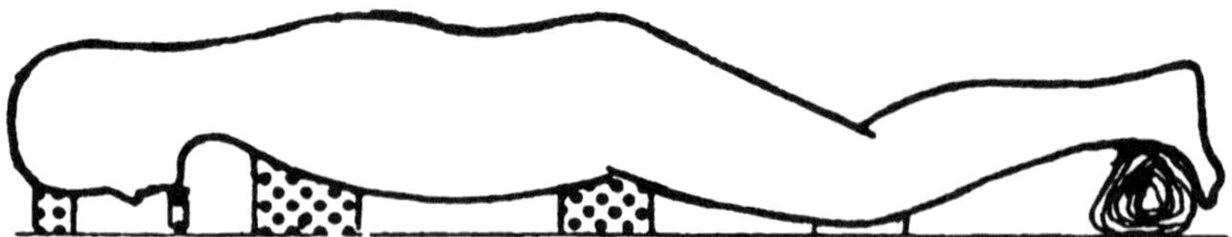

FIGURE 1.—When prone, patients ought to be supported by foam rubber pads under the upper thorax and pelvis. The head should be supported under the chin, cheeks, and forehead. It is essential that pressure on the eye bulbs be avoided at all times. (Courtesy of Mure M, Martling C-R, Lindahl SGE: Dramatic effect on oxygenation in patients with severe acute lung insufficiency treated in the prone position. *Crit Care Med* 25[9]:1539–1544, 1997.)

(Table 2). Care must be taken to anchor the endotracheal tube securely while the patient is prone, provide supports, and protect the eyes (Fig 1).

Results.—Overall, 12 of 13 patients responded to treatment in the prone position (Fig 2). Oxygenation indices increased each time that the 12 responding patients were treated in the manner, except for 1 patient whose oxygenation index did not improve the third time he was turned. In 5 patients the oxygenation indices decreased upon return to the supine position. The 2 patients who did not meet criteria for severe hypoxia responded moderately to the prone position. The single patient who failed to respond to the prone position, an alcoholic with severe liver disease, died of Gram-negative septicemia. The alveolar-arterial oxygen gradient decreased significantly when patients were in the prone position. Nine patients survived, and none of the deaths were attributed to impaired gas exchange.

Conclusion.—Twelve of 13 patients, including 11 with severe hypoxia, demonstrated significant improvement in impaired gas exchange when

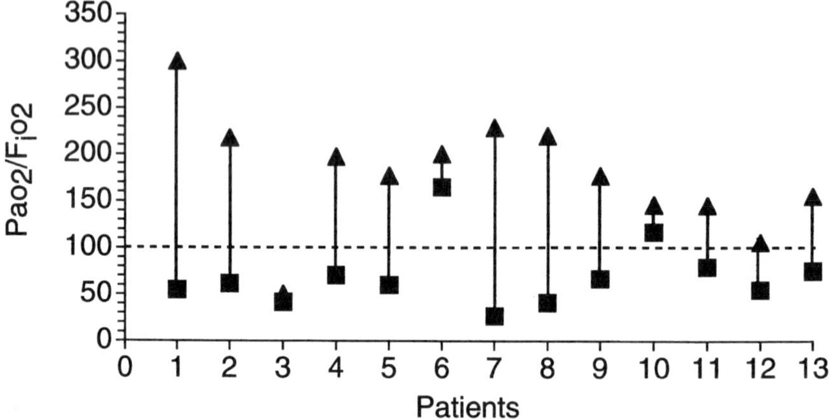

FIGURE 2.—Oxygenation index (Pa_{O_2}/F_{IO_2}) increased in 12 of the 13 patients when they were moved from the supine to the prone position. However, in patient 3, the oxygenation index was unchanged when the patient was turned prone. An oxygenation index of 100 torr (13.3kPa), the suggested level for severe hypoxia, is indicated by the *dashed line*. (Courtesy of Mure M, Martling C-R, Lindahl SGE: Dramatic effect on oxygenation in patients with severe acute lung insufficiency treated in the prone position. *Crit Care Med* 25[9]:1539–1544, 1997.)

treated in the prone position. Because extracorporeal membrane oxygenation was not required in any case, the prone position should be tried before other more complex modalities are ordered.

The Effects of Long-term Prone Position in Patients With Trauma-induced Adult Respiratory Distress Syndrome

Fridrich P, Krafft P, Hochleuthner H, et al (Univ of Vienna; Trauma Hosp "Lorenz Böhler," Vienna)

Anesth Analg 83:1206–1211, 1996 7–4

Introduction.—Prone positioning has been found to improve arterial oxygenation in some patients with acute respiratory failure, but there are no reports of the long-term effects of repeated turns between supine and prone position. Gas exchange, lung mechanics, and hemodynamic variables were evaluated prospectively in a group of patients with multiple trauma and severe adult respiratory distress syndrome (ARDS).

Methods.—During a 30-month study period, severe ARDS developed in 31 patients who met additional entry criteria: an Injury Severity Score of greater than 16 and PaO_2/fraction of inspired oxygen (FIO_2) less than 200 mm Hg at inverse ratio ventilation with positive end-expiratory pressure (PEEP) of greater than 8 cm H_2O for >24 hours. A protocol was followed in which sedated or paralyzed patients were turned from supine to prone at noon, then turned back to the supine position at 8 AM on the next day. The protocol was continued until either recovery or death as long as patients met entry criteria at the 11 AM evaluation.

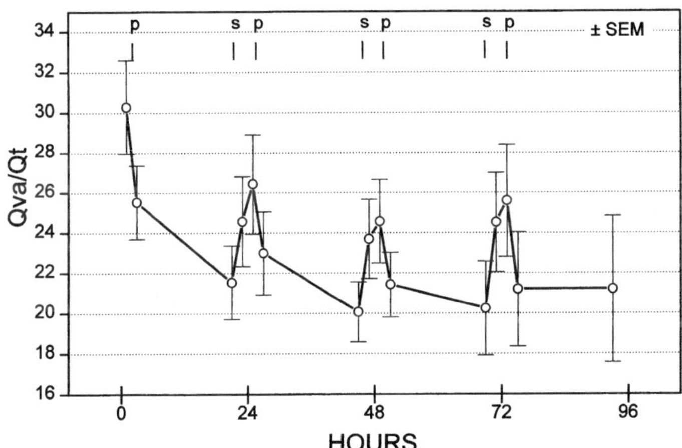

FIGURE 2.—Course of pulmonary venous admixture (*Qva/Qt*) during the first four study cycles. The "*s*" and "*p*" indicate the points of turning. (Courtesy of Fridrich P, Krafft P, Hochleuthner H, et al: The effects of long-term prone positioning in patients with trauma-induced adult respiratory distress syndrome. *Anesth Analg* 83[6]:1206–1211, 1996.)

Results.—Data from 20 patients were available for analysis. In this group the mean duration of ventilation was 30 days; a mean of 8 days was spent in the prone position. In addition to ARDS, renal failure was present in 2 patients and impaired liver function in 5. Documented cycles of prone/supine turning numbered 148; in 11, patients had to be returned early to the supine position (hemodynamic instability accounted for 6 cases). A significant improvement in oxygenation variables was observed each time the patients were placed prone. After the first turn from supine, mean PaO_2 increased from 97 to 152 mm Hg, mean intrapulmonary shunt (Qva/Qt) decreased from 30.3 to 25.5 (Fig 2), and the mean alveolar-arterial oxygen difference decreased from 424 to 339 mm Hg. Short periods in the supine position were needed for nursing care, medical evaluation, and interventions. Although the improvements gained during prone positioning were lost when patients were turned supine, a return to prone position within 4 hours allowed these gains to be reproduced. Eleven patients recovered quickly with use of the prone position, but 9 required 10 turns or more.

Conclusions.—Prone positioning of patients with trauma-induced severe ARDS led to significant improvements in lung function. Beneficial effects of the prone condition were lost to some extent when the supine position was required for a period. The turning maneuver must be performed carefully to avoid complications.

► Prone positioning for severly hypoxic patients with acute lung injury or adult respiratory distress syndrome has been touted as an effective form of therapy to improve ventilation and perfusion. Previous studies have suggested that prone positioning matches perfusion to the better ventilated dorsal aspects of the lungs. Although these studies (Abstracts 7–3 and 7–4) would further suggest an improvement in outcome, few randomized, controlled studies have reached this conclusion. Prone positioning requires intensive nursing care and quite often disrupts normal daily protocol within the intensive unit. Patients in these particular studies were positioned with foam pads (see Fig 1 of Abstract 7–3), which may or may not be optimal for diaphragmatic excursion. It would seem preferable to employ frames that are commonly used in the operating room for prone position cases (e.g., Jackson or Stryker frames) in order to facilitate nursing care and optimize functional residual capacity.

D.M. Rothenberg, M.D.

Sepsis/Acidosis

Randomised Comparison of Epinephrine and Vasopressin in Patients With Out-of-Hospital Ventricular Fibrillation

Lindner KH, Dirks B, Strohmenger H-U, et al (Univ of Ulm, Germany; Univ of Minnesota, Minneapolis)

Lancet 349:535–537, 1997 7–5

Introduction.—Intravenous epinephrine is the current drug of choice for treatment of ventricular fibrillation refractory to direct-current shock therapy. Since the observation of a large release of vasopressin immediately after cardiac arrest, there has been interest in the treatment value of vasopressin during cardiopulmonary resuscitation. Vasopressin is more effective than epinephrine in the restoration of cardiovascular function in cardiac arrest of long duration associated with severe hypoxia and acidosis. The effectiveness of vasopressin and epinephrine was compared in the treatment of out-of-hospital ventricular fibrillation in a prospective, randomized, double-blind trial.

Methods.—Forty consecutive patients treated for out-of-hospital cardiac arrest refractory to direct-current shocks were randomized to receive either IV epinephrine, 1 mg, or vasopressin, 40 U. Additional direct-current shock was delivered after drug administration. Resuscitation was continued to standard guidelines if the study drug was not effective.

Results.—Seven (35%) and 14 (70%) patients in the epinephrine and vasopressin groups, respectively, survived to hospital admission. Eleven patients in the epinephrine group and 16 patients in the vasopressin group had a return of spontaneous circulation for any length of time (not a significant difference). Four patients (20%) and 12 patients (60%) in the epinephrine and vasopressin groups, respectively, survived 24 hours. Of 11 patients alive at discharge, 3 (15%) were from the epinephrine group and 8 (40%) were from the vasopressin group. There were no between-group differences in neurologic outcome.

Conclusion.—A significantly greater proportion of patients who received vasopressin were successfully resuscitated, compared with patients who received epinephrine. Larger, multicenter trials are needed before vasopressin can be recommended in place of epinephrine in the treatment of ventricular fibrillation not responsive to direct-current cardioversion.

Vasopressin Pressor Hypersensitivity in Vasodilatory Septic Shock

Landry DW, Levin HR, Gallant EM, et al (Columbia Univ, New York)

Crit Care Med 25:1279–1282, 1997 7–6

Introduction.—Arginine vasopressin has little pressor effect in healthy individuals, but markedly increases arterial pressure in the presence of impaired sympathetic nerve function. The ability of vasopressin to main-

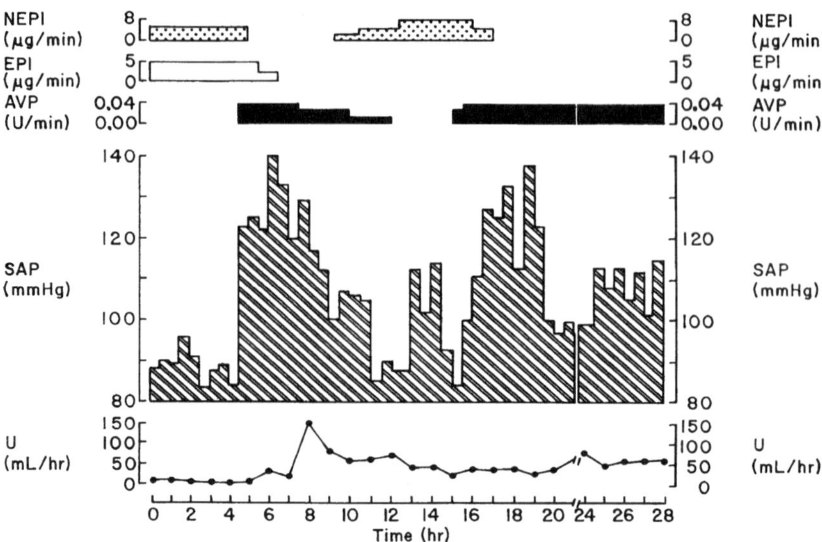

FIGURE 1.—Systolic arterial pressure (*SAP*) before and during vasopressin (*AVP*) administration in patient 1. *Abbreviations: NEPI*, norepinephrine; *EPI*, epinephrine; *U*, urine output. (Courtesy of Landry DW, Levin HR, Gallant EM, et al: Vasopressin pressor hypersensitivity in vasodilatory septic shock. *Crit Care Med* 25[8]:1279–1282, 1997.)

tain arterial pressure in 5 patients with vasodilatory septic shock who required vasopressor catecholamines was assessed.

Findings.—Exogenous vasopressin reduces cardiac output when delivered at adequately high doses; therefore, low doses were used in all patients. Vasopressin was first administered to a patient who had ventricular assist devices. Attending physicians administered vasopressin to the 5 study patients in open-label and unrandomized fashion. Arterial pressure increased significantly from 94 to 142 mm Hg within a few minutes of vasopressin administration because of a significant increase in systemic vascular resistance from 739 to 1,308 dyne·sec/cm^5. Catecholamine vasopressors were able to be discontinued in 4 patients after vasopressin administration. When vasopressin was the sole vasopressor, patients had hypotension when attempts were made to discontinue its administration on days 2–11. Reinstatement of vasopressin restored arterial pressure.

Conclusions.—Very low doses of vasopressin (0.01–0.05 unit/min) were effective in treating 5 patients with vasodilatory shock. This hypersensitivity to vasopressin contrasted with the blunted vasopressor response to norepinephrine. When administered together with catecholamines, vasopressin caused a greater pressure response than when given alone (Fig 1). Vasopressin should not be administered to patients with hypovolemic or cardiogenic shock because it reduces cardiac output. The therapeutic implications of vasopressin hypersensitivity in patients with vasodilatory shock are hard to determine. The ability of vasopressin to constrict coronary and mesenteric circulation calls for extreme caution in its use. Controlled trials are needed to determine the role of vasopressin in the management of patients with vasodilatory shock.

▶ The search continues for an effective vasopressor in the settings of vasodilatory shock and cardiopulmonary arrest. Although these preliminary studies (Abstracts 7–5 and 7–6) fail to show meaningful survival data, arginine vasopressin appears to be no worse than epinephrine or norepinephrine as supportive therapy.

D.M. Rothenberg, M.D.

Oxygen Delivery, Oxygen Consumption, and Gastric Intramucosal pH Are Not Improved by a Computer-controlled, Closed-Loop, Vecuronium Infusion in Severe Sepsis and Septic Shock

Freebairn RC, Derrick J, Gomersall CD, et al (Chinese Univ of Hong Kong)
Crit Care Med 25:72–77, 1997 7–7

Background.—The use of neuromuscular blocking agents such as vecuronium is common in ventilated patients in ICUs. Reported benefits include a reduction in oxygen consumption, an increase in oxygen delivery, and reduced barotrauma. However, none of these benefits have been confirmed in patients with severe sepsis or septic shock in the presence of deep sedation.

Methods.—Eighteen mechanically ventilated, heavily sedated patients with severe sepsis or septic shock were included in a prospective, randomized, placebo-controlled, cross-over trial. A closed-loop infusion of vecuronium or saline was administered. After the return of neuromuscular function, infusion with the other agent was administered.

TABLE 7.—Changes From Baseline of Respiratory Parameters

	p Value*	Average Percentage Change (~±SD) Vecuronium	Saline
Ct O_2	.098	1.1 ± 5.1	−1.1 ± 6.4
$\dot{D}O_2$	.334	5.3 ± 13.4	−3.7 ± 13.7
$\dot{V}O_2$	.350	1.1 ± 7.2	3.0 ± 17.2
Intramucosal pH	.365	0.2 ± 0.6	0.1 ± 5.9
HCO_3	.459	−2.1 ± 0.7	−1.7 ± 0.7
O_2 extr.	.288	5.7 ± 13.1	−2.5 ± 23.7

*One-tailed *t*-test.

Abbreviations: SD, standard deviation; *Ct* O_2, blood oxygen content: $\dot{D}O_2$, oxygen delivery; $\dot{V}O_2$, oxygen consumption; HCO_3, bicarbonate; O_2 *extr.*, oxygen extraction ratio.

(Courtesy of Freebairn RC, Derrick J, Gomersall CD, et al: Oxygen delivery, oxygen consumption, and gastric intramucosal pH are not improved by a computer-controlled, closed-loop, vecuronium infusion in severe sepsis and septic shock. *Crit Care Med* 25[1]:72–77, 1997.)

Findings.—At 40 minutes, vecuronium infusion achieved a first-twitch height of between 5% and 15%. Changes from baseline for static respiratory compliance after vecuronium infusion were significantly different from those after saline infusion. No significant differences in change from baseline were noted for systemic or pulmonary vascular resistance, oxygen delivery, oxygen consumption, oxygen extraction ratio, or intramucosal pH (Table 7).

Conclusion.—Closed-loop vecuronium infusion achieved the targeted level of paralysis and improved respiratory compliance in these patients. However, it did not change intramucosal pH, oxygen consumption, oxygen delivery, or oxygen extraction ratios. Neuromuscular blockade in deeply sedated patients in severe sepsis or septic shock does not significantly affect oxygen flux and should not be used as a routine method for improving tissue oxygenation in this population.

► There remains little doubt that neuromuscular blocking agents have a limited role in the ICU. This study could easily be applied to most clinical situations in which deep sedation and analgesia are often all that are necessary to control oxygen consumption. With the exception of improving respiratory compliance in cases such as status asthmaticus or minimizing muscle damage in cases of tetanus or status epilepticus, I am hard pressed to find an indication for prolonged use of this class of drugs.

D.M. Rothenberg, M.D.

A Guide for Predicting Arterial CO_2 Tension in Metabolic Acidosis

Fulop M (Albert Einstein College of Medicine, Bronx, NY)

Am J Nephrol 17:421–424, 1997 7–8

Introduction.—Patients with metabolic acidosis hyperventilate, which lowers alveolar and arterial carbon dioxide (CO_2) tensions and mitigates the severity of the acidemia. The relationship of partial pressure of carbon dioxide in arterial blood ($PaCO_2$) to plasma bicarbonate concentration [HCO_3-] has been observed in patients with renal failure, diabetic ketoacidosis, lactic acidosis, and diarrhea and has been used to formulate confidence bands to predict the average expected $PaCO_2$ at varying HCO_3- concentrations (Table 1). The $PaCO_2$ (in torr) in patients with metabolic acidosis has frequently been observed to be close to the 2-digit number to the right of the pH decimal point. The validity, possible usefulness, and physiologic basis for this observation were evaluated in 3 large groups of patients (from 3 different time periods) with diabetic ketoacidosis. The relationship between arterial CO_2 and the severity of acidemia was also examined.

Methods.—Pretreatment arterial blood pH and CO_2 tension levels were obtained in 262 episodes of diabetic ketoacidosis.

Results.—The relationship between measured arterial CO_2 tension levels and calculated plasma bicarbonate concentrations was similar to earlier findings. In 262 episodes with a blood pH of 7.10–7.37, down to a pH of

TABLE 1.—Relation Between Arterial CO_2 Tension and Plasma Bicarbonate Concentration in Metabolic Acidosis

Authors	Types of cases	n	$PaCO_2$* = a [HCO_3] + b			
			a	b	r	SE
Elkinton	Adults with renal failure	27	1.51	8.8	–	4.0
Albert et al.	Children with diarrhea, renal failure or DKA	60	1.54	8.36	0.97	1.1
Fulop et al.	Adults with DKA (original series)	29†	1.50	8.48	0.93	1.9
	1971–74 series‡	69	1.48	7.92	0.94	2.5
	1981–83 series‡	60	1.53	8.29	0.89	3.7
	1984–87 series‡	133	1.60	6.85	0.95	2.5
Ehlers et al.	Adults with DKA or lactic acidosis	58‡	1.51	7.45	0.89	3.5
Pierce et al.	Adults with cholera	12, plus 8 controls	1.11	12.38	0.98	1.5

*$PaCO_2$ in torr.
†Uncomplicated cases.
‡Episodes with blood pH 7.10–7.37.
(Courtesy of Fulop M: A guide for predicting arterial CO_2 tension in metabolic acidosis. *Am J Nephrol* 17:421–424, 1997. Reproduced with permission of S. Karger AG, Basel, publisher.)

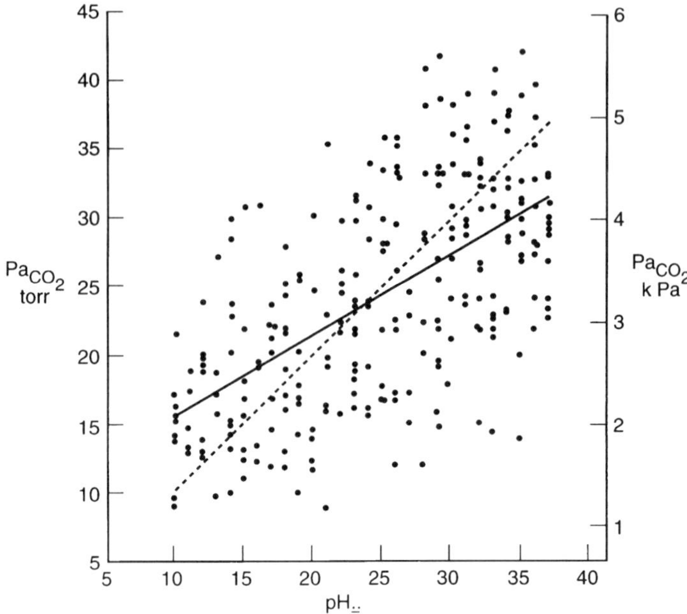

FIGURE 1.—Arterial CO_2 tension and blood pH in 262 episodes of diabetic ketoacidosis with pH 7.10–7.37. The abscissa term pH. . indicates the 2 digits to the right of the pH decimal point. The *solid line* indicates the regression equation for the data, $PaCO_2$ = 0.60 pH. . + 9.5 (r0.60, SE 6.4). The *dashed 45 = degree line* indicates identical $PaCO_2$ and pH. . values. (Courtesy of Fulop M: A guide for predicting arterial CO_2 tension in metabolic acidosis. *Am J Nephrol* 17:421–424, 1997. Reproduced with permission of S. Karger AG, Basel, publisher.)

7.10–7.15, the average $PaCO_2$ in torr often approximated the 2 digits to the right of the pH decimal point in the pH value (Fig 1).

Conclusions.—For patients with metabolic acidosis, this method provides a quick and easily remembered alternative guide for calculating the approximate expected $PaCO_2$. The foundation for this relation between $PaCO_2$ and blood pH may be the closely similar correlation between $PaCO_2$ and 1/cH+, which derives from the physiologically significant relation of alveolar ventilation to blood pH, and the inverse relation between $PaCO_2$ and alveolar ventilation.

► I have always had a *basic* objection to "shortcut" methods of arterial blood gas analyses, because use of whole blood buffer or base excess consistently leads to misinterpretation of mixed or chronic acid-base disturbances. Determining respiratory compensation in the setting of a metabolic acidosis is often a critical calculation, because failure to recognize an underlying respiratory acidosis may delay needed endotracheal intubation and mechanical ventilation.

Although simple (or simplistic) in design, this retrospective study fails the *acid* test of statistical analysis and produces nothing more than a scattergram (see Fig 1). Being within 5 torr of the measured value 52% of the time is reason enough to rarely use this equation.

D.M. Rothenberg, M.D.

Zidovudine-induced Fatal Lactic Acidosis and Hepatic Failure in Patients With Acquired Immunodeficiency Syndrome: Report of Two Patients and Review of the Literature

Sundar K, Suarez M, Banogon PE, et al (St. Luke's/Roosevelt Hosp Ctr, New York)

Crit Care Med 25:1425–1430, 1997 7–9

Introduction.—Various drugs have been associated with lactate accumulation, and a new class of therapeutic agents, the nucleoside analogs, is implicated in a syndrome of fulminant lactic acidosis and hepatic dysfunction. Two patients were described, both with HIV infection, who died of metabolic acidosis and hepatic failure after treatment with zidovudine.

Case Report 1.—A black man, 47, who had AIDS diagnosed a year ago, was hospitalized with fever, dyspnea, diarrhea, weakness, and constant right upper quadrant abdominal pain. He had been treated with zidovudine (500 mg daily) and trimethoprim-sul-

TABLE 1.—Blood Chemical and Hematologic Data in Patient 1

Chemistry	Day 1	Day 8	Day 9
Glucose, mg/dL (mmol/L)	67 (3.7)	71 (3.9)	265 (14.7)
Blood urea nitrogen, mg/dL (mmol/L)	7 (2.5)	6 (2.1)	7 (2.5)
Creatinine, mg/dL (μmol/L)	1.8 (137)	1.6 (122)	2.8 (213)
Anion gap	14	25	39
Lactate (mmol/L)*	—	17.9	29.4
pH	7.41	7.16	6.80
Pco_2, torr (kPa)	27 (3.6)	9 (1.2)	29 (3.8)
Po_2, torr (kPa)	96 (12.8)	121(16.1)	265 (35.3)
Bicarbonate, mEq/L (mmol/L)	17	3	4
Total bilirubin, mg/dL (μmol/L)	1.9 (33)	2.7 (46)	2.5 (43)
Asparate aminotransferase (U/L)	245	267	328
Alanine aminotransferase (U/L)	85	93	92
Alkaline phosphatase (U/L)	59	104	130
Albumin, g/dL (g/L)	3.1 (31)	2.9 (29)	2.6 (26)
Ammonia (μmol/L)	60	180	—
Prothrombin time (sec)	14.3	15.9	—
Partial thromboplastin time (sec)	26.2	61.3	—
Creatine kinase (U/L)	1053	1319	—
Lactate dehydrogenase (U/L)	3669	5808	—
Hematocrit (%)	32	29	29
White blood cell count ($\times 10^3$ cells/μL)	6.8	8.5	23.3
Neutrophil (%)	62	59	48
Platelet count ($\times 10^3$ thrombocytes/μL)	146	77	121

*The normal range for lactate is 0.7–2.1 mmol/L.

(Courtesy of Sundar K, Suarez M, Banogon PE, et al: Zidovudine-induced fatal lactic acidosis and hepatic failure in patients with acquired immunodeficiency syndrome: Report of two patients and review of the literature. *Crit Care Med* 25[8]:1425–1430, 1997.)

famethoxazole for the past 6 months. Abdominal US showed a markedly enlarged echodense liver. Laboratory data obtained on the day of admission and on hospital days 8 and 9 revealed development of a severe metabolic acidosis (Table 1), with an anion gap resulting from L-lactate accumulation. The patient exhibited a rapid decline in mental status and was transferred to the ICU. Despite antibiotic therapy, administration of IV fluids and dextrose, and bicarbonate infusions, his condition worsened and he died after repeated cardiac arrests. Autopsy demonstrated an enlarged liver (3 kg) with severe macrovesicular steatosis.

Case Report 2.—A Hispanic woman, 57, had similar symptoms at admission. She had been receiving zidovudine (1,200 mg daily) for 9 months but no other medications. Antibiotic treatment was started, and on hospital day 3 laboratory findings included severe metabolic acidosis with an anion gap of 33. The patient died after having cardiorespiratory arrest. Her liver showed no evidence of infection but was enlarged (5,100 g), with extensive macrovesicular steatosis.

Discussion.—This syndrome of zidovudine-induced hepatic steatosis and lactic acidosis is estimated to have an incidence of 1.3 per 1,000 person-years of antiretroviral use. The nucleoside analog therapy may interfere with mitochondrial metabolism, accounting for the lactate accumulation and the fat deposition in the liver.

► As more HIV-infected patients are being treated with nucleoside analogues, it is likely that intensivists will see more of this syndrome. Zidovudine should be added to the list of other agents causing type B lactate acidosis. Given the association of profound hepatic steatosis, it is unlikely that buffer therapy will have any benefit in the management of this syndrome.

D.M. Rothenberg, M.D.

Clinical and Bacteriologic Survey of Epidural Analgesia in Patients in the Intensive Care Unit

Darchy B, Forceville X, Bavoux E, et al (Centre Hospitalier de Compiègne, France)

Anesthesiology 85:988–998, 1996 7–10

Background.—For surgical patients, pain relief is often provided by several days of epidural analgesia. The infection rate is low. Patients in the ICU also frequently receive epidural analgesia. However, there are few data on the bacteriology of epidural analgesia in this setting. Infection rates and risk factors were prospectively studied among patients in the ICU receiving epidural analgesia for more than 2 days.

TABLE 3.—Characteristics of the 75 Epidural Analgesia Courses

No. of patients	75
EA duration (days) (mean ± SD) [range]	4.4 ± 1.8 [2–14]
EA indications	
Postoperative analgesia	62
Chest trauma	10
Pancreatitis	2
Acute leg ischemia	1
EA insertion site levels	
Thoracic	38
Lumbar	37
Reasons for EA withdrawal	
No longer indicated	61
Local discharge	12
Dural or vascular migration	0
Bacteremia during EA	2
Spinal space infection	0

Abbreviation: EA, epidural analgesia.

(Courtesy of Darchy B, Forceville X, Bavoux E, et al: Clinical and bacterial survey of epidural analgesia in patients in the intensive care unit. Anesthesiology 85:988–998 1996. Copyright American Society of Anesthesiologists, Inc. Used with permission of Lippincott-Raven Publishers.)

Methods.—The 75 patients were all free of clotting defects, septic or nonseptic shock, and bacteremia. The epidural catheter was inserted in the operating room for patients at high-risk for pulmonary problems postoperatively and in the ICU for patients with acute pain from chest trauma, pancreatitis, or acute leg ischemia. Epidural analgesia was withdrawn when it was no longer necessary and in case of a failed block, local discharge, dural puncture or catheter migration into an epidural vessel, bacteremia or septic shock, or signs of an epidural abscess or meningitis. All catheters were replaced under full aseptic technique, and dressings were changed every 24 hours. Patients with lumbar catheters received 0.25% bupivacaine, and those with thoracic catheters received morphine chlorhydrate. Evaluations for general signs of infection, inflammation at the insertion site, and neurologic signs of spinal space infection took place daily. Weekly monitoring included neurologic workups for 1 month after removal of the catheter. Patients with positive results of cultures of the epidural catheter underwent precontrast and postcontrast MRI scans at 15 and 30 days after catheter removal.

Findings.—Over the 15-month study period, 86 patients received epidural analgesia, which accounted for about 10% of the overall population and 36% of patients with potential indications. For the 75 asessable patients, the median duration of epidural analgesia was 4 days (Table 3). Of 27 patients with evidence of local inflammation, 9 had infections. All patients with both erythema and local discharge had infection. The infection rate was 12%—all 9 of these infections were local, but 4 of the patients also had epidural catheter infections. No patient had a spinal space infection. There were 9 positive swab cultures yielding a total of 12 types of microorganisms and 4 positive catheter cultures yielding 6 types of microorganisms. The most frequently identified organism was *Staphy-*

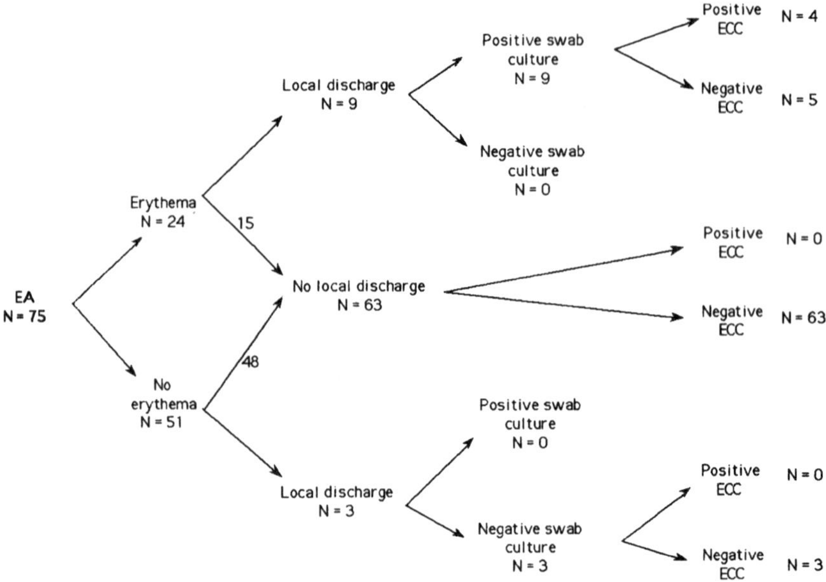

FIGURE 2.—Distribution of the 75 patients according to local signs and culture results. *Abbreviations: EA*, epidural analgesia; *ECC*, epidural catheter culture. (Courtesy of Darchy B, Forceville X, Bavoux E, et al: Clinical and bacteriologic survey of epidural analgesia in patients in the intensive care unit. *Anesthesiology* 85:988–998, 1996. Copyright American Society of Anesthesiologists, Inc. Used with permission of Lippincott-Raven Publishers.)

lococcus epidermidis. An epidural catheter culture was never positive in a patient with erythema alone or with no local signs (Fig 2). None of the 4 patients with positive epidural catheter cultures showed signs of epiduritis on follow-up MRI.

Conclusions.—Of patients in the ICU receiving epidural analgesia for more than 48 hours, 36% had local inflammation, 12% had local infections, 5% had epidural catheter infections, and none had a spinal space infection. The study did not have sufficient statistical power to prove the safety of this technique in terms of spinal space infections, however. The combination of erythema plus local discharge is 93% accurate in diagnosing positive epidural cultures. On its own, erythema is not a risk factor for colonization.

▶ The majority of patients in this study (83%) had their epidural catheters placed preoperatively, presumably under more sterile environmental conditions than those in whom the catheters were placed in the ICU. This raises the question of where the 4 patients who had infections had their catheters inserted. In addition, it would be interesting to note how many attempts it took to place individual catheters and whether an excessive number was associated with a higher infection rate. Finally, one could make an argument that a 5.3% incidence of epidural catheter-associated infection could be eliminated by simply avoiding the technique.

D.M. Rothenberg, M.D.
M. Wood, M.D.

Use of Neuromuscular Blockers in ICU

A Prospective, Randomized, Controlled Evaluation of Peripheral Nerve Stimulation versus Standard Clinical Dosing of Neuromuscular Blocking Agents in Critically Ill Patients
Rudis MI, Sikora CA, Angus E, et al (Henry Ford Health System, Detroit)
Crit Care Med 25:575–583, 1997 7–11

Introduction.—It has been suggested that monitoring with a peripheral nerve stimulator reduces neuromuscular blocking agent doses and decreases the risk of prolonged paralysis. Outcomes of critically ill, mechanically ventilated medical patients whose vecuronium doses were individualized by peripheral nerve stimulation vs. standard clinical assessment were compared in a prospective, randomized controlled investigation.

Methods.—Seventy-seven patients were randomly assigned to the treatment arm (dosing by peripheral nerve stimulation) or the control arm (dosing adjusted by standard clinical assessment). All patients received a loading dose and maintenance infusions of vecuronium. Doses of vecuronium were adjusted to 90% blockade (Train-of-Four) in the treatment group. The medical team was blinded to the Train-of-Four results and made dosing adjustments individualized to clinical response.

Results.—There were 35 patients in the control group and 42 in the treatment group. There were no between-group differences in initial doses and time to reach 90% blockage or clinical response. Significantly less drug was used in the treatment group, compared to the control group. The total cumulative amount of vecuronium for the episode of paralysis was 285.8 for the control group vs. 137.1 mg for the treatment group. Compared to the controls, patients in the treatment group recovered neuromuscular function and spontaneous ventilation significantly faster. Patients with combined renal and liver failure had a quicker recovery when they were in the treatment group than in the control group.

Conclusion.—Vecuronium dosing of mechanically ventilated critically ill medical patients by peripheral nerve stimulation resulted in smaller effective doses, lower cumulative drug doses, and improvement in the rate of recovery of neuromuscular function and spontaneous ventilation, compared to standard clinical dosing. Use of higher doses has cost and recovery ramifications that could be avoided by use of peripheral nerve stimulation.

► Some years ago, John Savarese, M.D.,[1] a noted authority on the use of neuromuscular blockers, stated that it should be considered a "relative overdose" to administer a neuromuscular blocker to a critically ill patient to the extent that all twitches during Train-of-Four monitoring are abolished.

This article scientifically confirms what Savarese and others have long suspected.

D.M. Rothenberg, M.D.

Reference

1. Fiamengo SA, Savarese JJ: Use of muscle relaxants in intensive care units. *Crit Care Med* 19:1457–1459, 1991.

Electrolyte/Renal Topics in Critical Care

Effects of Dopexamine on Creatinine Clearance, Systemic Inflammation, and Splanchnic Oxygenation in Patients Undergoing Coronary Artery Bypass Grafting

Berendes E, Möllhoff T, Van Aken H, et al (University of Münster, Germany)
Anesth Analg 84:950–957, 1997 7–12

Objective.—The synthetic catecholamine dopexamine acts via the dopaminergic receptor and β_2-adrenoreceptor agonism. It has mild positive inotropic effects caused by cardiac β_2-adrenoreceptor stimulation and potentiates endogenous norepinephrine via uptake-1 blockade. There is evidence that these effects lead to increased splanchnic and renal blood flow. Dopexamine's effects on renal function, splanchnic oxygenation, and systemic inflammation and the resultant acute phase response were studied in patients undergoing cardiopulmonary bypass (CPB).

Methods.—The study included 44 patients with a left ventricular ejection fraction of 0.5 or greater who were to undergo coronary artery bypass grafting. All patients were otherwise healthy and received standardized anesthesia. Instrumentation included an oximetric balloon catheter placed through the right hepatic vein and a gastric tonometer. After the patients were anesthetized and baseline values were obtained, they were randomized to receive either placebo or dopexamine by continuous infusion at a rate of 0.5, 1.0, or 2.0 µg/kg/min. Parameters monitored through 24 hours included hemodynamic variables; systemic oxygen delivery and consumption; arterial, mixed venous, and hepatic venous oxygenation; pHi; and mixed and hepatic venous plasma glucose, lactate, endotoxin, interleukin-6, serum amyloid A, and C-reactive protein concentrations. Also assessed were creatinine clearance values at 12 and 24 hours and endotoxin concentrations in the CPB prime solutions.

Results.—Patients receiving preoperative dopexamine at all infusion rates had increased cardiac output, stroke volume, systemic oxygen delivery, and mixed venous oxygen saturation. They also had decreased systemic and pulmonary vascular resistance. The highest dopexamine infusion rate increased heart rate, and the 2 highest rates reduced mean arterial pressure while increasing systemic oxygen consumption. Similar changes in hemodynamics and oxygenation were noted after surgery. The exception was a reduction in mean arterial pressure and an increase in cardiac output for patients receiving the highest infusion rate. By 6 hours in the

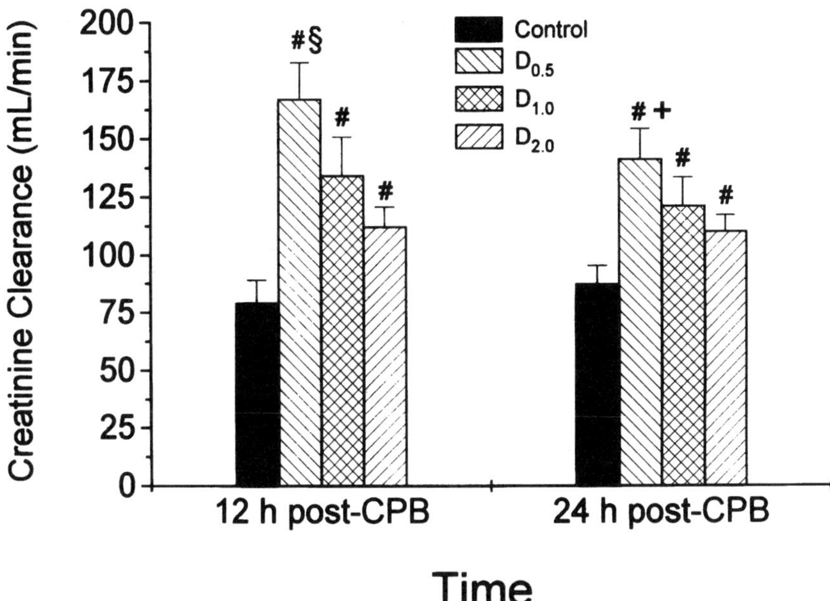

FIGURE 1.—Creatinine clearances in patients who underwent coronary artery bypass grafting 12 hours (**left**) and 24 hours (**right**) after admission to the ICU in patients receiving dopexamine and in control patients. $D_{0.5}$, 0.5 μg/kg/min dopexamine; $D_{1.0}$, 1.0 μg/kg/min dopexamine; $D_{2.0}$, 2.0 μg/kg/min dopexamine. Data represent mean plus or minus standard deviation. # $P \leq 0.025$ dopexamine group vs. control; + $P \leq 0.025$ $D_{2.0}$ vs. $D_{0.5}$; and §$P \leq 0.025$ $D_{2.0}$ vs. $D_{0.5}$ and $D_{1.0}$. *Abbreviation: CPB*, cardiopulmonary bypass. (Courtesy of Berendes E, Möllhoff T, Van Aken H, et al: Effects of dopexamine on creatinine clearance, systemic inflammation, and splanchnic oxygenation in patients undergoing coronary artery bypass grafting. *Anesth Analg* 84[5]:950–957, 1997.)

ICU, the hemodynamic values of the dopexamine group were similar to those of the control group. All 3 dopexamine groups had higher creatinine clearance levels than controls. This effect was most marked in patients receiving the lowest infusion rate (Fig 1).

Conclusions.—In patients undergoing CPB, dopexamine improves creatinine clearance while reducing systemic inflammation. It has no effect on splanchnic oxygenation. Counterbalancing its beneficial effects on systemic oxygenation, renal function, and systemic inflammation are hyperglycemia and lactic acidosis. The findings do not justify the routine use of continuous dopexamine infusion in otherwise healthy patients undergoing coronary artery bypass grafting.

▶ Dopexamine may be beneficial in other selective clinical situations such as in the 'septoid' patient (a term I've coined to encompass the patient with septic shock, sepsis, septicemia, or systemic inflammation response syndrome) who has myocardial depression. Perhaps the combination of norepinephrine and dopexamine will be more efficacious than norepinephrine and dopamine in supporting systemic pressure, in improving renal perfusion, and in decreasing the levels of circulating cytokines.

D.M. Rothenberg, M.D.

Postoperative Hyponatremia Despite Near-Isotonic Saline Infusion: A Phenomenon of Desalination

Steele A, Gowrishankar M, Abrahamson S, et al (Univ of Toronto)

Ann Intern Med 126:20–25, 1997 7–13

Background.—Postoperative hyponatremia is a potentially fatal but preventable problem occurring mainly in young women. Postoperative hyponatremia is often blamed on the infusion of excessive amounts of electrolyte-free water and on the effects of an antidiuretic hormone in preventing excretion. However, the authors' experience suggests electrolyte-free water is not necessarily involved in all cases of fatal postoperative hyponatremia. The occurrence of postoperative hyponatremia despite infusion of near-isotonic saline was documented in women undergoing gynecologic surgery.

Methods.—The prospective cohort study included a random sample of 22 women undergoing uterine surgery under general anesthesia. All patients were otherwise healthy and did not receive a diuretic. All received IV near-isotonic fluid—half as isotonic saline and half as Ringer lactate. Fluid volumes ingested and excreted were carefully measured. The estimated blood loss was less than 0.5 L.

Results.—Twenty-one of the patients had a decrease in plasma sodium concentration, and the average decrease was 4.2 mmol/L (Table 2). The lowest recorded plasma sodium concentration was 131 mmol/L. The volume of isotonic saline and Ringer lactate infused during 24 hours averaged 5.3 L. The urine volume averaged 2.5 L, which yielded a net water gain of 2.9 L. However, not all of the retained volume was electrolyte-free water. For the initial 17 hours after surgery, nearly every urine sample was hypertonic (Fig 1). Over 24 hours, the balance for both sodium and water was positive. After the gain of water and electrolytes was subdivided into isotonic and electrolyte-free water, there was a net gain of 1.8 L of isotonic saline and a gain of 1.1 L of electrolyte-free water. The isotonic saline led

TABLE 2.—Plasma Levels Before and After Surgery

Plasma Levels	Before Anesthesia	24 Hours after Anesthesia
Sodium, *mmol/L*	140 ± 0.5	136 ± 0.5*
Potassium, *mmol/L*	4.1 ± 0.1	3.8 ± 0.1
Chloride, *mmol/L*	106 ± 0.4	104 ± 0.5
Bicarbonate, *mmol/L*	22 ± 0.4	22 ± 0.5
Anion gap, *mEq/L*	12 ± 0.5	10 ± 0.3
Creatinine, *μmol/L (mg/dl)*	62 ± 2 (0.7 ± 0.02)	59 ± 3 (0.7 ± 0.02)
Blood urea nitrogen, *mmol/L (mg/dL)*	3.5 ± 0.2 (10 ± 0.6)	2.5 ± 0.3 (7 ± 0.8)
Glucose, *mmol/L (mg/dL)*	4.8 ± 0.1 (86 ± 2)	5.3 ± 0.4 (95 ± 8)

Note: Values are the mean plus or minus standard error.
*$P < 0.01$ by paired observations.
(Courtesy of Steele A, Gowrishankar M, Abrahamson S, et al: Postoperative hyponatremia despite near-isotonic saline infusion: A phenomenon of desalination. *Ann Intern Med* 126:20–25, 1997.)

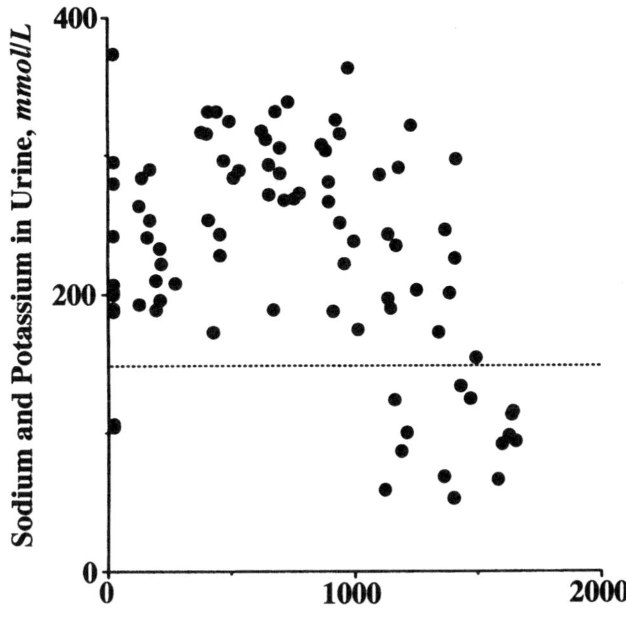

FIGURE 1.—Urinary excretion of sodium and potassium after surgery. A sodium plus potassium concentration greater than 150 mmol/L (*dotted line*) represents hypertonic urine and thus contributes to generation of hyponatremia. In contrast, values below this level represent excretion of hypotonic urine and thus a period when hyponatremia was being corrected. In samples obtained after 1,000 minutes (from 16 to 24 hours), the urine was hypertonic in some patients and hypotonic in others. (Courtesy of Steele A, Gowrishankar M, Abrahamson S, et al: Postoperative hyponatremia despite near-isotonic saline infusion: A phenomenon of desalination. *Ann Intern Med* 126:20–25, 1997.)

to the expansion of extracellular fluid volume, whereas the electrolyte-free water caused the hyponatremia.

Conclusions.—Retention of electrolyte-free water is not the only cause of acute postoperative hyponatremia. The excretion of electrolyte-free water generated by the kidney was prevented by the activity of an antidiuretic hormone. Partial desalination of the near-isotonic saline administered leads to a positive fluid balance for both fluid and electrolytes (Fig 2). The reduction in plasma sodium observed in this study resulted from electrolyte-free water, which made up approximately 3% of the total body water. Understanding the mechanisms of postoperative hyponatremia will aid in its prevention and treatment.

► This study helps in understanding the pathophysiologic process of postoperative hypotonic hyponatremia by proposing a dual mechanism: desalination from overexpansion of the extracellular space and concomitant electrolyte-free water retention secondary to antidiuretic hormone secretion. These effects may be more pronounced in healthy, premenstrual women who may retain more electrolyte-free water as a result of hormonal influ-

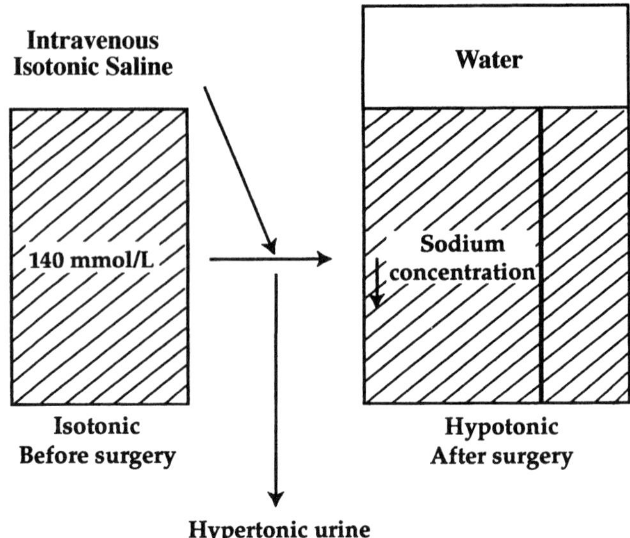

FIGURE 2.—The desalination process. *Hatching* represents isotonic saline in the extracellular fluid. The *rectangle* on the **left** represents the preoperative setting with a normal plasma sodium concentration (140 mmol/L). The *rectangle* on the **right** represents the postoperative state during which hypotonicity and edema have resulted from partial desalination of the infused near-isotonic saline. Expansion of extracellular fluid volume is caused by retention of isotonic saline. The desalination process involves administration of near-isotonic solutions and loss of hypertonic urine. An antidiuretic hormone causes retention of electrolyte-free water, which forms as a result of hypertonic urinary losses. Thus, 2 volumes are retained: the first volume (*larger hatched rectangle*) represents retained isotonic saline, which would not change the plasma sodium concentration. The second volume (*white rectangle*) represents retained electrolyte-free water (generated by excretion of hypertonic urine), which leads to hyponatremia and cell swelling. (Courtesy of Steele A, Gowrishankar M, Abrahamson S, et al: Postoperative hyponatremia despite near-isotonic saline infusion: A phenomenon of desalination. *Ann Intern Med* 126:20–25, 1997.)

ences. Previous studies documented postoperative deaths caused by acute hypotonic hyponatremia predominantly in this patient population who received hypotonic saline. Excessive administration of isotonic IV fluids intraoperatively solely to make urine appear may only exacerbate this clinical situation. Once again, here is another study that highlights the potential foolishness of using urinary output as a guide to renal or patient well-being.

D.M. Rothenberg, M.D.

▶ This is a very interesting study that followed an evaluation of hyponatremia occuring after surgery in five patients who died. Although this study examined postoperative hyponatremia in young patients, it can also be an important problem in elderly patients, especially those undergoing orthopedic surgery. The authors postulate that overexpansion of the extracellular volume occurred following induction of anesthesia in order to maintain an adequate blood pressure, leading to the excretion of a large volume of hypertonic urine. Hence, a prodigious urine output is not always a good thing!

M. Wood, M.D.

Anaritide in Acute Tubular Necrosis

Allgren RL, for the Auriculin Anaritide Acute Renal Failure Study Group (Scios, Inc., Mountain View, Calif; et al)

N Engl J Med 336:828–834, 1997 7–14

Purpose.—The hormone atrial natriuretic peptide (ANP) dilates afferent arterioles while constricting efferent arterioles, thus increasing the glomerular filtration rate and glomerular hydrostatic pressure. Animal models of acute renal dysfunction have shown that ANP can improve renal function. Anaritide, a 25-amino acid synthetic form of ANP, was tested for its effects in patients with acute tubular necrosis.

Methods.—The multicenter, randomized, double-blind, placebo-controlled trial included 504 adults with acute tubular necrosis caused by recent ischemic or nephrotoxic insults. Patients with other causes of acute renal dysfunction were excluded, as were those who had already had dialysis for their current episode of acute tubular necrosis. They were randomized to receive IV placebo or anaritide. Anaritide was given at an initial dose of 0.05 μg/kg/min, which was escalated to 0.20 μg/kg/min over 90 minutes, then continued at that level for the rest of the 24-hour

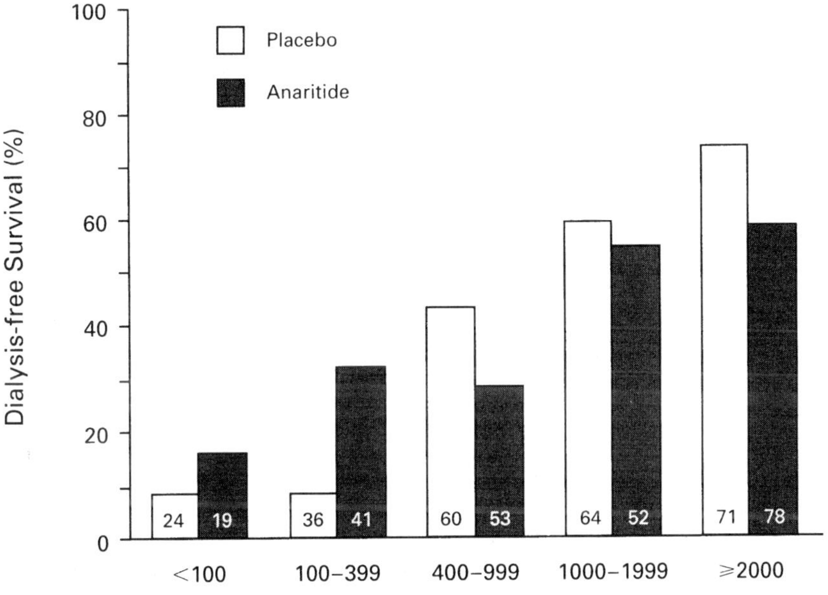

FIGURE 1.—Dialysis-free survival rates at 21 days in the anaritide and placebo groups, according to baseline urinary output. The *numbers* inside the bars indicate the number of patients in each subgroup. (Reprinted by permission of *The New England Journal of Medicine*, courtesy of Allgren RL, for the Auriculin Anaritide Acute Renal Failure Study Group: Anaritide in acute tubular necrosis. *N Engl J Med* 336:828–834. Copyright 1997, Massachusetts Medical Society. All rights reserved.)

treatment period. The 2 groups were compared on such measurements as urinary output and creatinine clearance, serum creatinine concentration, need for dialysis, and mortality. The patients received full supportive care, including low-dose dopamine or diuretics, as indicated.

Results.—Twenty-one-day dialysis-free survival rates were 43% in the anaritide group and 47% in the placebo group. Among patients with prospectively defined oliguria (urinary output less than 400 mL/day), the dialysis-free survival rate was 27% with anaritide vs. 8% with placebo. The benefits of anaritide were greatest for patients in the oliguric group who no longer had oliguria after treatment. For patients without oliguria, the dialysis-free survival rate was 48% with anaritide vs. 59% with placebo (Fig 1).

Conclusions.—In a large group of critically ill patients with acute tubular necrosis, anaritide treatment does not improve dialysis-free survival rates. However, it may improve survival rates for patients with initial oliguria and worsen survival rates for those who do not have oliguria. Future studies should stratify patients according to their urinary output.

▶ The results of this multicenter study show the beneficial effects of anaritide exclusively in a subset of patients with oliguria and acute tubular necrosis (ATN). This study supports previous work suggesting that interventional pharmacologic therapy aimed at converting oliguric acute renal failure to nonoliguric acute renal failure can increase dialysis-free survival rates. The hypotensive side effect of this drug may have contributed to the poorer response in patients without oliguria. Perhaps renal autoregulation changes differ between patients with ATN who have or do not have oliguria, yielding paradoxical responses to vasodilatory therapy.

D.M. Rothenberg, M.D.

Pulmonary Embolism

Low-Molecular-Weight Heparin in the Treatment of Patients With Venous Thromboembolism

Büller HR, and The Columbus Investigators (Univ of Amsterdam)

N Engl J Med 337:657–662, 1997 7–15

Introduction.—Compared with unfractionated heparin, low–molecular weight heparins have a longer half-life and a more suitable anticoagulation response that make them more appropriate for subcutaneous administration without laboratory monitoring in patients with venous thromboembolism. The effectiveness of low–molecular weight heparin in patients with pulmonary embolism or previous episodes of thromboembolism are not known. The clinical outcomes of recurrent venous thromboembolism, hemorrhage, and death during 12-week follow-up were evaluated in a large, open, international, randomized clinical trial designed to determine whether fixed-dose, subcutaneous low–molecular weight heparin and adjusted-dose, continuous intravenous unfractionated heparin have equivalent efficacy in unselected patients with symptomatic venous thromboembolism.

Methods.—One thousand twenty-one patients with symptomatic venous thromboembolism were randomly assigned to receive either fixed-dose, subcutaneous low–molecular weight heparin (reviparin sodium) or adjusted-dose, intravenous unfractionated heparin. Concomitant oral anticoagulation therapy with a derivative of coumarin was given over a period of 12 weeks. Nearly one third of patients had associated pulmonary embolism.

Results.—Among 510 patients treated with low–molecular weight heparin, 27 patients had 29 episodes of recurrent thromboembolism, compared with 30 episodes in 25 patients of the 511 patients treated with unfractionated heparin (5.3% vs. 4.9%). Of 93 instances of clinically important bleeding, 46 were in patients treated with low–molecular weight heparin and 47 were in patients treated with unfractionated heparin; 16 and 12, respectively, were major bleeding episodes. During the 12-week follow-up period, 75 patients died: 36 (7.1%) treated with low–molecular weight heparin and 39 (7.6%) treated with unfractionated heparin. The relative effect of the 2 treatment approaches were similar in primary outcome events: symptomatic deep-vein thrombosis or pulmonary embolism and major bleeding.

Conclusions.—Unmonitored, subcutaneous low–molecular weight heparin may be considered a safe and effective treatment for patients with venous thromboembolism. It is an appropriate alternative to unfractionated heparin in these patients.

A Comparison of Low-Molecular-Weight Heparin With Unfractionated Heparin for Acute Pulmonary Embolism

Simonneau G, for the THÉSÉE Study Group (Hôpital Antoine Béclère, Clamart, France; et al)

N Engl J Med 337:663–669, 1997 7–16

Introduction.—Low–molecular weight heparin seems to be at least as effective and safe as standard, unfractionated heparin in the treatment of deep-vein thrombosis. Data is scarce regarding the use of low–molecular weight heparin in the treatment of acute, symptomatic, pulmonary embolism. Six hundred twelve patients with symptomatic pulmonary embolism who did not require thrombolytic therapy or pulmonary embolectomy were randomly assigned to receive subcutaneous low–molecular weight heparin given in a fixed dose once daily, or an adjusted-dose, intravenous unfractionated heparin.

Methods.—In both sets of patients, oral anticoagulation therapy was initiated between the first and third days of the start of heparin therapy and was continued for at least 3 months on an open-label basis. Treatments were compared on day 8 and day 90 for major end points: recurrent thromboembolism, major bleeding, and death.

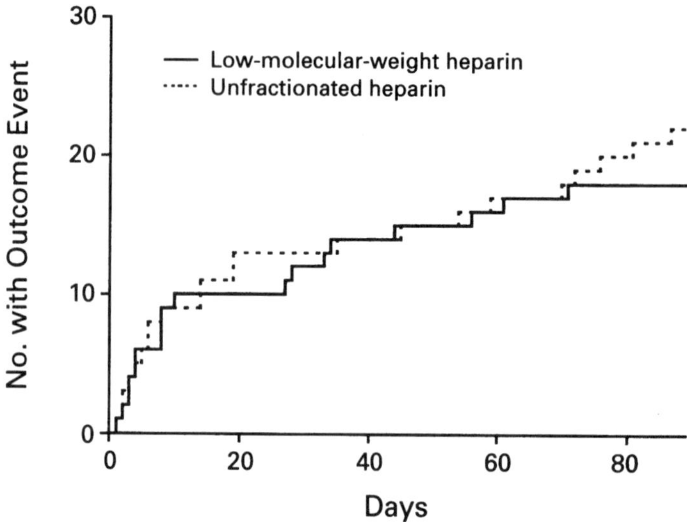

FIGURE 1.—Time-to-event analysis of the occurrence of recurrent thromboembolism, major bleeding, or death, studied as a combined outcome. *There was no significant difference between the treatment groups in the frequency of the combined outcome (P = 0.55 by the log-rank test). (Reprinted by permission of *The New England Journal of Medicine*, from Simonneau G, for the THÉSÉE Study Group: A comparison of low-molecular-weight heparin with unfractionated heparin for acute pulmonary embolism. *N Engl J Med* 337:663–669. Copyright 1997, Massachusetts Medical Society. All rights reserved.)

Results.—At least 1 end point was reached within the first 8 days of treatment in 9 of 308 (2.9%) patients treated with unfractionated heparin and in 9 of 304 patients treated with low–molecular weight heparin (3.0%). By day 90, these numbers were 22 (7.1%) and 18 (5.9%), respectively (Fig 1). Both treatment groups had similar risks of major bleeding throughout follow-up.

Conclusions.—Subcutaneous therapy with low–molecular weight heparin seemed to be as effective and safe as that with intravenous unfractionated heparin in the treatment of patients with acute pulmonary embolism.

► The use of low–molecular weight heparin (LMWH) appears likely to replace unfractionated heparin (UH) based on its lower incidence of heparin-induced thrombocytopenia and on its safety of administration, especially in an outpatient setting. Although the mode of anticoagulant action is similar for both LMWH and UH (i.e., activation of antithrombin), LMWH has a greater activity against factor Xa than it does against thrombin (UH has equivalent activity against both). Also, LMWH has less affinity for plasma proteins and endothelin, thereby producing a more predictable anticoagulant response than UH with better bioavailability, longer half-life, and less bleeding. These 2 studies (Abstracts 7–15 and 7–16), along with many others, validate the efficacy of LMWH in patients with deep-venous thrombosis or pulmonary embolism. The benefit of LMWH for patients at risk for developing postoperative deep-venous thrombosis or pulmonary embolism (i.e., after total hip or total knee replacement) has also been described. However, cases of epidural/spinal hematoma in patients undergoing regional anesthesia while receiving LMWH have been reported. Although less surgical bleeding has been cited, the longer half-life of LMWH warrants close observation in the postoperative period in patients having undergone regional anesthesia. This is particularly true in patients having received continuous catheter techniques. Guidelines for the use of regional anesthesia in patients receiving LMWH have been detailed in a recent review.[1] I recommend this additional article as essential reading.

D.M. Rothenberg, M.D.

Reference

1. Horlocker TT, Heit JA: Low–molecular weight heparin: Biochemistry, pharmacology, perioperative prophylaxis regimens, and guidelines for regional anesthetic management. *Anesth Analg* 85:874–885, 1997.

Diagnosis of Pulmonary Embolism With Magnetic Resonance Angiography

Meaney JFM, Weg JG, Chenevert TL, et al (Univ of Michigan, Ann Arbor)
N Engl J Med 336:1422–1427, 1997 7–17

Introduction.—Untreated pulmonary embolism has an estimated mortality of 30%, vs. 2.5% when treatment is initiated. Diagnosis can be difficult, however, because there is no reliable noninvasive imaging method. Patients with indeterminate findings on ventilation-perfusion scans require pulmonary angiography, an invasive and expensive approach. A new noninvasive method, gadolinium-enhanced pulmonary magnetic resonance angiography, was evaluated in a series of 30 patients.

Methods.—During an 8-month period, all consecutive patients referred for pulmonary angiography were considered for study inclusion. Twenty-three of 53 patients were excluded because of contraindications for MRI, mechanical ventilation, or lack of consent. The remaining 30 patients, all with clinically suspected pulmonary embolism, underwent magnetic resonance angiography during a single held breath. A gadolinium infusion was started 7–10 seconds before initiation of scanning. All patients were also studied with conventional pulmonary angiography, accepted as the "gold standard." The MRI scans were interpreted independently by 3 radiologists without knowledge of the findings on other imaging tests.

Results.—Standard pulmonary angiography detected pulmonary embolism in 8 of 30 patients. All 5 lobar emboli and 16 of 17 segmental emboli identified on standard angiograms were detected as well with magnetic resonance angiography. Two reviewers each reported 1 false-positive finding on an MRI study. Overall, 93% of the 720 vascular segments were adequately identified by magnetic resonance angiography. Compared with standard angiography, the 3 sets of MRI scans had sensitivities of 100%,

TABLE 1.—Sensitivity, Specificity, and Positive and Negative Predictive Values of Magnetic Resonance Angiography for Detecting Pulmonary Embolism, According to the Readings of Three Reviewers

Reading	Sensitivity	Specificity	Positive Predictive Value	Negative Predictive Value
	percent (95 percent confidence interval)			
Overall (consensus)	100	95 (87–100)	87 (74–100)	100
Reviewer 1	100	95 (87–100)	87 (74–100)	100
Reviewer 2	87 (75–100)	100	100	96 (89–100)
Reviewer 3	75 (57–93)	95 (87–100)	83 (68–98)	92 (82–100)

(Reprinted by permission of *The New England Journal of Medicine,* from Meaney JFM, Weg JG, Chenevert TL, et al: Diagnosis of pulmonary embolism with magnetic resonance angiography. *N Engl J Med* 336:1422–1427.)

87%, and 75% and specificities of 95%, 100%, and 95%, respectively (Table 1). Interobserver correlation was good.

Conclusions.—Compared with conventional pulmonary angiography, gadolinium-enhanced magnetic resonance angiography of the pulmonary arteries in this small series of patients had high sensitivity and specificity for the diagnosis of pulmonary embolism. Magnetic resonance angiography is also less costly and more acceptable to patients than pulmonary angiography.

► Technological advances in MRI as described in this study, may prove to be the most accurate, noninvasive method of diagnosing pulmonary embolism and possibly deep venous thrombosis. Much in the same fashion that MRI has revolutionized the diagnosis of thoracic aortic aneurysm and dissection, gadolinium-enhanced, single breath suspended MRI may replace ventilation-perfusion scanning (a technique with poor diagnostic accuracy), and alleviate the need to perform more costly and invasive pulmonary angiography.

D.M. Rothenberg, M.D.

► Postoperative pulmonary embolism remains an important perioperative complication in patients, for example, undergoing total knee replacement. The diagnosis is definitively made by pulmonary angiography and contrast venography, techniques that are complex and time consuming. This report of Meaney et al. describes a new noninvasive rapid technique that is sensitive and specific. Magnetic resonance imaging will be used more often to diagnose pulmonary embolism and may have an important effect on perioperative outcome.

M. Wood, M.D.

Other Critical Care Topics

Intrathecal Baclofen in Tetanus: Four Cases and a Review of Reported Cases

Dressnandt J, Konstanzer A, Weinzierl FX, et al (Univ of Munich)
Intensive Care Med 23:896–902, 1997 7–18

Introduction.—Tetanus is still associated with a high mortality rate, despite various treatment approaches geared toward improving outcome. Immunoglobulins have been instilled intrathecally to decrease the spread of tetanus toxin in the spinal cord, but recent reports are contradictory. Benzodiazepines are used to suppress the disinhibited excitatory neural mechanisms in the spinal cord and brain stem. Pancuronium is used to attain peripheral muscle relaxation. Most patients require mechanical ventilation. The γ-aminobutyric acid (GABA)-B agonist, baclofen, is not toxic and causes less sedation. Baclofen does not cross the blood-brain barrier easily, so it must be administered intrathecally. The concentration of baclofen infused at the lumbar or lower thoracic area diminishes in the cranial direction, and the half-life of baclofen in the CSF is 1–5 hours after intrathecal bolus. Four patients with tetanus treated with baclofen were described.

Patients.—All patients had generalized tetanus. They received 10,000 or more units of tetanus immunoglobulin and intrathecal baclofen. The intrathecal catheter tip was placed at the vertebral levels of T9–10. In 3 patients, doses of 500, 1,000, or 2,000 μg/day were effective, but 1,500 μg/day was insufficient for the fourth patient. The fourth patient required diazepam and mechanical ventilation throughout most of treatment.

> *Case Report.*—Woman, 52, who was a farmer had back pain, then trismus, then opisthotonus 4 weeks after an open foot injury. Diazepam and pancuronium were given for relaxation. On treatment day 12, these drugs were discontinued and baclofen (500 μg/day) therapy was initiated. Relaxation of the neck and head were good, but she still had trismus. She required mechanical ventilation. Flumazenil was administered intravenously on day 15 and she awakened immediately, was breathing spontaneously, and was able to move her extremities. She had increased trismus and elevated blood pressure and heart rate. She required 1 more day of mechanical ventilation after somnolence recurred, which decreased respiratory drive. The effects of sedation wore off, and she no longer required mechanical ventilation. Baclofen was continued for another 10 days. The dose was decreased to 150 μg/day on the day before the infusion was stopped. She had no further spasms. Blood pressure increased (within normal range) for 12 hours after lowering the baclofen dose. She was discharged on hospital day 43.

Conclusions.—Three of 4 patients with tetanus had sufficient muscle relaxation with intrathecal infusion of baclofen. A more cranial thoracic position at the level of T5–7 may have offered better suppression of spasms in the upper extremities at lower doses. Patients with severe tetanus may benefit from earlier baclofen infusion to prevent administration of large doses of benzodiazapines.

Management of Blood Pressure Instability in Severe Tetanus: The Use of Clonidine

Gregorakos L, Kerezoudi E, Dimopoulos G, et al (Chest Hosp of Athens, Greece; Polycliniki Hosp of Athens, Greece; PHEA Hosp of Athens, Greece)
Intensive Care Med 23:893–895, 1997 7–19

Introduction.—Autonomic hyperactivity, with its main feature of unstable blood pressure, occurs in most patients with tetanus and is associated with poor prognosis. Clonidine has recently been used to treat 2 patients with tetanus and blood pressure instability. The results are contradictory. The effectiveness of clonidine in the management of unstable blood pressure was evaluated in 27 patients with severe tetanus.

Methods.—All patients were graded IIB and were treated according to protocol. Seventeen patients were treated with clonidine, 2 µg/kg administered 3 times per day intravenously, and 10 did not receive clonidine. Patients received clonidine until blood pressure stability was fully restored. The dosage was gradually decreased, then stopped before discharge from the intensive care unit.

Results.—Seven of 27 patients (29.6%) died; 5 patients (50%) from the group not treated with clonidine and 2 (11.7%) from the clonidine-treated group. There were no between-group differences in age, weight, incubation period, duration of ICU stay, duration of ventilation, heart rate, and maximum and minimum systolic blood pressures.

Conclusions.—Overactivity of the autonomic nervous system is a life-threatening complication of tetanus that is currently thought to be caused by failure of inhibitory transmission. Mortality was significantly decreased with clonidine treatment in patients with severe tetanus and cardiovascular instability.

▶ I have only managed 2 cases of severe tetanus; however, I will never forget the challenges posed in attempting to pharmacologically control the marked degrees of autonomic hyperactivity. Minimal changes in noise or light levels, or the least bit of physical stimuli would cause marked swings in both heart rate and blood pressure. Concomitant use of vasopressors and vasodilators, in addition to industrial strength dosages of benzodiazepines and neuromuscular relaxants, were required to offset the tremendous hemodynamic instability. These 2 brief reports (Abstracts 7–18 and 7–19) offer reasonable approaches to caring for patients with this devastating infection.

D.M. Rothenberg, M.D.

Ocular Surface Disorders in the Critically Ill

Imanaka H, Taenaka N, Nakamura J, et al (Osaka Univ Hosp, Japan)

Anesth Analg 85:343–346, 1997 7–20

Introduction.—The incidence of ocular surface disorders in critically ill patients in the ICU, and factors causing the disorders were determined retrospectively. Fifteen additional patients were studied prospectively.

Methods.—Patients in the retrospective study had an ICU stay that exceeded 7 days. A member of the staff examined each patient's eyes once a day for the presence of conjunctivitis and corneal erosion. Variables recorded were age, prognosis, continuous IV administration of sedatives or muscle relaxants, and air conditioner settings. Standard eye care included ofloxacin eyedrops and erythromycin ointment every 8 hours.

The 15 consecutive patients studied prospectively had IV sedatives or muscle relaxants administered continuously for more than 48 hours. All were intubated and mechanically ventilated before study entry. These patients had cornea surfaces examined once a day, using fluorescein dye and slit-lamp biomicroscopy. Eye care was similar to that provided in the retrospective study. Eyelid taping was used in 4 patients who showed an increasing area of corneal erosion despite the eye care. Patients with and without corneal erosion during the study period were compared for potential causal factors.

Results.—Twenty-eight (20%) patients studied retrospectively had ocular surface disorders: conjunctivitis in 23 and corneal erosion in 5. Risk factors associated with ocular surface disorders were continuous sedation (35% vs. 15%) and continuous paralysis (39% vs. 11%). The incidence of ocular surface disorders was significantly higher among nonsurvivors (56%) than survivors (6%). Nine patients (60%) studied prospectively had corneal erosion, which developed in all cases within 1 or 2 days of continuous sedation or immobilization. There was a strong correlation between corneal erosion and the inability to completely close the eyelids. All patients whose eyelids were taped completely recovered from corneal erosion, but those with conventional lubrication showed no improvement in the established corneal erosion during the study period.

Conclusions.—Ocular surface disorders are common in ICU patients, and the incidence increases with sedation, paralysis, severity of illness, and longer ICU stay. Environmental factors such as air conditioner settings were not implicated, but lack of eye closure increased the risk for ocular surface disorders.

► It would seem prudent to include routine eye taping as part of daily care in patients with multiorgan system failure who are receiving positive pressure ventilation and are being treated with sedatives and/or neuromuscular relaxants. I do not believe that I would be *farsighted* in concluding that a *blinded* study is in order to assess the efficacy of eye taping with or without antibacterial or nonantibacterial ointment.

D.M. Rothenberg, M.D.

Initial Evaluation of Diaspirin Cross-linked Hemoglobin (DCLHb™) as a Vasopressor in Critically Ill Patients

Reah G, Bodenham AR, Mallick A, et al (Gen Infirmary at Leeds, England; Baxter Healthcare Corp, Round Lake, Ill)

Crit Care Med 25:1480–1488, 1997 7–21

Introduction.—Experimental studies have shown diaspirin cross-linked hemoglobin (DCLHb), a highly purified hemoglobin solution extracted from outdated volunteer-donated human erythrocytes, to be an effective blood substitute during resuscitation for hemorrhagic shock. Its vasopressor effect has been accompanied by indirect evidence of improved tissue perfusion, and DCLHb also appears to be a nitric oxide scavenger and a modulator of adrenoreceptor sensitivity. These favorable preliminary results led to an evaluation of the benefits of DCLHb in critically ill patients in shock.

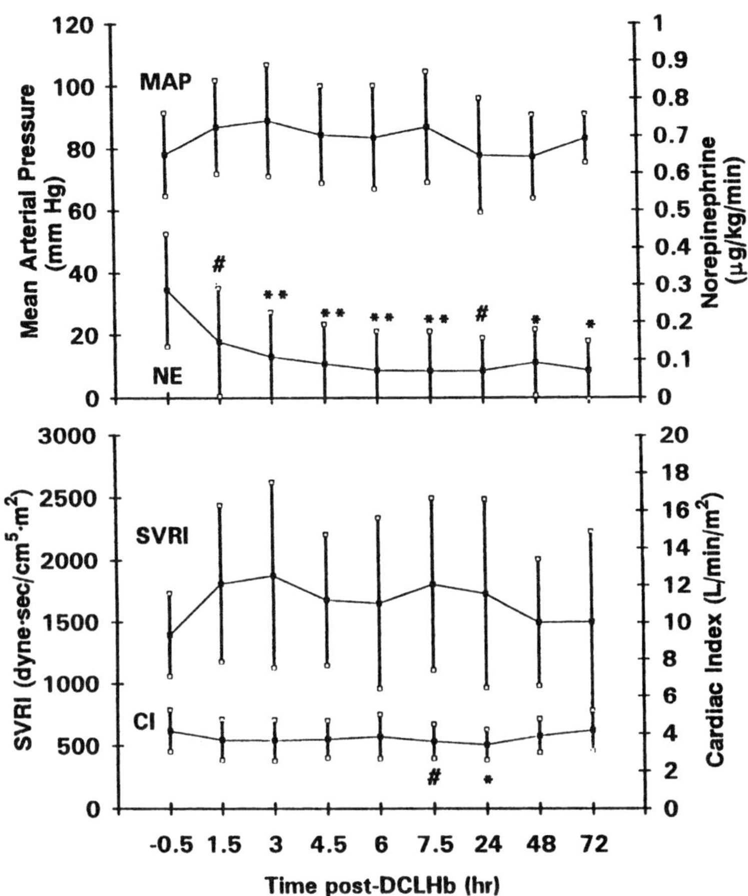

FIGURE 2.—**Top,** effects of diaspirin cross-linked hemoglobin (*DCLHb*) administration on norepinephrine requirements (*NE*) for 13 patients over a 72-hour period. Norepinephrine requirements were reduced while maintaining mean arterial pressure (*MAP*) at approximately preinfusion values. *Asterisk P* < 0.01; *pound sign, P* < 0.001; *double asterisk, P* < 0.0001. **Bottom,** effects of DCLHb on cardiac index (*CI*) and systemic vascular resistance index (*SVRI*). Cardiac index significantly decreased at 7.5 and 24 hours. Systemic vascular resistance index nonsignificantly increased during the first 24 hours after infusion. Asterisk indicates *P* < 0.01; *pound sign, P* < 0.001. The time points −0.5, 1.5, 3, 4.5, 6, and 7.5 hours correspond to preinfusion, post first infusion, post second infusion, post third infusion, post fourth infusion, and post fifth infusion, respectively. All values are expressed as mean ± SD. (Courtesy of Reah G, Bodenham AR, Mallick A, et al: Initial evaluation of diaspirin cross-linked hemoglobin [DCLHb] as a vasopressor in critically ill patients. *Crit Care Med* 25[9]:1480–1488, 1997.)

Methods.—The prospective, observational study enrolled 14 patients hospitalized in an ICU with clinical signs of shock. Each had either a low systemic vascular resistance index (SVRI) or was receiving increasing doses of vasopressors to maintain adequate mean arterial pressure (MAP). All patients had secondary organ dysfunction. Treatment with DCLHb (10 g/dL) consisted of a maximum of five 100-mL boluses administered over 15 minutes and 60–90 minutes apart. Reduction in the dose of norepinephrine was the main end point to assess the efficacy of DCLHb as a vasopressor.

Results.—All 14 patients exhibited an immediate vasopressor response within 5 minutes of receiving the initial bolus of DCLHb, an effect that lasted for 72 hours. Norepinephrine requirements were reduced (Fig 2) and cardiac index was significantly decreased at several time points. Throughout the 72-hour period, no significant changes were observed in MAP, heart rate, pulmonary arterial occlusion pressure, SVRI, central venous pressure, or urine output. Pulmonary vascular resistance index increased at 7.5 hours despite nonsignificant increases in mean pulmonary arterial pressure. Total plasma bilirubin levels increased significantly with DCLHb treatment but returned to baseline values within 5 days.

Conclusions.—The vasopressor effect of DCLHb was confirmed in this group of critically ill patients who required vasopressor therapy to maintain MAP. Patients responded within minutes of receiving the infusion, and norepinephrine requirements were reduced with each bolus infusion. The magnitude of response declined, however, with each subsequent bolus.

► Although there appears to be a potent vasopressor activity of DCLHb, the decreases in cardiac index and oxygen delivery associated with this therapy seem counterproductive to the oxygen-carrying capacity of this agent. Other than an increase in mean arterial pressure, no other clinical parameters assessing regional perfusion improve with this therapy. This would include no changes in serum creatinine, gastric intramucosal pH, or serum lactate levels. In this small study, toxicity appears to be limited to dilutional thrombocytopenia and hyperbilirubinemia. Future randomized clinical trials assessing DCLHb in other types of circulatory shock would be of interest.

D.M. Rothenberg, M.D.

Randomized, Double-blind Study of Intravenous Human Albumin in Hypoalbuminemic Patients Receiving Total Parenteral Nutrition

Rubin H, Carlson S, DeMeo M, et al (Northwestern Univ, Chicago)

Crit Care Med 25:249–252, 1997 7–22

Purpose.—Whether because of increased catabolism, decreased synthesis, or both, serum albumin increases in patients who have acute illness or who have undergone major surgery. In hospitalized patients, serum albumin is a useful predictor of mortality. However, it is uncertain whether serum albumin is a useful marker of nutrition. Most previous studies have shown no reduction in morbidity with the administration of human serum albumin to patients receiving total parenteral nutrition (TPN). The effects of IV albumin administration were investigated in hospitalized patients with hypoalbuminemia.

Methods.—The randomized, blind, placebo-controlled trial included 31 patients with a serum albumin concentration of less than 2.5 g/dL who were receiving at least 6 days of TPN. All were adults and free of metastatic cancer, cirrhosis, and nephrotic syndrome. Each patient received 6 or more days of therapy with either albumin or placebo. All were followed up through discharge or death. Albumin kinetics were evaluated as well.

Results.—The 2 groups were comparable in terms of hospital days that TPN was received and days that their assigned drug was received. Death occurred within 30 days for 1 patient in the placebo group and 2 in the albumin group. Sepsis occurred in 1 patient, and bacteremia occurred in 3 patients. Pneumonia occurred in 4 patients in the placebo group and in 7 in the albumin group; none of these differences were significant. All patients in the albumin group had an increase in serum albumin, including 1 patient who received albumin for only 6 days. The mean increase in serum albumin was 1.42 g/dL in the albumin group vs. 0.29 g/dL in the placebo group. Albumin metabolism increased from 17.4 to 20.5 g/day during the study. Overall, the results suggested that albumin was causing more harm than good, and the study was discontinued.

Conclusions.—Giving IV albumin to hospitalized patients with hypoalbuminemia does not appear to have any benefit. This is despite the fact that serum albumin increases during such treatment. Given the high cost of human serum albumin, the researchers recommend a reduction in its use for patients receiving TPN.

▶ This year a nationwide shortage of albumin occurred, which prompted many of us to cry out, "It's about time!" For too many years physicians have been administering albumin in a cavalier manner, with little if any data to support this practice. Arguments favoring its use over crystalloid resuscitation in the setting of acute lung injury (so as to minimize an increase in lung water) have never been substantiated. Furthermore, the use of exogenous albumin infusions to artificially raise serum albumin in hopes of improving the prognosis in critically ill patients is also unwarranted. If the lack of medical indications were not sufficient, then certainly the tremendous expense of albumin in an era of cost-containment should prohibit its use.

D.M. Rothenberg, M.D.

Heat Stroke: Opioid-mediated Mechanisms

Romanovsky AA, Blatteis CM (Univ of Tennessee at Memphis; Legacy Portland Hosps, Ore)

J Appl Physiol 81:2565–2570, 1996 7–23

Introduction.—A previous study in guinea pigs reported high mortality caused by heat stroke after the animals were subjected to intensive and prolonged intraperitoneal heating (IPH). Two paradoxical thermoregulatory phenomena accompanied this IPH-induced heat disorder: hyperthermia-induced vasoconstriction and hyperthermia-induced hypothermia. The hypothesis that the underlying mechanisms of these phenomena involve endogenous opioid agonists was tested.

Methods.—Experiments were conducted in 24 guinea pigs that were chronically implanted with an intraperitoneal thermode and intrahypothalamic thermocouple. Heat stroke was induced in the animals by IPH, performed by perfusing water at an inflow temperature of 45°C through the thermode. The study was designed to evaluate the effect of naltrexone (NTX), a wide-spectrum opioid-receptor antagonist, on the thermoregulatory symptoms of IPH-induced heat stroke. Naltrexone was administered via injection (0 or 50 μmol/kg subcutaneously) in pyrogen-free saline immediately before the beginning of IPH; some animals received NTX but had no IPH performed.

Results.—Heat stroke resulting from IPH had a high 48-hour mortality rate (50%) in control animals (0 μmol/kg subcutaneously). Responses to IPH included both the hyperthermia-induced hypothermia and hyperthermia-induced vasoconstriction. Skin vasodilation occurred at the onset of IPH, but subsequently changed to vasoconstriction despite high body temperature and continuing IPH. The hyperthermia induced by IPH (mean 1.8°C) was followed by a post-IPH fall in body temperature (mean −5.1°C). Animals treated with NTX did not exhibit hyperthermia-induced vasoconstriction, and the hyperthermia-induced hypothermia was reduced in this group (mean −1.8°C). None of the animals treated with NTX died. Naltrexone had little effect on body temperature regulation in the no-IPH group.

Conclusions.—The phenomena of both hyperthermia-induced vasoconstriction and hyperthermia-induced hypothermia appear to be opioid dependent, reflecting respectively, opioid-induced hemodynamic alterations and opioid-mediated inhibition of metabolism. Skin vasoconstriction and a posthyperthermia fall in body temperature may be markers of severity in heat stroke.

► The implications of this experimental study are important not only in the management of heat stroke but also potentially in the management of neuroleptic malignant syndrome and malignant hyperthermia.

D.M. Rothenberg, M.D.

Keeping Up With the Critical Care Literature

How to Keep Up With the Critical Care Literature and Avoid Being Buried Alive

Cook DJ, Meade MO, Fink MP (McMaster Univ, Hamilton, Ont; Univ of Toronto; Harvard Univ, Boston)

Crit Care Med 24:1757–1768, 1996 7–24

Introduction.—Relevant data in published medical literature offers information that can help improve decisions important in caring for patients. Well-informed intensivists need to be aware of current pathophysiologic investigations. Based on an estimated rate of 200,000 biomedical publications released per annum in 1979, it was calculated that if clinicians read

TABLE 2.—Combinations of Search Terms With the Best Sensitivity for Detecting Sound, Valid, Clinical Studies in the Prognosis, Diagnosis, and Management of Medical Problems

Article	Search Strategy	Sensitivity	Specificity
Prognosis	Incidence or "explode" mortality or follow-up studies or mortality (subheading) or prognos: (text word) or predict: (text word) or course (text word)	0.92	0.73
Diagnosis	"Explode" sensitivity, specificity or diagnosis and (subheading pre-explosion) or diagnostic use (subject heading) or sensitivity (text word) or specificity (text word)	0.92	0.73
Treatment	Randomized controlled trial (publication type) or drug therapy (subheading) or therapeutic use (subheading) or random: (text word)	0.99	0.74

Note: Colons indicate truncation. Truncation allows searching all terms beginning with the given prefix. For example, "random:" would drive a search looking for any of the following: "randomly," "randomized," "randomised," "randomization."

(Adapted with permission from Haynes RB, Wilczinski N, McKibbon A, et al: Developing optimal search strategies for detecting clinically sound studies in MEDLINE. *J Am Med Informatics Assoc* 1:447–458, 1994. Courtesy of Cook DJ, Meade MO, Fink MP: How to keep up with critical care literature and avoid being buried alive. *Crit Care Med* 24[10]:1757–1768, 1996.)

2 articles per day for a year, they would be 55 centuries behind in reading. Keeping aware of available literature is challenging and overwhelming.

Accessing the Literature.—The following are practical suggestions for accessing, utilizing, and storing the rapidly expanding literature on critical care medicine: (1) focus the clinical question (Table 2); (2) locate literature using bibliographic databases; (3) use original journal articles; (4) use systematic reviews with confidence (the Cochrane Data Base of Systematic Reviews is a large-scale, multidisciplinary product); (5) use textbooks with caution because they are often outdated on new approaches; (6) read the preappraised literature; (7) abandon advertisements; (8) throw away the throwaways; (9) teach yourself critical appraisal; (10) be wary of overinterpretation of substitute end points; (11) teach yourself basic clinical statistics; (12) engage in effective browsing; (13) store useful articles; (14) invest in informatics; and (15) implement evidence-based practice guidelines.

Conclusions.—The intensivist needs skills in efficient access, appraisal, and application of the literature on intensive care. It is possible for the busy practitioner to harness useful strategies for keeping up to date.

► I had to include this article for purely selfish reasons. Each year I promise to stay ahead of the YEAR BOOK's "article heaper," and each year I find myself needing a larger shovel! Now, however, I surely hold the secret to avoiding the "grave" implications of a publisher's *dead*line. No longer will I have to suffer endlessly through a morass of thousands of articles. Hallelujah! I've been saved! By the way, Tink, I was wondering if you are still trying to sell that piece of swamp land in Florida? I think I might be interested. In all seriousness, this article does offer exceedingly relevant information regarding how to improve computerized literature searches, the Cochrane Collaboration of Systematic Article Reviews, and medical informatics.

D.M. Rothenberg, M.D.

8 Pain Management

Acute Postoperative Pain Management

Postcesarean Analgesia With Both Epidural Morphine and Intravenous Patient-controlled Analgesia: Neurobehavioral Outcomes Among Nursing Neonates

Wittels B, Glosten B, Faure EAM, et al (Univ of Chicago; Univ of Washington, Seattle; Saint Francis Hosp, Blue Island, Ill; et al)

Anesth Analg 85:600–606, 1997 8–1

Introduction.—Morphine and meperidine share similar pharmacokinetics, but the accumulation of normeperidine (the active N-demethylated metabolite of meperidine) in maternal breast milk has been associated with significant neurobehavioral depression in nursing neonates. Postcesarean analgesia with morphine 4 mg and patient-controlled analgesia (PCA) meperidine or morphine were compared in a prospective, randomized, double-blind, controlled trial to determine whether neonatal neurobehavioral depression could be prevented when meperidine exposure was decreased in nursing infants.

Methods.—After cesarean delivery with epidural anesthesia, 2% lidocaine, and epinephrine 1:200,000, parturients received epidural morphine 4 mg after umbilical cord clamping. Women were randomly assigned to receive either PCA meperidine or PCA morphine. Nursing infants were assigned to 1 of 2 groups to observe the effect of PCA opioid in breast milk: the meperidine group (24 infants) and the morphine group (23 infants). Fifty-six bottle-fed infants acted as controls.

Results.—Infants in the morphine group were significantly more alert and oriented to animate human auditory cues on the third and fourth days of life than their meperidine and control group counterparts. During the first 48 hours post partum, the average PCA consumption was equivalent for the 2 opioids. Even with small doses, meperidine was associated with significantly poorer mental alertness and orientation, compared to morphine.

Conclusion.—Nursing infants exposed to morphine were more alert than those exposed to meperidine. Morphine is the PCA opioid of choice for women who are nursing and have undergone cesarean section.

▶ This study provides evidence that morphine is preferred over meperidine when providing IV PCA for postcesarean analgesia in nursing women. Perhaps the most interesting finding of this study is that infants in the morphine group were significantly more alert on the third day of life than infants in the control (i.e., bottle-fed) group. The authors noted that "bottle-fed infants may not have received the same degree of human attention and bonding as infants of nursing parturients," and that the greater alertness among the morphine-group infants on the third day of life was likely the result of "these differences in maternal constitutive factors."

D.H. Chestnut, M.D.

Analgesia After Caesarean Section: Patient-controlled Intravenous Morphine vs Epidural Morphine

Rapp-Zingraff N, Bayoumeu F, Baka N, et al (Maternité Régionale, Nancy, France; Hôpital Marin, Nancy, France)

Int J Obstet Anesth 6:87–92, 1997 8–2

Objective.—Epidural morphine offers better analgesia after cesarean section than previously used techniques, though it has some potentially serious side effects. Many studies have evaluated the use of IV morphine patient-controlled anesthesia (PCA) for this purpose. However, these studies have tended to compare different opioids and have rarely used a

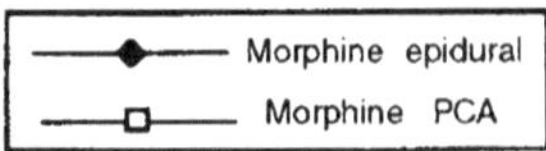

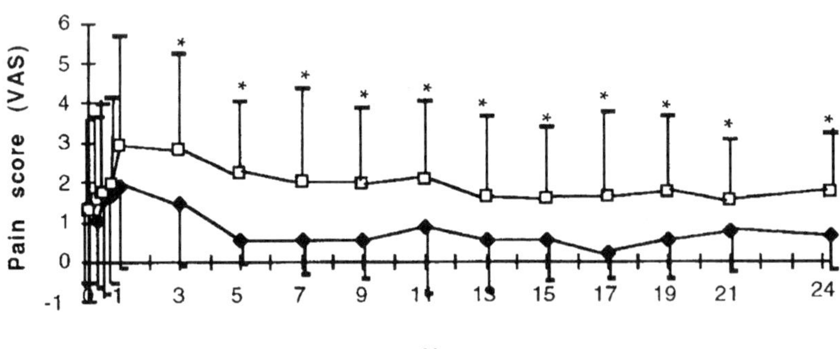

FIGURE 1.—Mean (±SD) pain scores (the hours during which there was a significant difference between groups are indicated, *$P < 0.05$). *Abbreviations: PCA,* patient-controlled anesthesia; *VAS,* visual analogue scale. (Courtesy of Rapp-Zingraff N, Bayoumeu F, Baka N, et al: Analgesia after caesarean section: Patient-controlled intravenous morphine vs epidural morphine. *Int J Obstet Anesth* 6:87–92. Copyright 1997, by permission of the publisher, Churchill Livingstone.)

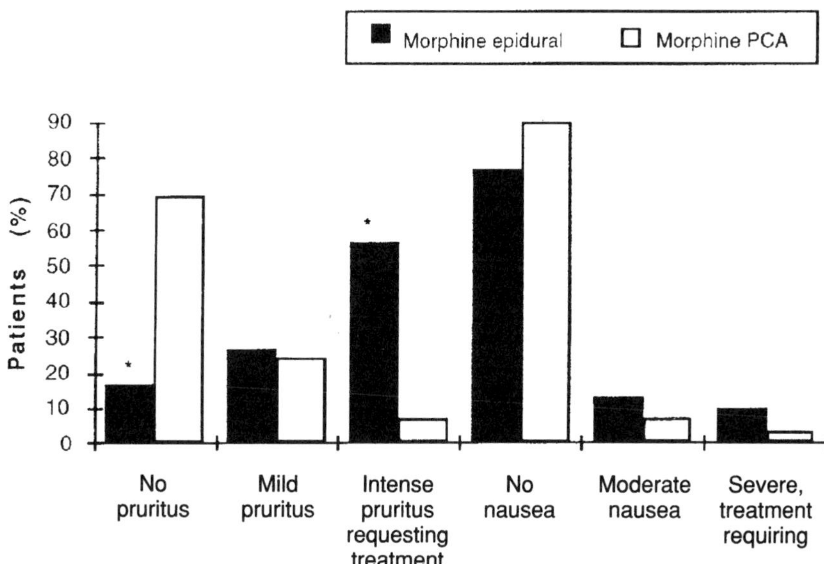

FIGURE 5.—Percentage of patients in each group reporting no, mild, or intense pruritus and nausea. $*P < 0.05$. *Abbreviation: PCA*, patient-controlled anesthesia. (Courtesy of Rapp-Zingraff N, Bayoumeu F, Baka N, et al: Analgesia after caesarean section: Patient-controlled intravenous morphine vs epidural morphine. *Int J Obstet Anesth* 6:87–92. Copyright 1997, by permission of the publisher, Churchill Livingstone.)

double-blind approach. A randomized, double-blind trial of PCA with morphine vs. epidural morphine after cesarean section was conducted.

Methods.—The trial included 60 ASA class I or II pregnant women scheduled to undergo elective cesarean section with regional anesthesia. After cesarean section with spinal anesthesia, the patients received either a single 5 mg morphine epidural bolus or a PCA. The morphine dose with PCA was 1 mg, with a lockout interval of 15 minutes and a maximum dose of 20 mg in 4 hours. The 2 approaches were compared for pain relief by visual analogue scale, comfort, satisfaction, and side effects.

Results.—Starting at the third hour, patients in the PCA group had higher pain scores (Fig 1); however, there was no significant difference in patient comfort. A quantitative measure of satisfaction during the first 24 hours suggested greater overall satisfaction in the epidural group, but there was no significant difference in qualitatively assessed comfort. The 2 groups were similar in hemodynamic and respiratory tolerance; none of the patients had an episode of respiratory depression or oxygen desaturation. Patients receiving epidural morphine were more likely to require specific treatment for pruritus. There was no difference in the incidence of nausea, vomiting, and sedation (Fig 5).

Conclusions.—In women who have undergone cesarean section, epidural morphine offers somewhat better analgesia than IV morphine PCA. However, pruritus is more of a problem with epidural morphine. Patient satisfaction with morphine PCA is good, despite the lesser degree of analgesia. The results suggest that PCA is a good alternative for patients who cannot receive epidural anesthesia, or who have had epidural anesthesia but cannot be monitored over the first 24 hours.

► As expected, epidural morphine provided slightly better analgesia than the PCA provided by IV morphine. However, more than half of the patients in the epidural morphine group requested treatment for intense pruritus. Given the frequency and severity of the pruritus, I am surprised that the satisfaction scores were slightly higher in the epidural morphine group than in the PCA group.

In my judgment, 5 mg represents an excessive dose of epidural morphine for postcesarean analgesia. In my experience, 3.5 mg of epidural morphine provides satisfactory postcesarean analgesia in most parturients with a transverse, lower abdominal skin incision. Unfortunately, even this smaller dose still results in a high incidence of pruritus.

D.H. Chestnut, M.D.

Patient-controlled Analgesia With Sufentanil: A Comparison of Two Different Methods of Administration

Sinatra RS, Sevarino FB, Paige D (Yale Univ, New Haven, Conn)

J Clin Anesth 8:123–129, 1996 8–3

Background.—Epidural patient-controlled analgesia (EPCA) combines the convenience of demand dosing with the analgesic potency of spinally acting opioids. Sufentanil's high potency, µ-receptor affinity and slow dissociation kinetics make it an ideal candidate for EPCA. A patient-controlled dosing paradigm was used to compare the safety and efficacy of epidural and IV sufentanil administration in a randomized, controlled, double-blind study of patients recovering from intra-abdominal gynecologic surgery.

Methods.—The study group consisted of 29 healthy women seen for elective nononcologic total abdominal hysterectomy with epidural anesthesia, who requested postoperative patient-controlled analgesia (PCA). Patients were randomly assigned to EPCA with sufentanil, IV PCA with sufentanil or IV PCA with morphine after surgery. Patients were observed for 24 hours after surgery. A visual analogue scale was used to measure analgesia and patient satisfaction. Pulmonary function was measured through respiratory rate, oxygen saturation, and forced expiratory flow. Sufentanil plasma levels were monitored in 8 patients.

Results.—The onset of analgesia with either method of sufentanil administration was more rapid than with morphine. Both methods of sufentanil administration produced equivalent levels of analgesia. The total administered dose and plasma sufentanil concentrations were similar in these 2 administration groups. More patients in the IV PCA sufentanil group had clinically significant oxygen desaturation. Although slower in onset, morphine analgesia was also satisfactory.

Conclusion.—Both IV and epidural administration of sufentanil provide rapid, effective postoperative analgesia for patients recovering from major abdominal surgery. There was a greater risk of oxygen desaturation with IV PCA administration than with EPCA administration of sufentanil.

▶ The results of this study indicate that epidural infusion of sufentanil behaves very much like epidural infusion of fentanyl, i.e., the analgesic effect is related predominantly to systemic uptake of the drug. There does not appear to be a substantial benefit to the epidural route compared with the IV route. It is still not clear whether intermittent bolus epidural injections of these drugs produces an appreciable spinal effect. In this study, there was a lower likelihood of respiratory depression with epidural administration than with IV administration. The same benefit would probably be seen with a subcutaneous infusion system.

S.E. Abram, M.D.

Preemptive Analgesia: Intraperitoneal Local Anesthetic in Laparoscopic Cholecystectomy—A Randomized, Double-blind, Placebo-controlled Study

Pasqualucci A, De Angelis V, Contardo R, et al (Univ of Udine, Italy; Univ of Perugia, Italy)

Anesthesiology 85:11–20, 1996 8–4

Background.—The clinical value of preemptive analgesia is debated. The optimum intensity, duration, and timing of analgesia relative to incision and surgery were further investigated.

Methods.—One hundred twenty patients undergoing laparoscopic cholecystectomy were studied. General anesthesia was induced in all. Topical peritoneal local anesthetic or saline was given immediately after the creation of a pneumoperitoneum and at the end of surgery. Four groups of 30 patients each were composed by random assignment. Patients in group A were given 20 mL 0.9% saline before and after surgery; group B, 20 mL 0.9% saline before surgery and 20 mL local anesthetic after surgery; group C, 20 mL local anesthetic before and after surgery; and group P, 20 mL local anesthetic before and 20 mL 0.9% saline after surgery.

Findings.—Pain intensity and analgesic requirements were significantly lower after postoperative bupivacaine, compared with placebo. Pain intensity and analgesic consumption also were lower in patients receiving bupivacaine preoperatively than in those receiving bupivacaine only after surgery. Patients given bupivacaine before surgery had significantly lower blood glucose and cortisol concentrations 3 hours after surgery (Fig 1).

Conclusions.—Intraperitoneal local anesthetic blockade given before or after surgery is more effective than placebo in preempting postoperative pain. Postsurgical pain intensity and the need for analgesic are lower in

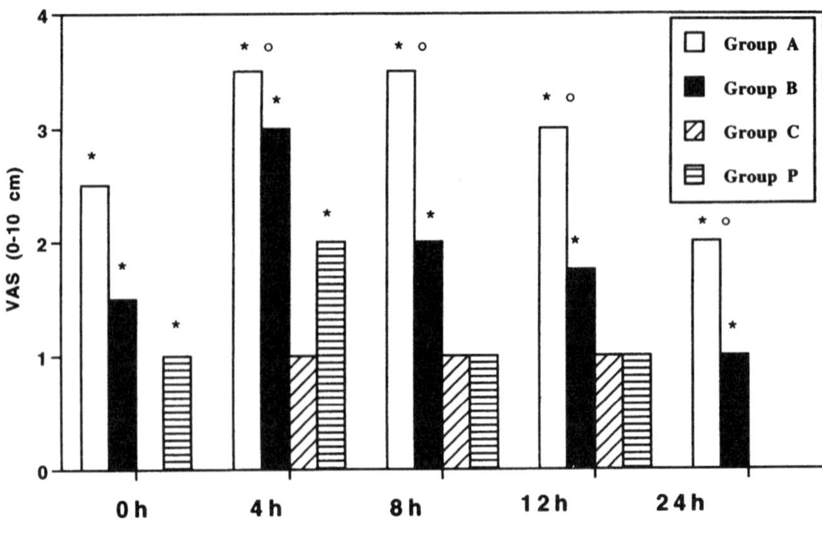

FIGURE 1.—Visual Analogue Scale (median). At 0 hours, Visual Analogue Scale was significantly lower in group C than in groups A, B, and P (*$P < 0.001$); no differences were detected among the other groups. At 4 hours, values for group C were significantly lower than for groups A, B, and P (*$P < 0.015$), and values for group P were lower than for group A (°$P < 0.001$). At 8, 12, and 24 hours, values for groups C and P were lower than for A and B (*$P < 0.001$); group A recorded higher values than B (°$P < 0.01$). Statistical analysis: Kruskal-Wallis test and Wilcoxon's rank sum test. (Courtesy of Pasqualucci A, De Angelis V, Contardo R, et al: Preemptive analgesia: Intraperitoneal local anesthetic in laparoscopic cholecystectomy—A randomized, double-blind, placebo-controlled study. *Anesthesiology* 85:11–20, 1996. Copyright American Society of Anesthesiologists, Inc. Used with permission of Lippincott-Raven Publishers.)

patients treated with local anesthetic before surgery than in those treated after surgery.

▶ This study shows that if you think ahead about how you are going to treat postoperative pain, you often can provide effective treatment by simple measures. Unfortunately, even today postoperative pain management remains a problem. "Customer" satisfaction reports continue to show that patients are not satisfied with their postoperative pain management.

M. Wood, M.D.

Intraperitoneal Bupivacaine for Analgesia After Laparoscopic Cholecystectomy

Mraović B, Jurišić T, Kogler-Majeric V, et al (Gen Hosp Sibenik, Croatia)
Acta Anaesthesiol Scand 41:193–196, 1997 8–5

Background.—The cause of pain after laparoscopic surgery is multifactorial. Visceral and shoulder pain is reported more commonly than parietal pain after laparoscopic cholecystectomy. The effects of intraperitoneal bupivacaine on such pain after laparoscopic cholecystectomy were investigated.

Methods.—Eighty patients of ASA physical status 1 and 2 were enrolled in the prospective, double-blind, randomized study. Immediately after pneumoperitoneum was obtained, 1 group of patients received 15 mL of 0.5% bupivacaine injected under direct vision into the hepatodiaphragmatic space near and above the hepatoduodenal ligament and above the gallbladder. Another 15 mL of bupivacaine was injected at the end of surgery. A second group of patients was given 15 mL of 0.9% saline solution in a comparable manner. Pain was assessed at 0.5, 4, 8, 12, and 24 hours after surgery using a visual analogue scale.

Findings.—Patients in the saline group had more intense pain at all time points. Between-group differences in pain were documented for up to 8 hours. Patients in the bupivacaine group had significantly lower analgesic consumption. There were no adverse effects.

Conclusions.—Intraperitoneal bupivacaine is effective in reducing pain after laparoscopic cholecystectomy. It is easy to administer and results in no adverse effects. Divided doses are recommended in this patient population, the first for analgesic effect to block shoulder pain and pain from surgical manipulation, and the second for visceral pain from the cholecystectomy wound.

▶ Most previous studies have been unable to demonstrate the analgesic efficacy of intraperitoneal bupivacaine following laparoscopy. The authors of this study argue that the site of instillation of anesthetic is important. More studies demonstrating substantial benefit are needed before this procedure can be recommended for widespread use. Nevertheless it may be worth trying in selected patients, such as those previously on high dose opioids.

S.E. Abram, M.D.

Preemptive Ketamine Decreases Postoperative Narcotic Requirements in Patients Undergoing Abdominal Surgery

Fu ES, Miguel R, Scharf JE (Univ of South Florida, Tampa)

Anesth Analg 84:1086–1090, 1997 8–6

Background.—Clinicians and researchers continue to seek effective preemptive treatment for postoperative pain. *N*-methyl-D-aspartic acid (NMDA) antagonists may be useful for preventing and treating such pain. The value of the preemptive administration of systemic ketamine, an NMDA antagonist with analgesic properties, was compared with that of postwound closure administration of ketamine in reducing postoperative pain.

Methods.—Forty patients undergoing abdominal procedures were randomly assigned to preemptive or postwound closure ketamine administration groups. The 20 patients in the first group received 0.5 mg/kg ketamine followed by a ketamine infusion of 10 μg·kg^{-1} before surgical incision and discontinued at abdominal closure. The 20 patients in the second group received 0.5 mg/kg of ketamine just after abdominal closure. After surgery, all patients were given IV morphine and were started on IV morphine patient-controlled analgesia after postanesthesia care unit discharge.

Findings.—Patients receiving preemptive ketamine consumed significantly less morphine on postoperative days 1 and 2. There were no significant differences in pain scores between the 2 groups throughout the study period.

Conclusions.—The preemptive administration of ketamine is more effective than postwound closure administration in reducing postoperative opioid requirements. The reduction of postoperative opioid requirements associated with preemptive administration persisted long after the normal expected duration of this agent.

▶ Most previous studies of the analgesic effect of ketamine for postoperative pain have involved postoperative administration of subdissociative doses. They have either shown no benefit or transient (<3 hours) analgesia. Theoretically, since ketamine is an N-methyl-D-aspartate (NMDA) antagonist, preoperative and intraoperative administration should block the development of spinally mediated hyperalgesia. This study provides evidence that there is indeed a preemptive effect. In addition to the potential for improved postoperative analgesia and reduced opiate requirements, NMDA antagonists may have the potential to reduce the incidence of long-term postoperative pain, such as intercostal neuralgia or post-amputation pain. Studies demonstrating such benefit would require large numbers of subjects.

S.E. Abram, M.D.

Epidural Analgesia Improves Outcome Following Pediatric Fundoplication: A Retrospective Analysis

McNeely JK, Farber NE, Rusy LM, et al (Med College of Wisconsin, Milwaukee; Children's Hosp, Milwaukee, Wis)

Reg Anesth 22:16–23, 1997 8–7

Background.—Severe gastroesophageal reflux in children may be life-threatening. Nissen fundoplication is commonly done in those at high risk. The effects of epidural versus IV opioid analgesia on the postoperative course of infants, children, and adolescents undergoing fundoplication were compared in the current study.

Methods.—One hundred fifty-five consecutive patients, aged 1 month to 19 years, were reviewed retrospectively. All underwent open fundoplication between January 1993 and October 1994. Seventy-two patients received perioperative analgesia with epidural opioids, and 83 received parenteral opioids. These 2 groups were comparable in age, weight, and associated preoperative medical diagnoses.

Findings.—The postoperative complication rates in the epidural and parenteral groups were 5.5% and 20%, respectively, which differed significantly. Four patients in the epidural group and 15 in the parenteral group needed mechanical ventilation for more than 24 hours. Patients receiving epidural analgesia had a shorter length of stay than those receiving parenteral analgesia and incurred about 20% less in hospital charges.

Conclusions.—The postoperative hospital course of children undergoing Nissen fundoplication may be modified significantly by the type of perioperative anesthesia or analgesia used. A prospective, randomized study is now warranted.

▶ While this study was retrospective and non-randomized, it should provide useful data since it contains large numbers, the study groups were comparable, and the postoperative assessment of both groups was rigorous. It adds further evidence for the contention that postoperative epidural analgesia improves outcomes for high risk patients, especially those undergoing upper abdominal or thoracic surgery. Previous evidence for such benefits has mainly come from adult experience,[1, 2] and this study demonstrates that high-risk children also have better outcomes with continuous regional analgesic techniques. Interestingly, the difference in outcome was most pronounced for patients under the age of 2 years.

One question that is not answered by this study is whether combined epidural local anesthetic plus opioid provides better outcomes than epidural opioid alone. There is experimental evidence that morphine exhibits greater efficacy (in addition to far greater potency) intrathecally than systemically. This is not true for fentanyl and sufentanil, which exhibit high efficacy whether given spinally or systemically. However, this study did not compare the systemic and neuraxial administration of a single opioid. All of the patients in this study received a combination of epidural opioid and local anesthetic, which perhaps provides the best prevention of stress-induced endocrine and metabolic changes.

S.E. Abram, M.D.

References

1. Yeager MP, Glass DD, Neff RK, et al: Epidural anesthesia and analgesia in high-risk surgical patients. *Anesthesiology* 66:729–736, 1987.
2. Rawal N, Sjöstrand U, Christoffersson E, et al: Comparison of intramuscular and epidural morphine for postoperative analgesia in the grossly obese: Influence on postoperative ambulation and pulmonary function. *Anesth Analg* 63:583–592, 1984.

Patient Experience of Pain After Elective Noncardiac Surgery

Lynch EP, Lazor MA, Gellis JE, et al (Harvard Med School, Boston; Univ of New Mexico, Albuquerque; Univ of California, San Francisco)

Anesth Analg 85:117–123, 1997 8–8

Background.—The intensity of postoperative pain is often underestimated and undertreated by health care providers. In this study, patients' experiences of postoperative pain were assessed after major elective surgery.

Study Design.—All patients admitted to Brigham and Women's Hospital between December 1992 and June 1993 for major elective, noncardiac surgery were eligible for inclusion in the study group. Data from 214 patients who underwent the 14 most common surgical procedures were analyzed for this study. Preoperative data were collected prospectively by questionnaire and included age, sex, use of narcotics, baseline pain score, pain chronicity, and level of anxiety. Postoperative data were collected prospectively by interview and included pain at rest, pain with movement, maximum pain scores on postoperative days 1–3, and mode of analgesia on postoperative day 1. Pain was assessed on a scale of 0 (none) to 10 (worst).

Findings.—The average pain score at rest was 2.6 on postoperative day 1 and decreased to 2.3 on postoperative day 3. The average pain score with movement was 4.5 on postoperative day 1 and decreased to 4.2 on postoperative day 3. The average maximum pain score through 24 hours was 6.3 on postoperative day 1 and decreased to 5.6 on postoperative day 3. Preoperative narcotic use and high baseline preoperative pain were significantly associated with increased postoperative pain at rest, pain with movement, and maximum pain. Epidural analgesia was the only type of analgesia significantly associated with decreased postoperative pain both at rest and with movement.

Conclusions.—After common major elective, noncardiac surgery, relatively high pain scores and minimal decreases in pain were seen during the first 3 postoperative days. These findings emphasize the need for more effective pain management continuing into the postoperative period to facilitate mobilization and recovery, as well as to increase patient comfort.

► This study emphasizes the need for extra effort in managing postoperative pain in patients with preexisting pain, particularly those who have been using opiates. As with many previous studies, this one demonstrates better pain control with epidural analgesia than with other techniques. It is not clear whether this benefit was related to the preemptive effect of intraoperative regional blockade or to the effect of postoperative epidural analgesia. Unfortunately, improved comfort is not a sufficient criterion to justify added costs associated with regional analgesic techniques in the current health care reimbursement system; we need to show improved outcomes that reduce health care costs to justify reimbursement for these added services.

S.E. Abram, M.D.

Epidural Morphine Plus Ketamine For Upper Abdominal Surgery: Improved Analgesia From Preincisional Versus Postincisional Administration

Choe H, Choi Y-S, Kim Y-H, et al (Chonbuk Natl Univ, Chonju, Republic of Korea)

Anesth Analg 84:560–563, 1997 8–9

Background.—Increased pain after surgery may result from CNS plasticity, which may be associated with the actions of *N*-methyl-D-aspartic acid (NMDA) receptors on neurons in the dorsal horn of the spinal cord. Because opioids act primarily on presynaptic receptors and decrease neurotransmitter release, and ketamine antagonizes NMDA receptors and prevents wind-up and long-term potentiation, the preoperative use of these 2 agents simultaneously may be effective in preventing CNS sensitization.

Methods.—Sixty patients in American Society of Anesthesiologists physical status class 1–2 undergoing upper abdominal surgery were included in the study. Ketamine, 60 mg, and morphine, 2 mg, were injected epidurally through an indwelling catheter inserted at the T7–8 interspace. The injections were performed before anesthesia induction in 30 patients (group 1) and immediately after the removal of a surgical specimen in 30 patients (group 2). Another 2 mg of morphine was administered when patients reported resting pain.

Findings.—The duration of analgesia was longer in group 1 than in group 2. Supplemental injections were needed in 56.7% of group 1 patients, compared with 90% of group 2 patients, a significant difference. The incidences of adverse effects were comparable.

Conclusion.—Preoperative analgesia with epidural morphine and ketamine is more effective than the postincisional administration of these drugs in the treatment of pain after upper abdominal surgery. Administering these drugs before surgery decreased the need for supplemental analgesics in this series.

► I selected this paper to highlight the issue of pre-emptive analgesia. I remain to be convinced; however, I do think that a major change we have seen over the last few years is that an integral part of the anesthetic plan is now the provision of acute postoperative pain relief and a consideration of how this should be provided before the start of anesthesia. Postoperative pain management is no longer an afterthought considered at the end of anesthesia, and that has to be a step forward.

M. Wood, M.D.

Single-Patient Data Meta-analysis of 3453 Postoperative Patients: Oral Tramadol Versus Placebo, Codeine and Combination Analgesics

Moore RA, McQuay HJ (Univ of Oxford, England)

Pain 69:287–294, 1997 8–10

Background.—Meta-analysis is popular because it can pool data from numerous studies with small sample sizes and thus allow a larger group for statistical analyses. The meta-analysis of individual patient data is associated with the least bias of any meta-analytic approach. Thus these authors performed meta-analysis of individual patient data from clinical trials of tramadol to determine this drug's role in postoperative pain management.

Methods.—Data were combined from studies involving 3,453 patients taking tramadol for postoperative pain (n = 9) or dental pain (n = 9). Drugs used in the studies included from 50 to 150 mg tramadol, 60 mg codeine, 650 mg aspirin plus 60 mg codeine, and 650 mg acetaminophen plus 100 mg propoxyphene. Patients rated their pain on a 4-point scale (0 = no pain; 3 = severe pain) and their pain relief on a 5-point scale (0 = no relief; 4 = complete). Each patient's total pain relief was calculated as the area under the curve for pain relief against time. Patients who achieved 50% or more of total pain relief with a drug were considered to have a response to treatment.

Findings.—In the studies of postoperative pain, tramadol was superior to placebo but less effective than aspirin with codeine and acetaminophen with propoxyphene (Fig 1). In the studies of dental pain, tramadol was

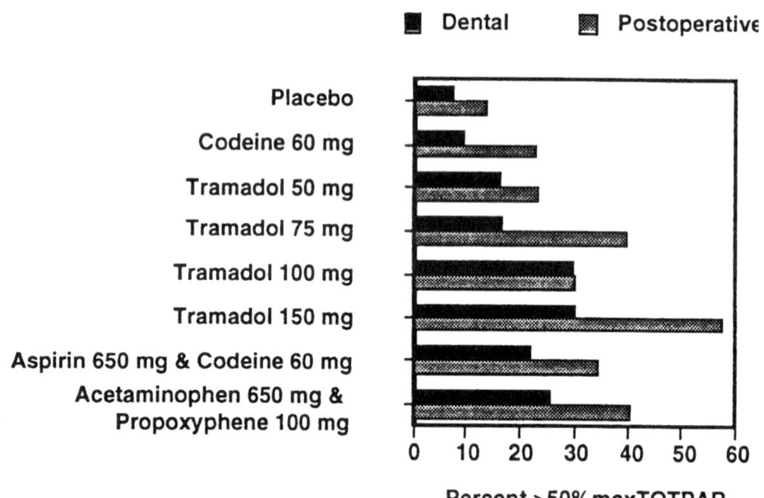

FIGURE 1.—Proportion of patients with more than 50% maximum total pain relief. (Courtesy of Moore RA, McQuay JH: Single-patient data meta-analysis of 3453 postoperative patients: Oral tramadol versus placebo, codeine and combination analgesics. *Pain* 69:287–294, 1997. Copyright 1997. Reprinted with kind permission of Elsevier Science-NL, Sara Burgerhartstraat 25, 1055 KV Amsterdam, The Netherlands.)

superior to all other treatments except 60 mg codeine. In both types of studies, tramadol-induced pain relief showed dose dependence, with 150 mg tramadol providing the best pain relief. Adverse effects, such as headache, nausea, vomiting, dizziness, and somnolence, were generally mild and tended to occur more often at higher doses.

Conclusions.—Compared with the other analgesics tested, tramadol was highly effective in controlling dental pain and had mixed results in controlling postoperative pain. Pain relief from tramadol differed substantially, depending on whether it was given for postoperative or dental pain. Thus, the results of these different types of studies were not directly comparable when evaluating the drug's efficacy.

► Although tramadol provides analgesia that is clearly superior to placebo, it does not appear to offer substantial advantages over other commonly used oral analgesics, either in terms of efficacy or side effects. The study did not assess differences in GI motility between tramadol and opioids. This may be an area of superiority for tramadol.

S.E. Abram, M.D.

Chronic Pain Syndromes/Problems/Therapy

Audit for Management of Low Back and Neuropathic Pain

Audit in Pain Clinics: Changing the Management of Low-Back and Nerve-Damage Pain

Davies HTO, Crombie IK, Macrae WA, et al (Univ of Dundee, South Africa; Gartnavel Gen Hosp, Glasgow, Scotland; Royal Victoria Infirmary, Newcastle, England)

Anaesthesia 51:641–646, 1996 8–11

Introduction.—Most outpatient pain clinics in the United Kingdom are run by anesthetists. The piecemeal development of pain services has resulted in variable and idiosyncratic approaches to pain management. A multicenter audit was conducted to enable pain clinicians from different centers to share their experiences and identify areas where pain management could be changed; then changes were implemented to benefit patients.

Methods.—Ten outpatient pain clinics in the United Kingdom, with 19 anesthetist consultants, 1 consulting psychiatrist, 1 clinical psychologist, and 2 anesthetic senior registrars, were assessed for their management of 1,236 patients with low back pain and nerve damage pain. The following commonly used treatments in the pain clinics were audited: antidepressants, anticonvulsants, strong opioids, sympathetic nerve blocks, local anesthetic or steroid injections, neuroablation, transcutaneous electrical nerve stimulation (TENS), acupuncture, physiotherapy, and psychological therapies. There were 3 stages of evaluation: (1) initial observations of current practice, (2) commitments made by clinics to change their use of treatments after active feedback of variations in practice, and (3) an assessment of the changes achieved. Data on an additional 1,791 patients was used to assess change.

Results.—Three treatments increased markedly in frequency as a result of audit feedback: (1) antidepressant drugs, (2) anticonvulsant drugs, and (3) TENS.

Conclusion.—The active feedback portion of the audit was successful in informing pain clinicians about their practices. There is reasonable evidence to support the benefits of using antidepressant and anticonvulsant drugs and TENS, but much of chronic pain management remains shrouded in mystery. What is needed are authoritative guidelines on the management of chronic pain against which local practice and local service provision may be assessed.

► This is an impressive article not only for what was done but also for what still needs to be done. The education and comments changed the management of low back pain and nerve-damaging pain and included, with just this process, a first step of much more use of antidepressant, anticonvulsant drugs, and TENS. One wants to know whether these changes actually improved outcome or worsened it. That is, were they captivated by a more rational process of care? We do not know if that more rational process of care is based on myth or whether there are outcome data in their patient population to substantiate that this was really an improvement in care. This issue brings the whole problem of writing clinical pathways. It is tough to devise a clinical pathway if there aren't outcome data to say what you do or that the changes you make in the pathway make a difference.

M.F. Roizen, M.D.

Neuropathic Pain

Randomised Double-blind Active-Placebo–controlled Crossover Trial of Intravenous Fentanyl in Neuropathic Pain

Dellemijn PLI, Vanneste JAL (Sint Lucas Andreas Ziekenhuis, Amsterdam; Sint Joseph Ziekenhuis, Veldhoven, The Netherlands)

Lancet 349:753–758, 1997 8–12

Introduction.—Opioid analgesics are administered to patients with neuropathic pain that is resistant to common pain-relieving agents, antidepressants, or anticonvulsants, but the effectiveness of opioids in such cases is limited. It is not known whether neuropathic pain relief with opioids results from an intrinsic analgesic effect on pain intensity, a change in mood that reduces the unpleasantness of pain, or a sedative effect. A randomized double-blind trial assessed relief of pain intensity and pain unpleasantness with IV infusions of fentanyl.

Methods.—The crossover study used 2 consecutive infusions: fentanyl plus diazepam (active placebo) or fentanyl plus saline (inert placebo). Diazepam was selected because it modulates the patient's emotional experience while lacking intrinsic analgesic effects. Eligible patients had continuous unilateral neuropathic pain of 3 types: nociceptive nerve pain,

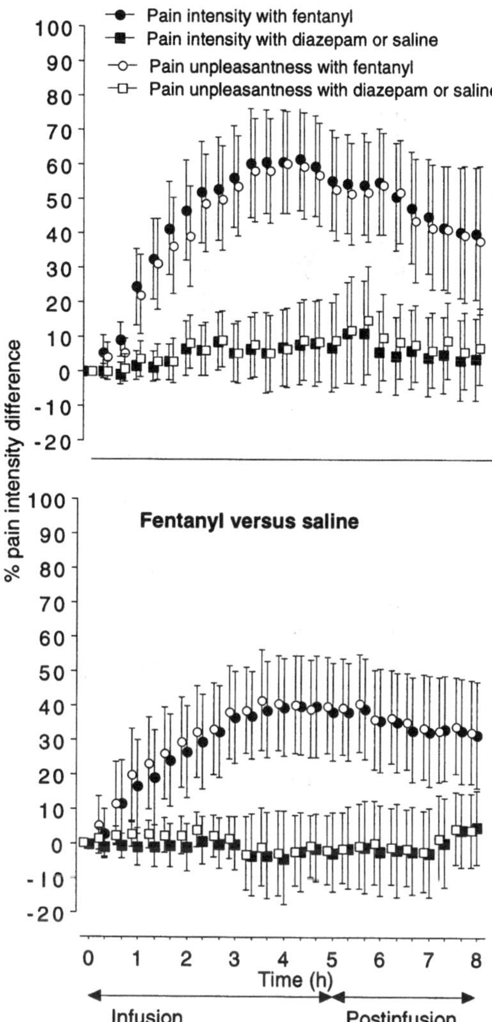

FIGURE 2.—Time course of changes in pain relief. *Error bars* are 95% confidence interval. A negative score indicates an increase in pain. (Courtesy of Dellemijn PLI, Vanneste JAL: Randomised double-blind active-placebo–controlled crossover trial of intravenous fentanyl in neuropathic pain. *Lancet* 349:753–758. Copyright by the Lancet Ltd., 1997.)

deafferentation pain, and mixed neuropathic pain. Medication was infused at a constant rate for a maximum of 5 hours. Pain, sedation, and side effects of the agents were evaluated from start of infusion for 8 hours. Patients were asked to rate pain intensity and pain unpleasantness on a scale from 0 to 100.

Results.—Of 53 patients, 27 were randomly assigned to receive fentanyl plus diazepam, and 26 to receive fentanyl plus saline; 50 completed the

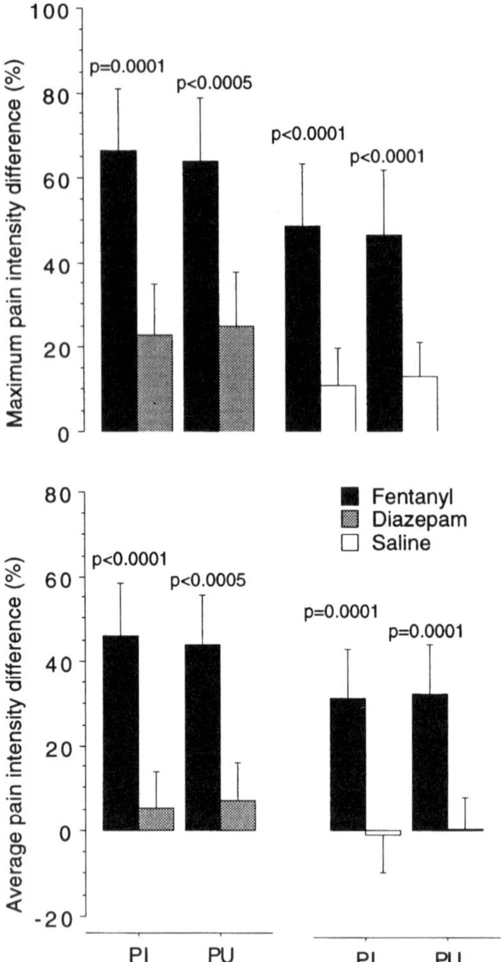

FIGURE 3.—Maximum and average pain relief. *Error bars* are 95% confidence interval. A negative score indicates an increase in pain. *Abbreviations: PI*, pain intensity; *PU*, pain unpleasantness. (Courtesy of Dellemijn PLI, Vanneste JAL: Randomised double-blind active-placebo–controlled crossover trial of intravenous fentanyl in neuropathic pain. *Lancet* 349:753–758. Copyright by the Lancet Ltd., 1997.)

study. Pain intensity and unpleasantness were similar at baseline in the 2 groups. Forty-four patients were severely and 6 moderately depressed. Fentanyl provided increased relief of pain intensity and pain unpleasantness, with superiority to diazepam evident at 60 minutes and superiority to saline at 100 minutes (Fig 2). Both the maximum and average relief of pain intensity and pain unpleasantness were greater with fentanyl (Fig 3) than with diazepam or saline. Fentanyl's beneficial effects were independent of the type of neuropathic pain and the degree of sedation. Although significantly more side effects were reported with fentanyl than with diazepam or saline, none of these effects were severe. There was a significant correlation between total number of adverse events and maximum relief of pain.

Conclusions.—Patients with different types of neuropathic pain of noncancer origin had pain relief from an infusion of fentanyl. The opioid appears to have an intrinsic analgesic effect, rather than acting by sedation or modulation of a patient's perception of pain.

► Neuropathic pain can be notoriously difficult to treat, and the use of opioids is controversial. As the authors state, because neuropathic pain is not a single clinical entity, the response of different neuropathic syndromes to opioids may vary. They therefore investigated 3 different types of neuropathic pain. Intravenous fentanyl had an analgesic effect in patients with different kinds of neuropathic noncancer pain, whereas benzodiazepines did not appear to produce significant relief of pain in this group of patients. However, the type of neuropathic pain did not predict whether the patient might respond to fentanyl.

M. Wood, M.D.

The Effects of Pre-emptive Treatment of Postherpetic Neuralgia With Amitriptyline: A Randomized, Double-blind, Placebo-controlled Trial

Bowsher D (Walton Hosp, Liverpool, England)

J Pain Symptom Manage 13:327–331, 1997 8–13

Background.—Previous research has indicated that administering amitriptyline 3–6 months after the onset of acute herpes zoster infection can improve pain control in the later course of the infection. This study involved an even earlier dose of amitriptyline—beginning within 48 hours of rash onset—to determine its effect on later postherpetic neuralgia.

Methods.—Acute shingles was diagnosed in 80 patients (71% women, 39% men) 60 years of age or older. Treatment was split into 2 groups with further subgroups. Amitriptyline, 25 mg, was given to 38 patients either alone (n = 29) or with acyclovir (n = 9), and placebo was given to 34 patients, either alone (n = 17) or with acyclovir (n = 17). Both active drug and placebo administration began within 48 hours of the diagnosis and continued for 90 days. The outcome measure was the prevalence of pain at 6 months.

Findings.—There were 8 dropouts, 6 because of noncompliance (3 in each treatment arm) and 2 who were lost to follow-up. For the remaining 72 patients, Table 2 shows that early dosing with amitriptyline significantly reduced the frequency of pain at 6 months, with an odds ratio of 2.9:1. Pain control was best (89%) in the patients who received amitriptyline in conjunction with acyclovir.

Conclusions.—The long-term prevalence of postherpetic neuralgia was significantly reduced by beginning a course of 25 mg amitriptyline within 48 hours of rash onset. Improvement continued even after the 90-day drug dosing period ended. Six patients taking amitriptyline did not have pain

TABLE 2.—Patients Commencing Amitriptyline or Placebo at Onset of Herpes Zoster

n	Regimen	Pain lost by 1 month	Pain lost between 2 and 3 months	Cumulative total pain free at 3 months	Pain lost between 4 and 6 months	Cumulative total pain free at 6 months
38	All amitriptyline	18 (47%)	10 (26%)	28 (73.7%)	4 (10.5%)	32 (84.2%)
9	Amitriptyline + acyclovir	5 (55%)	2 (22%)	7 (77.8%)	1 (11%)	8 (89%)
29	Amitriptyline only	13 (45%)	8 (27.5%)	21 (72.4%)	3 (10.3%)	24 (82.75%)
34	All placebo	13 (38%)	8 (23.5%)	21 (61.75%)	1 (3%)	22 (64.7%)
17	Placebo + acyclovir	3 (17.6%)	5 (29.4%)	8 (47%)	1 (6%)	9 (53%)
17	Placebo only	10 (59%)	3 (17.6%)	13 (76.5%)	0	13 (76.5%)

Note: Odds ratio for all amitriptyline vs all placebo pain free at 6 months, 2.9:1. Chi-square and Fischer's exact test for all amitriptyline vs all placebo pain free at 6 months, 0.05.

(Reprinted by permission of Elsevier Science, from Bowsher D: The effects of pre-emptive treatment of postherpetic neuralgia with amitriptyline: A randomized, double-blind, placebo-controlled trial. *J Pain Symptom Manage* 13:327–331, 1997. Copyright 1997 by the U.S. Cancer Pain Relief Committee.)

control by 6 months. Perhaps a higher dose or an increased dosing period could improve results in this group. These results indicate that early administration of low-dose amitriptyline plus an antiviral drug is useful for elderly patients who develop shingles.

▶ The use of amitriptyline for pain of herpes zoster is generally deferred until the postherpetic phase. It is encouraging to find that it may have some benefit in reducing the incidence of postherpetic neuralgia when administered during the acute phase. Recent evidence that amitriptyline has NMDA receptor blocking activity may explain its salutary effect. To date, there is little evidence that nerve blocks administered during the acute eruption reduce the incidence or severity of chronic postherpetic pain.

S.E. Abram, M.D.

Severity of Skin Lesions of Herpes Zoster at the Worst Phase Rather Than Age and Involved Region Most Influences the Duration of Acute Herpetic Pain

Higa K, Mori M, Hirata K, et al (Fukuoka Univ, Japan; Kitakyushu Municipal Hosp, Japan)

Pain 69:245–253, 1997 8–14

Introduction.—Reactivation of varicella-zoster virus after chickenpox causes herpes zoster (HZ). Severe, acute herpetic pain (AHP) related to HZ remains a problem and can progress into post-herpetic neuralgia. A retrospective study of patients with HZ-related pain sought to determine which factor—age, involved regions, and severity of skin lesions at the worst phase—most influenced duration of AHP.

Methods.—Patients were referred because of severe AHP that persisted despite large doses of nonsteroidal anti-inflammatory drugs. All inpatients were treated with sympathetic nerve blocks employing intermittent injections of 1% mepivacaine 4–6 mL at least 4 times daily. In cases of moderate to mild pain, nerve block were given daily on an outpatient basis. Treatment was continued until the pain disappeared. Skin lesions were graded at the worst phase and treated with vidarabine or acyclovir.

Results.—Treatment for 1,489 of 2,000 consecutive patients referred for HZ-related pain from 1973 to 1991 was started within 14 days; skin lesions were clearly described in 1,431 of these patients. Duration of AHP in the 807 women and 624 men was analyzed with respect to age, involved region, severity of skin lesions, and use of antiviral drugs. Without taking into account the severity of skin lesions, the duration of AHP was significantly longer for patients older than 60 than for those younger than 40. When duration of AHP was analyzed according to severity of skin lesions, all 8 decennial age groups (age 19 or younger to 80 or older) showed highly significant differences with increase in the severity of skin lesions. Duration of AHP was also significantly longer with increase of severity of lesions in all regions (trigeminal, cervical, thoracic, and lumbosacral).

Severe skin lesions were present significantly more often in patients older than 60 and in those with trigeminal involvement. Multiple stepwise regression analysis of the duration of AHP with respect to age, involved region, severity of skin lesions, and use of antiviral drugs revealed that the greatest influence was severity of lesions at the worst phase; antiviral drugs appeared to have no influence on duration of AHP.

Conclusion.—The severity of skin lesions in patients with HZ had the greatest influence on duration of AHP; age and involved regions had lesser influence, whereas antiviral drugs appeared to have no influence. Results of treatment of AHP should be analyzed according to severity of skin lesions at the worst phase.

► This study provides some interesting data with respect to 2 issues:

1. It establishes severity of skin lesions as the principle factor affecting duration of acute pain. Older patients and patients with trigeminal involvement both tend to have more severe lesions and have longer duration of acute phase pain.
2. It fails to show any significant benefit from antiviral drugs in their ability to shorten pain in the acute phase. However, as the authors point out, antiviral drugs were generally started late in these patients.

Our understanding of the efficacy of early interventions in the control of acute phase pain and the prevention of postherpetic neuralgia is hindered by the lack of controlled studies. It is still unclear whether early treatment with antiviral drugs or with sympathetic or neuraxial blocks has any impact on the duration of the acute phase pain or the development of chronic neuropathic pain. Future studies, it seems, will probably need to stratify patients according to the severity of skin lesions as well as to site of involvement and age.

S.E. Abram, M.D.

Effect of Adrenergic Receptor Activation on Post-Herpetic Neuralgia Pain and Sensory Disturbances

Choi B, Rowbotham MC (Univ of California, San Francisco)

Pain 69:55–63, 1997 8–15

Background.—Post-herpetic neuralgia (PHN) begins with an episode of herpes zoster or shingles and can lead to a chronic neuropathic pain syndrome. The role of sympathetic nervous system activation in the pain of PHN has never been defined. If PHN nociceptor afferents acquire the ability to respond to adrenergic agonists, PHN pain should increase after administration of an adrenergic agonist. A double-blind study was performed to determine the effect of administration of normal saline, epinephrine, or phenylephrine into the painful area and a mirror-image unaffected area in patients with chronic PHN.

Methods.—Study participants had pain persisting in areas affected by shingles more than 3 months after rash healing and were otherwise healthy. In session A, mirror-image normal skin was injected with saline in the morning and PHN skin was injected with an adrenergic agonist in the afternoon. In session B, mirror-image normal skin was injected with an adrenergic agonist in the morning and PHN skin was injected with saline in the afternoon. Subjects were randomly assigned to the order of their double-blinded sessions. The 2 sessions were separated by at least 48 hours.

Results.—Injection of either saline or adrenergic agonist into normal skin produced mild, transient pain, without allodynia and without affecting the overall intensity of PHN pain. Injection of either saline or adrenergic agonist into PHN skin produced equivalent transient pain that was more intense than that produced in the normal skin. After injection of the adrenergic agonist into PHN skin, overall PHN allodynia and pain severity were significantly higher than after saline injection, with a peak 10–15 minutes after injection.

Conclusion.—Injection of adrenergic agonists, but not normal saline, into PHN skin increased overall PHN pain and allodynia in adjacent skin. Injections of either saline or adrenergic agonists into normal, mirror-image skin did not affect PHN pain or allodynia. This increase in PHN pain with administration of adrenergic agonists is consistent with the acquisition of adrenergic sensitivity after nerve injury. The transient and modest nature of this increase in pain and allodynia is consistent with clinical reports that chronic PHN does not usually respond to sympathetic blockade.

▶ Although this study provides evidence that adrenergic agonists may produce a modest increase in pain of PHN, it does not offer proof that resting sympathetic tone is responsible for maintaining ongoing pain or that sympathetic blocks play a therapeutic role in this condition. The authors note that systemic uptake of local anesthetics may reduce nociceptor discharge. It is also likely that placebo response is responsible for pain relief after many injections. Although some patients experience transient relief from local anesthetic blockade of the sympathetic chain, there is little evidence that such blocks produce any lasting benefit.

S.E. Abram, M.D.

Psychological Dysfunction in Patients With Reflex Sympathetic Dystrophy

Ciccone DS, Bandilla EB, Wu W (New Jersey Med School, Newark)
Pain 71:323–333, 1997 8–16

Background.—Reflex sympathetic dystrophy (RSD) is a neuropathic pain syndrome associated with allodynia, edema, abnormal vasomotor and sudomotor activity, dystrophic soft-tissue changes and impaired motor function after a minor injury. It can lead to permanent disability. Because symptom severity appears to be out of proportion to the initial injury, some have speculated that RSD is nonorganic in origin. The psychologic correlates of RSD were analyzed to determine whether patients with this disease have an unusual pattern of psychologic dysfunction compared with patients with localized neuropathic pain and patients with chronic back pain. Patients with localized neuropathy were selected because they also have neuropathic pain, but their symptoms are believed to be proportionate to a known organic cause. Patients with chronic back pain were selected because they have pain and disability presumed to be disproportionate, but this pain is not neuropathic.

Study Design.—The records of 253 consecutive referrals to a tertiary pain center were reviewed, and 25 patients were assigned to the RSD group, 44 to the chronic back pain group, and 21 to the local neuropathy group. Patients were assessed by the frequency of their medical visitations, length of disability, demographic survey, pain survey, Sickness Impact Profile, Hopkins Symptom Checklist, Disease Conviction scale of the Illness Behavior Questionnaire, Beck Depression Inventory, Cognitive-Somatic Anxiety Questionnaire, and a validated survey of childhood trauma.

Results.—With stringent diagnosis criteria and an analysis of covariance to control for differences in symptom duration and age among the study groups, no evidence was found to indicate that patients with RSD were psychologically unique. Patients with RSD were extremely similar to those with local neuropathy in symptom reporting, illness behavior, and psychologic distress. Patients with RSD had more disability days in the preceding 6 months than had those with local neuropathy. The back pain group had more diffuse pain reports and more nonspecific medical symptoms than had either the RSD or local neuropathy group. A validated survey of childhood trauma found abuse and trauma to be evenly distributed among all 3 study groups.

Conclusions.—Patients with RSD dystrophy are not similar to patients with chronic back pain but are quite similar to patients with local neuropathy. The findings of this study raise doubts about the proposed psychologic causes of RSD. The burden of proof would now appear to be on those who favor a nonorganic explanation to provide evidence of psychologic involvement in the etiology of RSD.

► Controlled studies that assess the presence of personality disorders or psychologic dysfunction among patients with RSD have uniformly failed to show differences between patients with RSD and patients without chronic pain or patients with other painful disorders. Despite such evidence, patients with this diagnosis are often labeled as having a "typical RSD personality" or as having a "nonorganic" source of reported pain. Patients faced with such skepticism from their health care providers are likely to to become frustrated and angry, further reinforcing the negative attitudes of their physicians. This particular study is unique because it rules out differences in demographic variables and assesses a large number of variables, including symptom reporting, illness behavior, psychologic distress, and history of childhood trauma. It still fails to show differences between patients with RSD and those with neuropathic pain for any of the variables assessed.

S.E. Abram, M.D.

The Long-term Outcome of Microvascular Decompression for Trigeminal Neuralgia

Barker FG II, Jannetta PJ, Bissonette DJ, et al (Massachusetts Gen Hosp, Boston; Univ of Pittsburgh, Pa; Southwest Ohio Neurosurgery, Piqua)
N Engl J Med 334:1077–1083, 1996 8–17

Introduction.—A syndrome characterized by paroxysmal facial pain, trigeminal neuralgia (or tic douloureux) can be treated with carbamazepine. Operative treatments include neurectomy of trigeminal nerve branches outside the skull, percutaneous ablations, injection of glycerol, or physical compression. Most reports provide only short-term follow-up information about several surgical procedures of treating trigeminal neuralgia. Patients with trigeminal neuralgia who had microvascular decompression of the trigeminal nerve root during a 20-year-period were studied.

Methods.—Microvascular decompression of the trigeminal nerve for medically intractable trigeminal neuralgia was provided to 1,185 patients. The procedure involved a small retromastoid craniectomy, through which the trigeminal nerve is examined microsurgically for vascular compresion at or near its point of entry into the brain stem. Repositioning with stents was accomplished with any compressive arteries and some veins. Patients filled out questionnaires annually on the presence and nature of any facial pain and the details of any subsequent treatment for tic.

Results.—The median follow-up for the 1,185 patients was 6.2 years. Most postoperative recurrences of tic were in the first 2 years after surgery. Recurrences of tic occurred with 30% of patients, and 11% had second operations for the recurrences. Excellent final results were found for 70% of patients 10 years after surgery. These patients reported they were free of pain without medication for tic. Another 4% indicated they had occasional pain, but did not require long-term medication. The annual rate of recurrence of tic was less than 1% 10 years after surgery. In 82% of patients, immediate postoperative relief from tic was complete; in 16%, it was partial and in 2%, relief was absent. Significant predictors of eventual recurrence were female sex, venous compression of trigeminal root entry zone, symptoms lasting more than 8 years, and lack of immediate postoperative cessation of tic. If a trigeminal ganglion lesion had been created with radiofrequency current before microvascular decompression, patients were more likely to have burning and aching facial pain. A patient's likelihood of having a cessation of tic after microvascular decompression was not lessened by a previous ablative procedure. Complications included 2 deaths before the operation (0.2%) and one brain stem infarction (0.1%). Ipsilateral hearing loss occurred in 16 patients (1%).

Conclusion.—Microvascular decompression is a safe and effective treatment for trigeminal neuralgia. The long-term success rate is high.

► This study is a good example of the potential value of nonrandomized, uncontrolled clinical outcome studies. Obviously it is not feasible to randomly assign patients to treatments as diverse as craniotomy, neurolytic injection, and balloon compression. Nevertheless, careful collection of data over long periods in large numbers of patients provides substantial amounts of useful data regarding the rational selection of treatment options.

Although it may seem very aggressive to treat otherwise healthy patients with a non-life-threatening disease with a craniotomy, the high success rates and low morbidity, particularly the low incidence of sensory loss, make this an attractive option for patients in whom medical therapy has failed because of inadequate response or intolerable side effects.

Carbamazepine was cited in this study as the most commonly used medication. It is associated with a high incidence of side effects, occasional serious complications, and a moderately high rate of loss of efficacy over time. Gabapentin is being reported more frequently as an alternative treatment. It is clearly a safer and better tolerated drug. It remains to be seen whether it is as efficacious as carbamazepine.

S.E. Abram, M.D.

Difference in Pain Relief After Trigger Point Injections in Myofascial Pain Patients With and Without Fibromyalgia

Hong C-Z, Hsueh T-C (Univ of California Irvine, Orange; Natl Cheng-Kung Univ, Taiwan)

Arch Phys Med Rehabil 77:1161–1166, 1996 8–18

Background.—Myofascial pain syndrome (MPS) is characterized by chronic muscle pain caused by myofascial trigger points (TrPs), localized sensitive spots in taut skeletal muscle fiber bands. Myofascial trigger points are associated with both local and referred pain, restricted range of motion (ROM), and a local twitch response (LTR). Fibromyalgia syndrome (FMS) is characterized by chronic pain involving multiple regions. Some patients have both MPS and FMS. Injection is often used to inactivate TrPs. A prospective study was performed to examine the effect of TrP injection on pain intensity, pain threshold and ROM in patients with MPS or MPS and FMS.

Methods.—The study group consisted of 18 female patients with active MPS TrPs in the upper trapezius muscle on 1 or both sides. Nine of these patients had MPS and 9 had MPS and FMS. Patients received myofascial TrP injection with 0.5% xylocaine for pain relief, followed by spray and stretch therapy. Pain intensity, pain threshold, and ROM were measured before, immediately after, and 2 weeks after the TrP injections. Post-injection soreness was also assessed.

Results.—In patients with MPS only, pain intensity, pain threshold, and ROM were significantly improved immediately after injection. In the patients with MPS and FMS, only ROM was significantly improved immediately after injection. By 2-week follow-up, both groups had equivalent significant improvement in all 3 therapeutic response parameters. Postinjection soreness occurred faster, was more severe, and lasted longer in patients with MPS and FMS.

Conclusion.—In this study of trigger point injection for myofascial pain in patients with and without fibromyalgia, TrP injection was useful in the treatment of both groups. However, pain relief was delayed in patients with both MPS and FMS. Postinjection soreness was also more severe in patients with MPS and FMS.

► Most discussions of the management of the fibromyalgia indicate that trigger point injections are of little or no use. Although this study indicates that there is little immediate benefit from trigger point injections among patients with fibromyalgia, it suggests that there is some delayed benefit.

Fibromyalgia differs considerably from MPS. Patients with fibromyalgia have bony tenderness in addition to diffuse muscle tenderness. There is a large preponderance of women with this condition, many of whom are in the 35–50 age range. Myofascial pain syndrome, on the other hand, is characterized by muscle tenderness only and generally involves fewer sites. Palpation of TrPs typically produces referred pain, whereas pressure on tender points in patients with fibromyalgia is associated with local pain.

It has been proposed that fibromyalgia is associated with malfunction of intrinsic pain suppression mechanisms rather than with local muscle pathology. However, the results of the study suggest that injection of tender points in patients with fibromyalgia may be a worthwhile part of a comprehensive pain management program

S.E. Abram, M.D.

A Systematic Review of Antidepressants in Neuropathic Pain

McQuay HJ, Tramèr M, Nye BA, et al (Univ of Oxford, England; The Churchill, Oxford, England)

Pain 68:217–227, 1996 8–19

Background.—Antidepressants are used in the treatment of neuropathic pain, but their use remains somewhat controversial. A systematic review of randomized, controlled trials of antidepressant treatment for neuropathic pain was conducted to address the effectiveness and safety of this therapeutic approach.

Methods.—MEDLINE and the Oxford Pain Relief Database were used to locate reports of randomized, controlled trials of antidepressants for the treatment of chronic neuropathic pain. The reference lists of included papers and review articles were searched for additional reports. Unpublished reports, abstracts, reviews, drugs that were withdrawn during development, and studies of less than 10 patients were excluded. Each possible report was read by each author and scored for quality.

Results.—Twenty-one placebo-controlled treatments in 17 randomized, controlled trials involving 10 antidepressants were included in the review. In 6 of 13 diabetic neuropathy studies, the odds ratio showed significant benefit compared with placebo. The combined odds ratio was 3.6 with a number needed-to-treat (NNT) for benefit of 3. In 2 of 3 postherpetic neuralgia studies, the odds ratio showed significant benefit, with a combined odds ratio of 6.8 and an NNT of 2.3. In 2 atypical facial pain studies, the combined odds ratio for benefit was 4.1, with an NNT of 2.8. Tricyclic antidepressants did not significantly differ from each other but were significantly more effective than benzodiazepines. Paroxetine and mianserin were not as effective as imipramine. For 11 of 21 treatments, there were dichotomous data on minor adverse effects, with an NNT of 3.7. Data on major adverse effects were available from 19 studies, with an NNT of 22.

Conclusion.—Antidepressants are effective in the relief of neuropathic pain. Compared with placebo, of 100 patients with neuropathic pain who take antidepressants, 30 will obtain more than 50% relief from pain, 30 will have minor adverse reactions, and 4 will withdraw from treatment because of major adverse effects. The data from these reports are insufficient to determine whether antidepressants or anticonvulsants are more effective in the treatment of neuropathic pain, or which should be the drug of first choice. Further research is required to determine which of these drugs are most effective in the treatment of neuropathy.

▶ This study documents the benefit of antidepressants in some chronic pain states and provides a good assessment of the chances of beneficial vs. adverse effects. Several questions remain to be answered: Are selective serotonin reuptake inhibitor–type antidepressants effective for neuropathic pain? In which conditions are antidepressants most helpful compared with anticonvulsants? Are combinations of antidepressants and anticonvulsants more effective than either drug alone? What is the mechanism of analgesic action of antidepressants? Is it simply the result of norepinephrine or serotonin reuptake inhibition, or are other mechanisms at work, such as *N*-methyl-D aspartate receptor antagonism?

S.E. Abram, M.D.

Effect of Sympathetic Nerve Block on Acute Inflammatory Pain and Hyperalgesia

Pedersen JL, Rung GW, Kehlet H (Hvidovre Univ, Denmark; Pennsylvania State Univ, Hershey)

Anesthesiology 86:293–301, 1997 8–20

Background.—Sympathetic nerve blocks relieve pain in some chronic pain states, but the role of the sympathetic nervous system in acute inflammatory pain has not been well studied. To determine the role of the sympathetic nervous system in acute pain and hyperalgesia, the effect of a unilateral lumbar sympathetic plexus block on pain after heat injury was investigated in healthy volunteers.

Methods.—A randomized, single-blinded study was performed with 21 healthy male and 3 healthy female volunteers, aged 22–46. Bupivacaine injection was used to induce a lumbar sympathetic nerve block, and saline injection was used to induce a contralateral placebo block in the volunteers. The sympathogalvanic skin response and skin temperature were used to assess the quality and duration of the blocks. Bilateral heat injuries were created on the medial surfaces of the calves 45 minutes after blocks. Pain intensity, pain threshold, and secondary hyperalgesia were recorded before and after block and 1, 2, 4, and 6 hours after heat injury.

Results.—Of the 24 participants, 8 were excluded because of somatic block or incomplete sympathetic block. There were no significant differences in the effects of sympathetic block and placebo block on pain or mechanical allodynia during injury, or in pain thresholds, pain response to heat, or areas of secondary hyperalgesia after heat injury.

Conclusion.—There were no significant differences between sympathetic block and placebo block in pain intensity, mechanical allodynia, pain threshold, or secondary hyperalgesia. Sympathetic nerve block did not reduce acute clinical pain in healthy skin, nor hyperalgesia after a heat injury.

► This study confirms the finding of previous investigations that failed to show sensitization of normal nociceptors by activations of the sympathetic nervous system. There is some evidence that increased sympathetic tone can produce sensitization of mechanoreceptors, and it is postulated that heightened mechanoreceptor activity, plus sensitization of wide dynamic range neurons in the dorsal horn, is responsible for mechanical allodynia in some cases of reflex sympathetic dystrophy.

Another mechanism by which sympathetic efferent discharge can increase pain perception involves increased firing arising ectopically from injured nerves. Over 20 years ago, it was shown that the rate of spontaneous firing originating from a neuroma can be increased by either stimulation of the sympathetic chain or by topical application of norepinephrine. Still another possible mechanism for activation of nociceptors by sympathetic efferent discharge is by ephaptic transmissions of the inductions of neuronal depolarization of nociceptive afferents by sympathetic efferents. It is presumed that such abnormal transmission takes place at injured nerve segments, where Schwann cells or myelin sheaths have been injured.

S.E. Abram, M.D.

Phantom Pain and Sensation Among British Veteran Amputees
Wartan SW, Hamann W, Wedley JR, et al (Guy's Hosp, London)
Br J Anaesth 78:652–659, 1997 8–21

Background.—Virtually all patients undergoing amputation have various types of persisting phantom sensations. The relationship between such sensations and phantom pain remains unclear. The reported frequency of chronic phantom limb pain has a vast range—from 1% to 98%. The incidence and time course of phantom limb and stump pain in long-standing amputees, the possible relationship between phantom sensation

TABLE 6.—Methods Used for Treatment of Phantom Pain and Patient Satisfaction

Treatment type	Amputees received treatment	Amputees were satisfied with treatment
TENS	26 (36%)	11 (42.3%)
Operation on the stump	12 (16.6%)	5 (41.6%)
Injections of the stump	11 (15%)	1 (9%)
Sympathectomy	8 (11%)	3 (37.5%)
Acupuncture	3 (4%)	0
Others	15 (20.8%)	0
Nothing	8 (11%)	N/A*

Abbreviation: Others, Cryotherapy, cordotomy, nerve block, ointments, and hitting the stump with a wooden mallet.

*All respondents who were offered no treatment returned the question "Were you satisfied with your treatment?" unanswered

(Reprinted by permission of the BMJ Publishing Group, from Wartan SW, Hamann W, Wedley JR, et al: Phantom pain and sensation among British veteran amputees. *Br J Anaesth* 78:652–659, 1997.)

and phantom pain, and the choice and efficacy of treatment were investigated in the current study.

Methods and Findings.—Five hundred ninety veterans with amputations were surveyed by mail. The response rate was 89%. Fifty-five percent of the subjects reported phantom limb pain, and 56%, stump pain. Phantom pain and phantom sensation were highly correlated. The intensity of phantom sensation significantly predicted the time course of phantom pain. The condition worsened in only 3% of subjects with phantom pain. One hundred forty-nine subjects with phantom pain had discussed the pain with their family physicians. Forty-nine of these subjects were told there was no available treatment. Satisfactory methods for controlling phantom limb pain included transcutaneous nerve stimulation (TENS), analgesics, and nonsteroidal anti-inflammatory drugs (NSAIDs) (Tables 6 and 7).

TABLE 7.—Medication Used for Phantom Pain Treatment and Patient Satisfaction

Type of medicine	Respondents using it	Respondents satisfied
Simple analgesics	96 (53%)	45 (47%)
Compound analgesics	67 (37%)	42 (63%)
NSAID	27 (15%)	20 (74%)
Anticonvulsants	12 (6.6%)	3 (25%)
Opioids	10 (5.5%)	4 (40%)
Antidepressants	2 (1%)	0
Alcohol	42	31 (74%) (helpful)

Abbreviations: Simple analgesics, paracetamol; *compound analgesics,* paracetamol and opioid; *NSAID,* nonsteroidal antiinflammatory drugs; *anticonvulsants,* carbamezapine; *antidepressants,* amitriptyline

(Reprinted by permission of the BMJ Publishing Group, from Wartan SW, Hamann W, Wedley JR, et al: Phantom pain and sensation among British veteran amputees. *Br J Anaesth* 78:652–659, 1997.)

Conclusions.—Phantom pain is a major problem among long-standing amputees, with 47% reporting continuing pain. Equally common was stump pain, which is more treatable. Treatment with TENS, analgesics, and NSAIDs appears to be beneficial.

► There are several important lessons to be learned from this survey. It is helpful to be able to reassure patients with phantom limb pain that the condition is unlikely to become progressively worse. It is also useful to know that low-risk interventions such as oral analgesics and TENS are likely to provide some benefit. Finally, it is helpful to have confirmation of the view that many pain physicians have observed: that nerve blocks are rarely of lasting benefit.

S.E. Abram, M.D.

Oral Ketamine Therapy in the Treatment of Postamputation Stump Pain
Nikolajsen L, Hansen PO, Jensen TS (Aarhus Univ, Denmark)
Acta Anaesthesiol Scand 41:427–429, 1997 8–22

Background.—Hyperactivity of N-methyl-D-aspartate (NMDA) receptors may play a role in stump pain after amputation. Ketamine, an anesthetic agent with NMDA receptor-blocking properties, has been shown to decrease neuropathic pain in experimental models and to reduce wind-up-like pain, allodynia, and spontaneous pain in clinical studies. However, the use of a ketamine has been associated with adverse effects. The successful use of ketamine in a patient who experienced no adverse effects was reported.

> *Case Report.*—Man, 61, required treatment for severe pain in both stumps after bilateral amputation at the knee level 5 months earlier. Ketamine was given intravenously to the patient in a double-blind, saline-controlled fashion. Stump pain was relieved for 31 hours after the infusion, with a reduction of the allodynic area and of wind-up-like pain and an increase in pressure-pain thresholds. After this double-blind session, ketamine was given orally. Ketamine, 50 mg dissolved in juice, was given 4 times per day. The patient had no adverse effects and developed no tolerance during the 3-month treatment.

Conclusions.—Oral ketamine may be effective in the treatment of postamputation stump pain. An observation period of longer than 3 months may be needed to determine conclusively the safety of the drug and the possibility of tolerance development.

► This is not the first case report to document clinical benefit from NMDA antagonists in general and ketamine in particular for patients with central or neuropathic pain. It is unique, however, in that it demonstrates benefit from oral ketamine. Before this technique can be recommended, it would be helpful to determine the oral bioavailability of the drug. A placebo response to the orally administered drug cannot be ruled out, since the bitter taste may have enabled patients to discern active drug from placebo.

S.E. Abram, M.D.

Randomised Trial of Epidural Bupivacaine and Morphine in Prevention of Stump and Phantom Pain in Lower-Limb Amputation

Nikolajsen L, Ilkjaer S, Christensen JH, et al (Univ of Aarhus, Denmark)

Lancet 350:1353–1357, 1997 8–23

Introduction.—The development of phantom pain has been associated with severe preamputation pain. Previous studies have shown that the rate of phantom pain was lower among patients receiving epidural treatment for pain before the amputation; however, these studies have had small sample sizes, insufficient randomization, and nonblinded assessment of treatment and pain. Extra hospital costs are associated with the administration of an epidural treatment before rather than at the time of amputation. To clarify whether postoperative stump and phantom pain is reduced by preoperative pain treatment with epidural bupivacaine and morphine, a randomized, double-blind trial was conducted.

Methods.—There were 60 patients scheduled for lower-limb amputation who were randomly assigned to receive either morphine (0.16–0.28 mg/hr) and epidural bupivacaine (0.25%, 4–7 mL/hr) for 18 hours before and during the operation (blockade group), or epidural saline and oral or IM morphine (control group). There were 29 patients in the blockade group and 31 in the control group. General anesthesia was administered to all patients for the amputation. After 1 week, and then after 3, 6, and 12 months, all patients were asked about stump and phantom pain. Consumption of opioids, intensity of stump and phantom pain, and rate of stump and phantom pain were measured.

Results.—In the blockade group, the median duration of preoperative epidural blockade was 18 hours, and in the saline group, it was 18.5 hours. In both groups, the combined median duration of postoperative epidural pain treatment was 166 hours. Phantom pain was seen in 14 patients (52%) in the blockade group and in 15 (56%) in the control group after 1 week. At 3 months, phantom pain was seen in 14 patients in the blockade group (82%) vs. 10 patients in the control group (50%). At 6 months, phantom pain was seen in 13 patients in the blockade group (81%) vs. 11 in the control group (55%). At 12 months, phantom pain was seen in 9 patients in the blockade group (51%) and in 11 patients in the control group (69%). In both groups at all 4 postoperative interviews, intensity of stump and phantom pain and consumption of opioids were similar.

Conclusions.—Phantom or stump pain is not prevented by preoperative epidural blockade started a median of 18 hours before the amputation and continued into the postoperative period. Preoperative ischemic pain and postoperative stump pain, however, are reduced with epidural pain treatment.

► Although this is a negative study, it is important because it had been suggested that epidural analgesia before amputation might reduce phantom pain after limb amputation, and highlights the importance of performing controlled randomized trials followed by publication of outcome, even if negative.

M. Wood, M.D.

Sudomotor Function in Sympathetic Reflex Dystrophy

Birklein F, Sittl R, Spitzer A, et al (Friedrich-Alexander-Universität Erlangen, Germany)
Pain 69:49–54, 1997 8–24

Background.—Reflex sympathetic dystrophy (RSD) can develop after limb trauma or peripheral nerve lesion. It is associated with motor, sensory, and autonomic disturbances. The autonomic symptoms consist of vasomotor and sudomotor disturbances. To investigate the pathophysiology of RSD, basal and stimulated sudomotor activities were examined in affected and unaffected limbs.

Methods.—There were 9 male and 18 female study participants with RSD. At the time of the study, their average age was 50 years, and the median duration of disease was 8 weeks. The patients were seated comfortably in a temperature- and humidity-controlled room and allowed to acclimatize for 2 hours. Skin temperature was recorded. Two small chambers were then affixed to hairy skin on both the affected and unaffected limbs, and dry nitrogen gas was passed through at a constant rate. The relative humidity of this gas was measured to assess sweating. After baseline assessment, thermoregulatory-induced sweating was triggered by having the subjects drink hot tea and by irradiation with infra-red. The thermoregulatory sweat test (TST) is thought to monitor preganglionic sympathetic neuronal mechanisms. Sudomotor stimulation was also carried out via transcutaneous carbachol application. The quantitative sudomotor axon reflex test (QSART) is believed to involve postganglionic mechanisms.

Results.—Nineteen affected arms and 8 affected legs were investigated. The average skin temperature was significantly higher on the affected side. Despite this significant temperature difference, there was no significant difference in basal sweat levels between the affected and unaffected sides. Both the TST and the QSART led to significantly greater sweat responses on the affected side, with shorter latency periods.

Conclusion.—When sudomotor responses were examined in the hairy skin of the limbs of reflex sympathetic dystrophy patients, baseline sweat response was the same for affected and unaffected limbs, despite an increased temperature on the affected side. Both reduced latency and increased sweat production were manifested on the affected side by both the TST and QSART procedures. This may be explained by increased blood flow caused by decreased vasoconstrictor activity in the affected limb. An increased sudomotor drive may also be present. This would imply that vasoconstrictor and sudomotor efferents are differentially affected by RSD.

▶ It is not surprising that this study showed differences between vasomotor and sudomotor function. It has been demonstrated previously that injury to an extremity, particularly if it involves nerve injury, results in dysregulation of regional autonomic function. Characteristic of this dysregulation is the loss of temperature regulatory function, which involves both vasomotor and sudomotor activity in the affected limb.

S.E. Abram, M.D.

Pain in Guillain-Barré Syndrome

Moulin DE, Hagen N, Feasby TE, et al (Univ of Western Ontario, London; Univ of Calgary, Alta)

Neurology 48:328–331, 1997 8–25

Introduction.—The various pain syndromes observed in patients with Guillain-Barré syndrome (GBS) may frequently go unrecognized and may be undertreated. The character, intensity, and frequency of pain in GBS and the response to treatment were evaluated in a longitudinal survey.

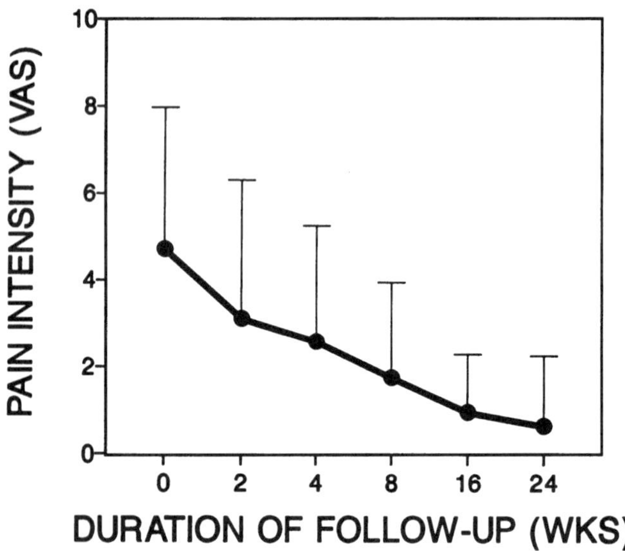

FIGURE 1.—Mean pain intensity (+SD) over time in 55 patients with Guillain-Barré syndrome. *Abbreviation*: *VAS*, Visual Analogue Scale. (Courtesy of Moulin DE, Hagen N, Feasby TE, et al: Pain in Guillain-Barré syndrome. *Neurology* 48:328–331, 1997. Copyright American Academy of Neurology. Used with permission of Lippincott-Raven Publishers.)

TABLE 2.—Pain Syndromes Observed in Guillain-Barré Syndrome

Back and leg pain	34 (61.8%)
Dysesthetic extremity pain	27 (49.1%)
Myalgic-rheumatic extremity pain	19 (34.5%)
Visceral pain	11 (20%)
Pressure palsy (ulnar nerve)	1 (2%)
Headache caused by dysautonomia	1 (2%)

Note: $n = 55$.

(Courtesy of Moulin DE, Hagen N, Feasby TE, et al: Pain in Guillain-Barré syndrome. *Neurology* 48:328–331, 1997. Copyright American Academy of Neurology. Used with permission of Lippincott-Raven Publishers.)

Methods.—Fifty-five consecutive adult patients with GBS were evaluated within 48 hours of admission and at 2, 4, 8, 16, and 24 weeks regarding character and intensity of pain, treatment, and response to pain intervention. A Visual Analogue Scale (VAS, 0–10 cm) and the Present Pain Intensity of the McGill Pain Questionnaire were used to help determine pain intensity and response to pain intervention. The VAS was correlated with the Disability Grading Scale.

Results.—Forty-nine of 55 patients (89.1%) reported pain during the course of illness. The mean intensity of pain on admission was 4.7 on the VAS. Of patients with pain, 26 (47.3%) described pain that was considered distressing, horrible, or excruciating (VAS 7.0) (Fig 1). Patients reported the most common pain syndromes to be deep aching back and leg pain and dysesthetic extremity pain (Table 2). On admission and throughout the evaluation period, pain intensity was poorly correlated with neurologic disability. Opioid analgesics were required by 41 patients (74.5%). Sixteen (29%) patients needed parenteral morphine for adequate pain relief.

Conclusions.—Moderate to severe pain is a frequent and early symptom in patients with GBS. Aggressive treatment is needed. Back and leg pain usually diminishes in the first 8 weeks, but dysesthetic extremity pain can be persistent in 5% to 10% of patients, despite motor recovery and use of analgesics.

► We tend to think of Guillain-Barré syndrome as a purely motor disorder, and are likely to ignore the fact that severe pain is a common symptom of this disorder. This article is valuable because it documents the high incidence of pain among patients with Guillain-Barré syndrome who are often unable to communicate their discomfort. However, the information regarding pain in this condition is not new. Twenty years ago, Ernest Henschel published a remarkable account of his personal experience with this condition.[1] That article should be required reading for anyone who cares for ventilator patients.

S.E. Abram, M.D.

Reference

1. Henschel, EO: The Guillain-Barré syndrome: A personal experience. *Anesthesiology* 47:228–231, 1977.

Alfentanil, But Not Amitriptyline, Reduces Pain, Hyperalgesia, and Allodynia From Intradermal Injection of Capsaicin in Humans

Eisenach JC, Hood DD, Curry R, et al (Wake Forest Univ, Winston-Salem, NC)

Anesthesiology 86:1279–1287, 1997 8–26

Background.—The intradermal injection of capsaicin in humans produces brief pain, followed by hyperalgesia and allodynia. Spinal N-methyl-D-aspartate (NMDA) mechanisms mediate the latter effects. Recently, amitriptyline was found to antagonize NMDA receptors. The current study determined the effect of amtitriptyline alone and with alfentanil on hyperalgesia and allodynia resulting from intradermal capsaicin injection.

Methods.—Forty-six healthy persons volunteered for the study. Intradermal injections of capsaicin, 100 µg, were given alone or before and after systemic injection of 4 mg midazolam, 25 mg amitriptyline, alfentanil by computer-controlled infusion, or amitriptyline plus alfentanil.

Findings.—The injection of capsaicin resulted in acute pain, followed by hyperalgesia and allodynia. Alfentanil decreased these pain responses in a plasma-concentration–dependent fashion. Reductions in hyperalgesia and allodynia were associated with decreases in acute pain. By itself, amitriptyline had no effect. It did not potentiate alfentanil. The latter produced concentration-dependent nausea, the effect reduced by amitriptyline.

Conclusions.—The reduction in hyperalgesia and allodynia after intradermal injection of capsaicin by systemically administered opioids may be secondary to decreased nociceptive input by acute analgesia. The current findings do not support the use of acute systemic amitriptyline for acute pain, hyperalgesia, and allodynia, although the role of chronic therapy and spinal administration are currently under investigation.

▶ The fact that amitriptyline produces analgesia in patients with chronic neuropathic pain but not in patients with acute nociceptive pain suggests NMDA antagonism as a possible analgesic mechanism. Eisenach's previous findings with intrathecal amitriptyline in animal studies of spinal sensitization also point toward such a mechanism. We have begun to rethink our previous theories that tricyclic antidepressants produce analgesia through inhibition of serotonin and norepinephrine reuptake. Some of the most effective serotonin reuptake inhibitors, including many of the newer antidepressants, are relatively ineffective in producing analgesia for conditions that are often improved by tricyclics.

S.E. Abram, M.D.

Cancer Pain

A Survey of Pain in Patients With Advanced Cancer

Twycross R, Harcourt J, Bergl S (Univ of Oxford, England; Churchill Hosp, Oxford, England)

J Pain Symptom Manage 12:273–282, 1996 8–27

Background.—The majority of patients with advanced cancer have pain and many have multiple pains. A group of patients with advanced cancer were evaluated to examine the number of pains, their causes, and the impact of treatment.

Methods.—The study group consisted of 111 patients with advanced cancer who were referred to the Sir Michael Sobell House, a specialist palliative care unit associated with the medical school at Oxford University. The patients were assisted in completing a 4-page initial Wisconsin Brief Pain Inventory (BPI) and then asked to complete it on their own once a week for the next 4 weeks.

Results.—At the initial assessment, there were 370 pains recorded, for a median of 3 pains per patient. Of the 111 patients, 85% had more than 1 pain and 40% had 4 or more pains. The causes of pain were cancer in 46%, debility in 29%, treatment in 5%, concurrent disorder in 8%, and no stated cause in 12%. Although 68% of these patients completed 2 BPIs, only 41% completed 5 BPIs. After 4 weeks of palliative treatment, the median number of pains had decreased to 1.5, although 78% had more than 1 pain. Only 20% had 4 or more pains at this time. The intensity of pain also decreased. Among those who completed 5 BPIs, 22% were pain free and 29% had acceptable pain relief, whereas 20% had unacceptable pain levels at the end of 4 weeks of treatment. At initial assessment, there were highly significant correlations between all 7 interference with activities and enjoyment of life factors and present, worst, and average pain intensities. After 4 weeks, these correlations were lost, suggesting that interference factors may not be useful as assessments of satisfactory pain management. Many patients did not complete their BPIs, suggesting that the BPI is not short enough for repeated clinical evaluation.

Conclusion.—A large group of patients with advanced cancer referred to a specialist palliative care center completed BPIs for a 4-week period. Most of these patients had multiple pain sites, with cancer responsible for only about half of the pain. With treatment, the numbers and the intensity of pain decreased, but almost 30% of patients continued to have unacceptable levels of pain. The BPI was too long for repeated clinical evaluation, and the BPI short form was not complete enough. A diary card for repeated evaluation of pain relief and pain management is currently under development.

► Of particular note in this study is the finding that nearly one third of patients continued to have severe pain 1–4 weeks after initiation of treatment. This is particulary disturbing because this statistic comes from a respected cancer pain management program. Older reports have indicated that 90% of cancer pain can be controlled fairly easily with simple measures such as oral opioids. This result may be a function of referral patterns, with the most difficult problems being referred to the authors' institution. On the other hand, it may be related to more honest reporting of unresolved pain.

It is also interesting that only half of the reported pain complaints were the result of direct effects of tumor. Most patients had multiple causes of pain, requiring careful assessment of the various components and the availability of a wide range of treatment options.

S.E. Abram, M.D.

High-Dose Epidural Infusion of Opioids for Cancer Pain: Cost Issues

Manfredi PL, Chandler SW, Patt R, et al (Univ of Texas, Houston)

J Pain Symptom Manage 13:118–121, 1997 8–28

Background.—Many variables influence the choice of intraspinal opioids for the treatment of cancer pain. Cost issues associated with this choice were illustrated in a case report.

> *Case Report.*—Man, 38, required treatment for pain from uncontrollable metastatic large-cell adenocarcinoma of unknown primary origin. The patient's pain persisted despite trials of 2 opioid agonists, upward titration of parenteral opioids until the occurrence of dose-limiting side effects, and the addition of adjuvant analgesics. Pain was reduced but still significant after a trial of epidural fentanyl and bupivacaine. Sufentanil was substituted for fentanyl, ultimately resulting in complete pain relief until the patient died 18 days after hospital discharge. However, the associated charges to the patient were high, which was not immediately evident to the treatment team. The daily average wholesale price (AWP) for sufentanil alone was $698. By contrast, the AWP of equianalgesic doses of epidural preservative-free morphine prepared by the hospital pharmacy was as little as $4 per day.

Conclusions.—Epidural infusion of the more expensive opioids, such as sufentanil, should not be used until there is an adequate trial with morphine, particularly in patients requiring high doses of systemic opioids with a life expectancy of more than a few days. Hospital pharmacies should weigh the risks and financial benefits of preparing morphine solutions from bulk powder to decrease patient charges and hospital costs.

▶ There is evidence from animal studies that more potent opioids such as sufentanil may be more efficacious than less potent drugs such as morphine or meperidine. There is also considerable evidence that highly lipid soluble drugs such as fentanyl and sufentanil have little added benefit when infused epidurally as opposed to intravenously. Since the cost of epidural sufentanil in a very tolerant patient is so high, it might be reasonable to utilize the intrathecal route, enabling the use of substantially lower doses, especially when combined with very low doses of bupivacaine. A subcutaneous port or even a tunneled subarachnoid catheter is a reasonable alternative for a patient whose expected lifespan is measured in days. For patients whose life expectancy is in months, an implanted intrathecal infusion pump would be a cost-effective option, particularly if a 5- to 10-fold reduction in drug dose were possible.

S.E. Abram, M.D.

Spinal Epidural Metastasis: Implications for Spinal Analgesia to Treat "Refractory" Cancer Pain

Appelgren L, Nordborg C, Sjöberg M, et al (Sahlgrenska Univ, Gothenburg, Sweden; Univ of Gothenburg, Sweden; Mölndal Hosp, Gothenburg, Sweden)

J Pain Symptom Manage 13:25–42, 1997 8–29

Background.—Although studies suggest that spinal compression by an epidural metastasis commonly results in refractory cancer pain, this relationship has not been investigated specifically. The hypothesis that epidural metastasis is a common cause of refractory cancer pain and that its presence may affect the efficacy and complication rates of intraspinal pain treatment was tested.

Methods.—Two hundred one consecutive patients with cancer pain receiving intrathecal pain treatment between 1985 and 1993 were studied retrospectively. Fifty-seven patients underwent metrizamide myelography, CT, MRI, laminectomy, or neurohistopathologic evaluation.

Findings.—Seventy percent of the patients had epidural metastases, and about 58% had spinal stenosis. Seven patients had total occlusion and 26 had partial occlusion of the spinal canal. Catheter insertion complications, daily dosages, and complications of the intrathecal pain treatment were affected by the presence of epidural metastasis only when it was associated with spinal canal stenosis. During intrathecal therapy, the patients with confirmed epidural metastasis and total spinal canal stenosis needed significantly greater daily doses of opioids and intrathecal bupivacaine. This group also had significantly greater rates of radicular pain at injection and poorer distribution of analgesia than patients without epidural metastasis and spinal canal stenosis. However, the rate of postdural puncture headache occurrence was significantly lower in patients with partial spinal stenosis (4%) and total spinal stenosis (14%) than in those without such stenosis (29%). Four patients had unexpected paraplegia caused by a collapse or by accidental injury during an attempted dural puncture procedure.

Conclusions.—About 70% of these patients with systemic cancer referred to a pain unit had epidural metastases associated with refractory pain. The presence of epidural metastasis affected catheter insertion complications, daily dosages, and complications of the intrathecal pain treatment only when it was related to spinal canal stenosis and thus to compression of the cauda equina or spinal cord or both.

► The presence of epidural metastatic disease is an extremely important issue when deciding whether to initiate neuraxial drug administration techniques. As this study indicates, treatment efficacy as well as the complication rate is greatly affected by the presence of tumors within the spinal canal. The simple expedient of obtaining an MRI scan before initiating an expensive, invasive, and potentially risky form of therapy represents time and money well spent. In this population, we often forego the usual precautions we take for patients without cancer because the pain is so severe and the duration of potential complications in the terminally ill is brief. This study points out the fallacy of such reasoning.

S.E. Abram, M.D.

The Inappropriate Use of the Epidural Route in Cancer Pain

Mercadante S, Agnello A, Armata MG, et al (Buccheri La Ferla Fatebenefratelli Hosp, Italy; Home Palliative Care Unit, Palermo, Italy)

J Pain Symptom Manage 13:233–237, 1997 8–30

Background.—Authorities continue to debate the optimal use of the epidural route in the treatment of cancer pain. The current paper describes the inappropriate use of the epidural route in 3 patients needing home palliative care and further discusses the issues involved in the use of the epidural route for cancer pain treatment.

Discussion.—The patients treated by the epidural route developed severe clinical problems because of its use. Simpler measures, such as oral and subcutaneous opioids, provided adequate analgesia and a better quality of life for these patients.

There is no proof that epidural analgesia is better than the oral route, and technical problems can occur. Bupivacaine-opioid epidural administration may be beneficial in some patients. Additional patients may benefit from treatment through the intrathecal route. When appropriate support for ongoing management of spinal administration is not available, spinal opioid treatment is inappropriate. Educating hospital and home nursing staff, family members, and other caregivers is important for successful treatment. Because systemic opioids adequately relieve pain in most patients and oral therapy is feasible for most of the clinical course, the WHO guidelines should be widely distributed among health care workers.

► The fact that, in the cases presented, epidural analgesia was ineffective and that systemic opiates provided reasonable analgesia does not necessarily indicate that the decision to use epidural analgesia was inappropriate. The epidural anesthetics may have been ineffective because of technical errors or inappropriate choices of drugs and dosages. Theoretically, the early institution of regional analgesic techniques can lead to reduced spinal sensitization ("windup") and a more comfortable course throughout the terminal phases of a painful disease. Errors of omission, that is, the persistence in trying to manage intractable pain with opiate regimens that are ineffective when more effective regional analgesic or neurolytic techniques are available, are probably far more common than the perceived errors of commission illustrated here. Perhaps the best solution to such problems is a multidisciplinary approach to cancer pain management in which all appropriate disciplines are involved early in the course of a painful terminal illness.

S.E. Abram, M.D.

Long-term Intrathecal Infusion of Morphine in the Home Care of Patients With Advanced Cancer

Gestin Y, Vainio A, Pégurier AM (Montpellier Cancer Inst Val d' Aurelle, France)

Acta Anaesthesiol Scand 41:12–17, 1997 8–31

Introduction.—Concern about infections and other complications may make physicians leery of giving intrathecal morphine to patients with chronic cancer pain. However, recent data suggest that intrathecal morphine offers better pain relief and fewer side effects at a lower dose than epidural morphine. The authors' cancer center has had long experience with the use of intrathecal morphine. They reported their recent experience with intrathecal morphine for patients with cancer pain.

Methods.—The review included 50 patients with refractory cancer pain treated by continuous intrathecal morphine infusion. There were 29 men and 21 women (mean age, 56 years). All had nociceptive or mixed nociceptive-neuropathic pain that was at least partially opioid sensitive and had not responded to other forms of pain treatment. The patients were treated from 1991 to 1994, with morphine infusion given through an external pump with patient-controlled boluses. The intrathecal catheter was inserted by a lateral puncture technique under strict aseptic conditions. The patients' therapy was managed on an outpatient basis, with control visits at 4- to 6-week intervals. A telephone/fax service was available for emergencies. A total of 5,602 days of morphine therapy was analyzed.

Results.—Intrathecal morphine infusion continued for an average of 142 days. The average morphine dose was 5.4 mg/day, with a mean starting dose of 2.5 mg/day and a mean final dose of 9.2 mg/day (Table 3). All patients achieved moderate or better pain relief, enough to permit discontinuation of oral or parenteral opioids. There were no clinical episodes of infection and no cases of respiratory depression during intrathecal morphine treatment. Six patients with temporary external catheters had CSF leakage followed by postspinal headache. This complication did not occur when the lateral lumbar puncture technique was used for long-term treatment. There were 2 cases of catheter crushing associated with a

TABLE 3.—Duration of Treatment and Mean Daily Doses of Intrathecal Morphine in 40 Patients Having an Implanted Catheter

Primary site	Number of patients	Mean follow-up (days)	Mean starting dose (mg)	Mean final dose (mg)	Mean dose (mg)
Lung	10	108	2.39	6.63	4.62
Rectum	7	191	2.98	6.31	7.75
Gynaecological	6	95	2.72	19.76	5.83
Prostate	4	240	2.98	10.20	8.25
Breast	3	118	1.80	5.93	5.57
Gastro-intestinal	3	130	5.61	6.71	5.97
Other	7	116	1.23	21.06	10.84
Total	40	142	2.54	9.15	5.38

(Courtesy of Gestin Y, Vainio A, Pégurier AM: Long-term intrathecal infusion of morphine in the home care of patients with advanced cancer. *Acta Anaesthesiol Scand* 41:12–17, 1997.)

collapsed vertebra and 1 of catheter perforation associated with lumbar puncture.

Conclusion.—Intrathecal morphine infusion appears to be an option for long-term management of severe cancer pain. This technique provides good analgesia with a low rate of side effects and maintenance of patient autonomy. The use of low morphine doses minimizes the severity of central side effects.

▶ The lack of serious infections in this series is remarkable and encouraging. The intrathecal route of administration has clear advantages over the epidural route, in terms of both analgesic efficacy and lack of catheter fibrosis and occlusion. The cost of fully implanted infusion systems is a deterrent to their use in terminal patients.

S.E. Abram, M.D.

Transdermal Fentanyl in the Long-term Treatment of Cancer Pain: A Prospective Study of 50 Patients With Advanced Cancer of the Gastrointestinal Tract or the Head and Neck Region

Grond S, Zech D, Lehmann KA, et al (Univ of Cologne, Germany)
Pain 69:191–198, 1997 8–32

Background.—For patients with advanced cancers of the head and neck or abdomen, parenteral analgesics are often needed for pain control. Less invasive alternatives for drug delivery are transdermal therapeutic systems (TTSs). A pilot study found that a combination of patient-controlled analgesia (PCA) and transdermal fentanyl provided safe and rapid pain relief, although the conversion ratio from IV to transdermal fentanyl was too low. A open, prospective study, using an improved conversion table, of TTS-fentanyl for long-term treatment of cancer pain was reported.

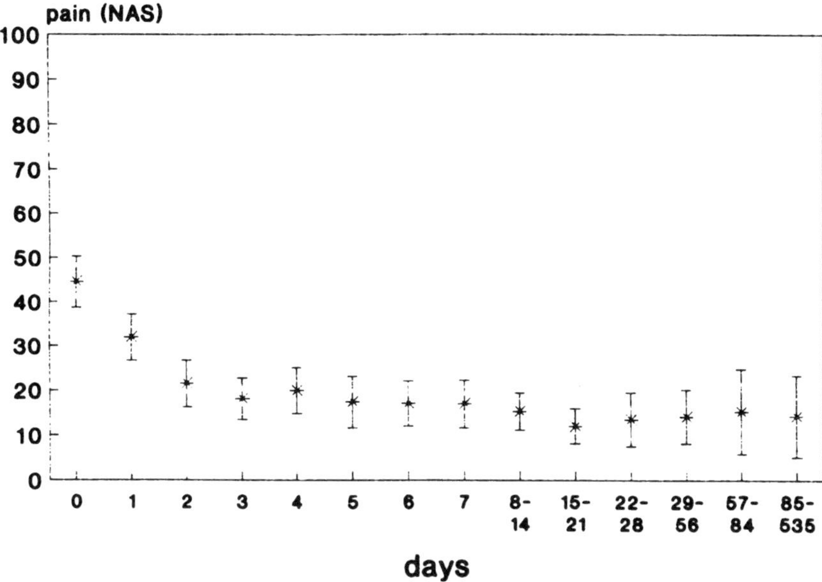

FIGURE 1.—Pain intensity prior to treatment (day 0), during the titration phase (days 1–7), and during long-term treatment (days 8–535). Mean pain scores and their 95% confidence intervals (CIs) are presented. Due to graphical analyses of the CIs, pain scores during the titration phase and long-term treatment were significantly reduced in comparison with the ratings before the study (CI did not overlap) and represented adequate analgesia by transdermal therapeutic system–fentanyl (all CIs entirely below 30). (Reprinted from *Pain*, Grond S, Zech D, Lemann KA, et al: Transdermal fentanyl in the long-term treatment of cancer pain: A prospective study of 50 patients with advanced cancer of the gastrointestinal tract or the head and neck region. *Pain* 69:191–198. Copyright 1997, with kind permission from Elsevier Science–NL, Sara Bugerhartstraat 25, 1055 KV Amsterdam, The Netherlands. Courtesy of Mantha S, Thisted R, Foss J, et al: A proposal to use confidence intervals for visual analog scale data for pain measurement to determine clinical significance. *Anesth Analg* 77:1041–1047, 1993.)

Methods.—The study included 50 patients requiring opioid treatment for severe pain resulting from gastrointestinal tract or head and neck cancers. After initial dose titration with PCA, all patients received long-term therapy with transdermal fentanyl. The dosage of fentanyl that the patient self-administered by PCA over the first 24 hours was used as the basis for the delivery rate of the first TTS-fentanyl system. The patients were permitted oral or subcutaneous morphine as rescue medication. The fentanyl patches remained in place for 48 to 72 hours. When they were removed, the patch size was changed, if necessary, based on the patient's pain score and use of supplementary morphine. Pain was assessed on a 101-point numeric analogue scale. Daily side effects were assessed as well.

Results.—The patients continued treatment for a mean of 66 days, to a maximum of 535 days. Mean pain intensity decreased from 45 at baseline, to 19 during the titration phase, to 15 during long-term treatment (Fig 1). The average TTS-fentanyl delivery rate was 5.9 mg/day (Table 3), and the average plasma fentanyl concentration during long-term treatment was 3.2 ng/mL (Fig 3). Moderate respiratory depression occurred in 3 patients, but there were no other serious side effects. The patients required supple-

TABLE 3.—Mean Daily Doses of PCA-fentanyl, TTS-fentanyl, and Supplemental S.C. Morphine and Mean Plasma Concentrations of Fentanyl (n = 50)

Day	PCA-fentanyl (mg/day)		TTS-fentanyl (mg/day)		s.c. morphine (mg/day)		Fentanyl concentration (ng/ml)		Patients
	Mean ± SD	Range	Mean ± SD	Range	Mean ± SD	Range	Mean ± SD	Range	*N*
0 (Prior study)	—	—	—	—	56.0 ± 43.8*	8.3–240			*50*
1 (PCA)	1.6 ± 0.9	0.1–3.9	—	—	—	—	1.5 ± 2.6	0.0–16	*50*
2 (TTS + PCA)	1.2 ± 1.0	0.0–4.9	2.4 ± 1.4	0.6–6.0	—	—	2.9 ± 3.5	0.2–21.8	*50*
3 (TTS + PCA)	1.0 ± 1.2	0.0–5.4	2.4 ± 1.4	0.6–6.0	—	—	2.4 ± 1.5	0.2–8.3	*50*
4 (TTS)	—	—	3.1 ± 2.3	0.6–10.8	7.3 ± 10.1†	0–40	3.1 ± 4.3	0.0–20.4	*48*
5 (TTS)	—	—	3.5 ± 2.2	0.6–10.8	6.0 ± 9.5†	0–30	2.2 ± 1.4	0.1–5.8	*48*
6 (TTS)	—	—	3.6 ± 2.5	0.6–13.2	5.6 ± 8.0†	0–30	2.6 ± 3.0	0.3–12.5	*45*
7 (TTS)	—	—	3.7 ± 2.6	0.6–13.2	6.1 ± 7.6†	0–30	2.7 ± 2.6	0.2–9.1	*44*
8 (TTS)	—	—	3.8 ± 2.7	0.6–13.2	2.6 ± 4.1†	0–20	2.8 ± 1.7	0.1–8.9	*42*
8–535 (TTS)	—	—	4.8 ± 3.5	0.6–19.2c	5.3 ± 5.9†	0–160‡	3.2 ± 2.3	0.0–14.5	*42*

*The opioid dose taken prior to study (day 0) is calculated as intramuscular morphine equivalent dose.
†The s.c. dose is presented. Oral applications were converted to s.c. doses using a ratio of 3:1.
‡The range of all single values, and not the range of patient means is presented.
Abbreviations: PCA, patient-controlled analgesia; *TTS,* transdermal therapeutic system; *s.c.,* subcutaneous.
(Reprinted from *Pain,* Grond S, Zech D, Lehmann KA, et al: Transdermal fentanyl in the long-term treatment of cancer pain: A prospective study of 50 patients with advanced cancer of the gastrointestinal tract or the head and neck region. *Pain* 69:191–198. Copyright 1997, with kind permission from Elsevier Science–NL, Sara Bugerhartstraat 25, 1055 KV Amsterdam, The Netherlands.)

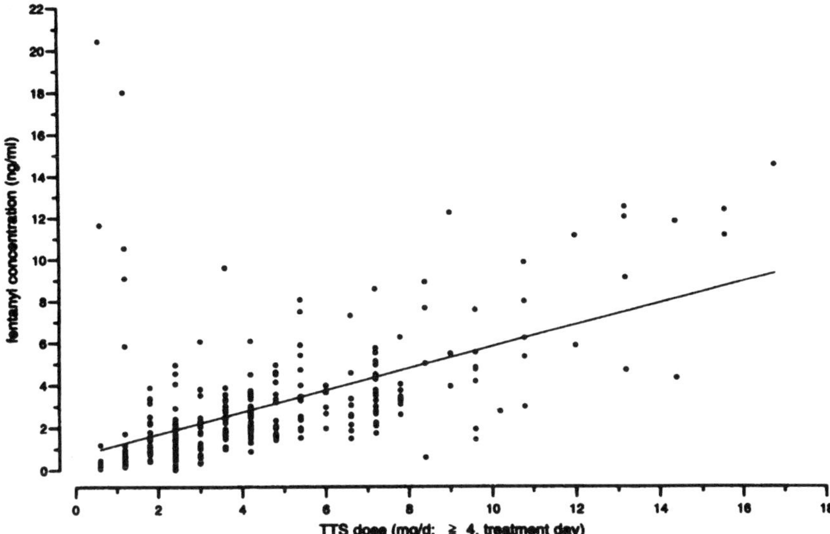

FIGURE 3.—Fentanyl plasma concentrations in relation to transdermal therapeutic system (TTS)-fentanyl dose. Because of patient-controlled analgesia with fentanyl at days 2 and 3 values of these days are not included. The correlation between TTS dose and plasma fentanyl concentration was statistically significant (linear regression analysis: Y = 0.51 × X + 0.66, $r = 0.55$, $P = 0.001$, $n = 285$). (Reprinted from *Pain*, courtesy of Grond S, Zech D, Lehmann KA, et al: Transdermal fentanyl in the long-term treatment of cancer pain: A prospective study of 50 patients with advanced cancer of the gastrointestinal tract or the head and neck region. *Pain* 69:191–198. Copyright 1997, with kind permission from Elsevier Science–NL, Sara Bugerhartstraat 25, 1055 KV Amsterdam, The Netherlands.)

mentary morphine on 40% of days, most often given orally . The patients were highly compliant with and accepting of TTS-fentanyl. Quality-of-life scores improved significantly (Table 6).

Conclusion.—For patients with advanced cancer, a combination of PCA and TTS-fentanyl is an effective treatment for cancer pain. Transdermal fentanyl is noninvasive, easy to administer, and well-accepted by patients. Its major disadvantage is slow pharmacokinetics, which makes it difficult

TABLE 6.—Moderate or Severe Impairment of Quality of Life Indices

Moderate or severe reduction of	Patients prior to study ($n = 50$)	% Days of titration period ($n = 285$)	% Days of long-term treatment ($n = 2979$)
Activity	76	24	21
General state of health	74	21	21
Mobility	64	23	18
Mood	80	22	20

(Reprinted from *Pain*, Grond S, Zech D, Lehmann KA, et al: Transdermal fentanyl in the long-term treatment of cancer pain: A prospective study of 50 patients with advanced cancer of the gastrointestinal tract or the head and neck region. *Pain* 69:191–198. Copyright 1997, with kind permission from Elsevier Science–NL, Sara Bugerhartstraat 25, 1055 KV Amsterdam, The Netherlands.)

to adjust the dose rapidly in the face of changing analgesic needs. Comparative studies of transdermal fentanyl and slow-release morphine are needed.

▶ This study provides a useful scheme for conversion of patients from morphine to transdermal fentanyl. The rationale for such a change is the phenomenon of improved efficacy when switching from a drug with lower intrinsic activity (defined as fraction of receptor occupancy needed to produce a given effect), such as morphine, to a drug with a higher intrinsic activity, such as fentanyl. There are animal data to suggest that fentanyl and sufentanil are more efficacious than meperidine or morphine when noxious stimulus intensity is high. In addition, there is evidence that tolerance development is less of a problem with drugs of higher intrinsic activity.[1]

One must keep in mind, however, that patients are not laboratory animals, and there is tremendous variation in how people respond to drugs. An example is the fact that 1 patient in this study had pain that could not be controlled with 7.2 mg/day of transdermal fentanyl but was well controlled on 240 mg/day of oral time-release morphine.

S.E. Abram, M.D.

Reference

1. Paronis CA, Holtzman SG: Development of tolerance to the analgesic activity of mu agonists after continuous infusion of morphine, meperidine or fentanyl in rats. *J Pharmacol Exp Ther* 262:1–9, 1992.

Transdermal Fentanyl Versus Sustained-Release Oral Morphine in Cancer Pain: Preference, Efficacy, and Quality of Life

Ahmedzai S, for the TTS-Fentanyl Comparative Trial Group (Univ of Sheffield, England)

J Pain Symptom Manage 13:254–261, 1997 8–33

Background.—Although opioids are often used successfully to treat cancer pain, their side effect profile has significant repercussions on a patient's quality of life. Other drugs to control cancer pain are constantly being evaluated, and one such drug is fentanyl. These authors evaluated the effects of transdermal fentanyl patches compared with those of oral morphine on pain control and patient preferences.

Methods.—Adult patients (112 men and 90 women, mean age 62 years) with cancer who were receiving large doses of opioids for analgesia and were taking a stable morphine dose for 48 hours or longer were recruited for the study. Half of the patients (n = 101) were randomized to receive transdermal fentanyl (by patches) for 15 days, then 15 days of sustained-release oral morphine at their typical dose. The other 101 patients received morphine first, then fentanyl. Pain control at the start of the study, at crossover, and for any breakthrough pain was titrated by immediate-release oral morphine. The transdermal fentanyl patches delivered from 25 to 300 μg fentanyl per hour, with doses based on the patient's morphine

TABLE 5.—Commonest Adverse Events Recorded During Treatment

Event	Fentanyl	Morphine
Abdominal pain	18	0
Constipation	6	15
Diarrhea	35	7
Dyspnea	10	5
Nausea	32	23
Somnolence/ drowsiness	17	19
Sweating	12	5
Vomiting	18	18

(Reprinted by permission of Elsevier Science, Inc., from Ahmedzai S, for the TSS-Fentanyl Comparative Trial Group: Transdermal fentanyl versus sustained-release oral morphine in cancer pain: Preference, efficacy, and quality of life. *J Pain Symptom Manage* 13:254–261, 1997. Copyright 1997 by the U.S. Cancer Pain Relief Committee.)

dose. Quality of life was assessed by instruments of the World Health Organization (WHO) and the European Organization for Research and Treatment of Cancer (EORTC).

Findings.—Oral morphine and transdermal fentanyl were equally effective in controlling cancer pain. Significantly more patients taking fentanyl had to use immediate-release morphine to control breakthrough pain (54% vs. 42%), although the incidence of breakthrough pain in either group was not high (1.64 days for fentanyl and 1.2 days for morphine). Fentanyl caused significantly less daytime drowsiness, but significantly more sleep disturbances. Furthermore, constipation was significantly less in the fentanyl group. Side effects (Table 5) were more common in the fentanyl group. Yet, at the end of the study, significantly more patients indicated that fentanyl had caused fewer interruptions in their personal and family lives and was easier to take than morphine. Scores on the WHO and EORTC quality of life assessments showed no significant differences between the 2 drug treatments.

Conclusions.—At equipotent doses, transdermal fentanyl patches were as effective as oral morphine in controlling cancer pain. The quality of life did not differ significantly between the 2 drug treatments, although patients taking fentanyl had less constipation and less daytime drowsiness but more sleep disturbances and overall side effects. In general, patient satisfaction with fentanyl was higher than it was with oral morphine.

► Although there was a significantly higher patient preference and a slightly better side effect profile for transdermal fentanyl than there were for oral morphine the overall differences between the 2 analgesic delivery systems were not great. One factor that was not assessed in this study was cost. There are considerable regional differences in the cost of these preparations. If the cost differential for a particular institution is substantial, the less expensive option will generally be tried first. Another long-acting opioid that was not assessed in this study is methadone. Although somewhat more difficult to dose adjust, it is generally as effective as sustained-release morphine or transdermal fentanyl, and it is far less expensive than either.

S.E. Abram, M.D.

Pilot Study Evaluating Local Anesthetics Administered Systemically for Treatment of Pain in Patients With Advanced Cancer

Chong SF, Bretscher ME, Mailliard JA, et al (Univ of Nebraska, Omaha; Mayo Clinic and Found, Rochester, Minn; Sioux Community Cancer Consortium, Sioux Falls, SD; et al)

J Pain Symptom Manage 13:112–117, 1997 8–34

Objective.—Many cancer patients are unable to get adequate pain relief from opioids. Oral anesthetics have been shown to be effective in the management of diabetic neuropathy and advanced cancer pain. Preliminary information about analgesic efficacy, toxicity, and tolerability of mexiletine and flecainide in patients with advanced cancer was reported.

Methods.—Mexiletine (200 mg orally every 8 hours) or flecainide (100 mg orally every 12 hours) was administered to 20 patients with an Eastern Cooperative Oncology Group performance status of 3 or higher and with cancer pain inadequately controlled by opioids. Patients filled out questionnaires about pain and toxicity.

Results.—Days on study varied from 3 to 532. One patient who initially received mexiletine was later given flecainide. Thirteen patients received treatment for less than 24 days because of unrelieved pain and unchanged opioid requirements. Four patients who received treatment for 57–94 days had no change in pain scores or opioid requirements. Two patients had a definite benefit, and 2 patients had some benefit from treatment. Mexiletine caused significant nausea and gastrointestinal distress in 5 of 8 patients. One patient receiving flecainide had palpitations, and 1 had gastrointestinal symptoms and a prolonged QT wave.

Conclusions.—Seventeen patients received no benefit from oral mexiletine or flecainide. One patient receiving mexiletine and 1 receiving flecainide had definite benefits, and 2 patients receiving flecainide had some benefits. Mexiletine caused severe adverse reactions in 5 of 8 patients.

► Sodium channel blockers are generally used for peripheral neuropathic pain. Spontaneous peripheral nerve firing originating from experimentally induced neuromas in animals is effectively silenced by moderate systemic doses of lidocaine. It is not surprising, therefore, that the number of responding patients would be low in a cohort whose only characteristic was pain related to metastatic cancer. The rational way to assess efficacy of oral sodium channel blockers is to select patients with evidence of peripheral neuropathy, prescreen with intravenous lidocaine to determine whether their pain is responsive to sodium channel block, and then assess the benefit of oral drugs. It is surprising that flecainide was selected for use in this study because it is associated with a relatively high incidence of sudden fatal arrhythmias in postmyocardial infarction patients and is approved by the Food and Drug Administration only for life-threatening arrhythmias.

S.E. Abram, M.D.

A Randomized, Controlled Trial of Intravenous Clodronate in Patients With Metastatic Bone Disease and Pain

Ernst DS, Brasher P, Hagen N, et al (Tom Baker Cancer Centre, Calgary, Alta; Cross Cancer Inst, Edmonton, Alta)

J Pain Symptom Manage 13:319–326, 1997 8–35

Background.—Bone pain is common in patients with advanced malignant disease. Unfortunately, it also is common for these patients to have suboptimal pain relief, mainly because of dose-limiting side effects of the drugs used to treat the pain. These investigators studied the bone resorption inhibitor clodronate for its effectiveness in pain control for patients with metastatic bone disease and refractory pain.

Methods.—The study involved 59 patients 37–85 years old (mean age 63 years) with cancer who had bone metastases. All had bone pain refractory to opioids, nonsteroidal anti-inflammatory drugs, and local radiotherapy. Patients used analgesic diaries to record their pain symptoms. They were allowed to continue their regular opioid analgesics and to use immediate-action opioids for breakthrough pain. Daily morphine equivalent doses were calculated based on all analgesics the patient took. Patients used visual analog tests to rate their general pain, pain at rest, and pain with movement. In this 2-period crossover study, patients received either 600 or 1,500 mg intravenous clodronate followed 14 days later by an intravenous infusion of placebo, or they received placebo first, followed by active drug. Assessments were made at the end of the second 14-day period.

Findings.—Of the initial 59 patients, 46 were evaluable because of dropouts. Results with the 2 doses of clodronate were combined because preliminary analyses showed no change in effect with dosage. Both patients and investigators expressed a significant preference for clodronate over placebo for pain relief (patients 57% vs. 26% and investigators 65% vs 22%, respectively). Visual analog data were scored for the first period only because of a carryover effect. Although general pain scores in the clodronate group decreased 22 ± 7.2 mm over 14 days, this decrease was not significant compared with placebo (13.2 ± 7.5 mm loss over 14 days). Similarly, scores for pain at rest and pain with movement with clodronate were almost half of those with placebo (pain at rest 14 vs 8.5, pain with movement 24 vs 15, respectively), but the difference was not statistically significant. Furthermore, analgesic requirements decreased with clodronate. The daily morphine equivalent dose (mean value 451 mg) was significantly less for clodronate (−6.4 ± 2.9) than it was for placebo (24 ± 14.9).

Conclusions.—In conjunction with the patient's regular opioid dose, intravenous clodronate was superior to placebo in reducing refractory bone pain. Clodronate was more popular with patients and investigators alike. Further studies of this drug should assess the most effective dose and the optimal dosage schedule in controlling metastatic bone pain.

▶ Although the analgesic efficacy of clodronate in patients with pain associated with bone metastasis was not dramatic, it is significantly better than placebo, and bisphosphonates may be helpful for individual patients whose bone pain is poorly controlled with analgesics alone. Other options to consider are subcutaneous or intranasal calcitonin, radiation, chemotherapy, hormonal therapy, and stabilization of pathologic fractures.

S.E. Abram, M.D.

Individualized Use of Methadone and Opioid Rotation in the Comprehensive Management of Cancer Pain Associated With Poor Prognostic Indicators

Vigano A, Fan D, Bruera E (Grey Nuns Community Health Ctr, Edmonton, Alta)

Pain 67:115–119, 1996 8–36

Introduction.—Neuropathic pain and opioid tolerance are both difficult-to-manage problems in cancer patients. Neuropathic pain may be resistant to opioid analgesia, whereas opioid tolerance develops in a substantial percentage of patients receiving parenteral opioids. Incidental pain and somatization are poor prognostic factors in patients with cancer pain. The use of methadone and opioid rotation in a patient with complicated neuropathic pain was reported.

> *Case.*—Man, 45, was admitted to a palliative care unit for control of pain in his back, radiating to his legs. The pain, which was considered to be neuropathic in nature, was related to a renal cell carcinoma that had metastasized to the spine. Pain management was complicated by the presence of incidental pain components and an adjustment disorder with a component of somatization. The patient was treated with methadone, but tolerance and toxic effects quickly developed. The patient was then rotated to methadone, with a decrease in the morphine equivalent daily dose (MEDD) from 1,050 to 36. Methadone provided good pain relief for 4 months, when the pain got worse in association with myoclonus and sedation. This necessitated a switch over back to hydromorphone, which increased the MEDD from 480 to 4,950. Treatment with hydromorphone continued for 2 weeks and was complicated by intractable nausea and sedation. When the patient was rotated back to methadone, the MEDD dropped to 24 (Fig 1). Methadone provided good pain control without opioid toxicity.

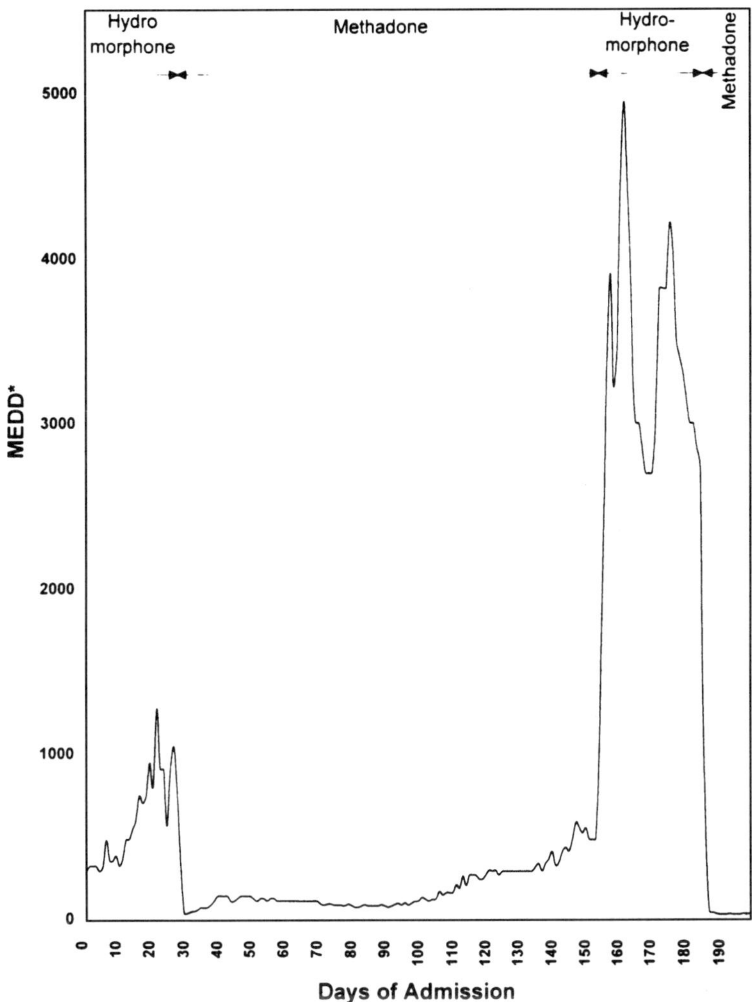

FIGURE 1.—Morphine equivalent daily dose (*MEDD*) mg/24 hr. (Reprinted from *Pain* courtesy of Vigano A, Fan D, Bruera E: Individualized use of methadone and opioid rotation in the comprehensive management of cancer pain associated with poor prognostic indicators. *Pain* 67:115–119, 1996.)

Discussion.—This experience with the use of methadone and opioid rotation for management of cancer pain associated with poor prognostic factors demonstrates the importance of individualized opioid titration, especially with methadone. It also shows the value of opioid rotation when there is inadequate analgesia at the point at which opioid-related toxicity develops. The authors review potential mechanisms of opioid tolerance and its reversal.

▶ This report illustrates the unpredictable responses of individuals to different opioids. It is not safe to assume that development of treatment resistance to 1 opioid drug results in resistance to all opioids. Similarly, the side effects of different opioid drugs in a given patient may vary greatly. It is generally reasonable to try several different drugs before giving up on the entire class.

S.E. Abram, M.D.

Other Topics in Chronic Pain Medicine

Postoperative Analgesic Effect of Intrathecal Neostigmine and Its Influence on Spinal Anaesthesia

Klamt JG, Slullitel A, Garcia IV, et al (Faculty of Medicine of Ribeirão, Preto, Brazil)

Anaesthesia 52:547–551, 1997 8–37

Background.—The combination of intrathecal neostigmine and local anesthetic may improve the quality of spinal anesthesia and prolong postoperative analgesia. The effects of intrathecal neostigmine on the characteristics of spinal anesthesia and its postoperative analgesic efficacy and safety were assessed.

Methods.—Thirty-six patients undergoing anterior and posterior vaginoplasty under spinal anesthesia were enrolled in the double-blind, placebo-controlled trial. By random assignment, the patients received normal saline, 1 mL; morphine, 100 μg in 1 mL of saline; or neostigmine, 100 μg in 1 mL of saline intrathecally just before hyperbaric 0.5% bupivacaine, 4 mL, was injected spinally.

Findings.—The mean time to first analgesic administration was prolonged significantly by intrathecal neostigmine and morphine compared with saline. The number of patients needing subcutaneous morphine to complement the analgesia provided by the IM nonsteroidal anti-inflammatory drugs and the mean administration times also differed among groups; 8 patients in the saline group (mean administration time, 8 hours), 1 in the morphine group (18 hours), and 2 in the neostigmine group (8 and

TABLE 4.—Incidence of Adverse Events of Intrathecal Saline (1 mL), Morphine (100 μg), or Neostigmine (100 μg injection) in Patients Submitted to Spinal Anesthesia With Hyperbaric Bupivacaine (0.5%, 4 mL)

	Saline	Morphine	Neostigmine
Hypotension SBP < 90 mmHg	5	5	1
Hypertension SBP > 150 mmHg	0	0	2
Vomiting during surgery	2	3	8*
Evacuation during surgery	0	0	4
Profuse sweating, distress, agitation	0	0	2
Pruritus	0	5	0

Note: Results are expressed as number of patients.
*Significantly different from the saline and morphine groups by the Fisher Exact Test ($P < 0.05$).
Abbreviation: SBP, systolic blood pressure.
(Reprinted from Klamt JG, Slullitel A, Garcia IV, et al: Postoperative analgesic effect of intrathecal neostigmine and its influence on spinal anesthesia. *Anaesthesia* 52[6]:547–551. Copyright 1997 by permission of the publisher, WB Saunders Company Limited, London.)

12.9 hours, respectively) needed subcutaneous morphine. The analgesic efficacy was similar in the patients given morphine and neostigmine. Neither intrathecal morphine nor neostigmine modified the characteristics of spinal anesthesia. Intrathecal neostigmine was associated with severe nausea and vomiting, sweating, and distress during surgery. However, patients given neostigmine had less hypotension (Table 4).

Conclusions.—Intrathecal neostigmine provided analgesia for about 12 hours, and the analgesia was maintained easily with nonsteroidal anti-inflammatory drugs in these patients undergoing anterior and posterior vaginoplasty under spinal anesthesia. Although the severity of the adverse effects associated with intrathecal neostigmine may limit its value as the sole analgesic, a smaller dose may be just as effective and may have less intense or no adverse effects.

► Given the high incidence of nausea associated with the use of intrathecal (IT) neostigmine, it would appear that the principal benefit of the technique will result from its combination with other drugs such as morphine and clonidine. In animals, IT cholinergics are synergic with opiates and α-2 agonists, and they tend to counteract the hypotension associated with IT clonidine. It is not clear whether this drug will be useful for long-term infusion in patients with chronic pain.

S.E. Abram, M.D.

Effect of Neonatal Circumcision on Pain Response During Subsequent Routine Vaccination

Taddio A, Katz J, Ilersich AL, et al (Hosp for Sick Children, Toronto; Toronto Hosp; Univ of Toronto)

Lancet 349:599–603, 1997 8–38

Background.—Preliminary research suggests that pain in the neonatal period may have long-lasting effects on future infant behavior. Whether neonatal circumcision affects pain response at 4- or 6-month vaccination compared with uncircumcised babies was investigated, and the effects of circumcision pretreatment with lidocaine-prilocaine cream (EMLA) were determined.

Methods and Findings.—Eighty-seven infants were studied prospectively. One group was uncircumcised, 1 group had been randomly assigned to EMLA pretreatment for pain in circumcision, and 1 group had been assigned to placebo before circumcision. The 3 groups were comparable in birth and infant characteristics at the time of vaccination, including age and temperament scores. Multivariate analysis showed significant differences in percentage facial action, percentage cry time, and Visual Analogue Scale pain scores at vaccination. Univariate analyses were significant for all outcome measures. Babies receiving placebo before circumcision had higher difference scores than uncircumcised babies for percentage facial action, percentage cry duration, and Visual Analogue Scale pain scores. All

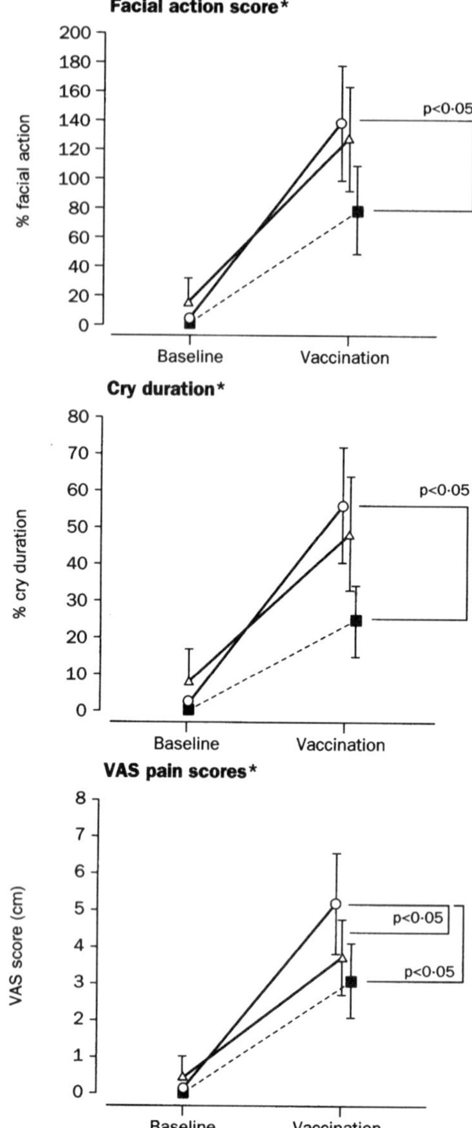

FIGURE.—Top, middle, and **bottom,** infant pain response to vaccination for infants in all groups. *Values shown as mean (95% confidence interval). *Abbreviation: VAS,* Visual Analogue Scale. (Courtesy of Taddio A, Katz J, Ilersich AL, et al: Effect of neonatal circumcision on pain response during subsequent routine vaccination. *Lancet* 349:599–603, 1997. Copyright by *The Lancet* Ltd., 1997.)

outcome measures showed a significant linear trend, with pain scores increasing from uncircumcised infants to those pretreated with EMLA to those given placebo before circumcision (Figure).

Conclusions.—Pain responses to routine vaccination are stronger in circumcised babies than in uncircumcised ones. Preoperative EMLA treatment can attenuate this pain response. Such treatment is recommended to alleviate neonatal pain during circumcision.

► I thought that this was a fascinating study that raises many questions on the development of CNS pain mechanisms in infants. It also shows that first-class clinical research can be done at low financial cost—what is needed are good ideas.

M. Wood, M.D.

The Pathologic Effects of Intrathecal Betamethasone

Latham JM, Fraser RD, Moore RJ, et al (Royal Adelaide Hosp, Australia; Inst of Med and Veterinary Science, Adelaide, Australia; Univ of Newcastle, Australia)

Spine 22:1558–1562, 1997 8–39

Purpose.—Many recent studies have addressed the safety and efficacy of epidural steroid. In Australia, there have been reports of arachnoiditis and other adverse effects of methylprednisolone (Depo-Medrol). In response, drug manufacturers have recommended that steroid preparations not be used epidurally. Arachnoiditis may result from intrathecal, rather than epidural, administration of methylprednisolone. No studies have examined the safety of intrathecal betamethasone (Celestone Chronodose). Intrathecal betamethasone was studied for its histopathologic effects in sheep.

Methods.—Experiments were performed in 23 adult merino sheep. After lumbar puncture at the L6–S1 level, differing volumes of Celestone Chronodose or normal saline were injected into the subarachnoid space. Six weeks later, the animals were killed for histopathologic examination of the spinal cord, meninges, and nerve roots.

Results.—Saline injection, in a volume of up to 16 mL, caused no pathologic abnormalities. Neither were there any pathologic changes in 11 sheep injected with 1 mL (5.7 mg) of Celestone Chronodose. This was true even in animals receiving repeated steroid injections at weekly intervals. Histologic changes consistent with arachnoiditis did occur in 1 of 6 sheep injected with 2 mL of Celestone Chronodose and in 3 of 3 sheep injected with volumes greater than 2 mL.

Conclusion.—Extrapolated to humans, the results suggest that 1 and probably 2 mL doses of betamethasone, in the form of Celestone Chronodose, can be safely injected intrathecally. Arachnoiditis is unlikely to occur at this dose; however, complications become more likely at higher doses. Caution is needed to avoid intrathecal injection of steroid during epidural injection, especially if spinal stenosis or fibrotic partial obliteration of the epidural space is present.

▶ The use of epidural steroids in Australia has all but ceased, not because of scientific data regarding the safety and efficacy of the technique but because of sensationalistic adverse publicity by the popular press. The evidence that the current preparations of steroid suspensions commonly used for the treatment of sciatica are harmful when injected epidurally is practically nil. Similarly, there is practically no evidence that a single accidental injection of triamcinolone diacetate or methylprednisolone acetate intrathecally will cause harm. Nevertheless, the medicolegal climate in Australia is such that the technique will probably not be reinstituted until another safe preparation is introduced.

It is unfortunate that the authors did not publish the constituents of Celestone Chronodose and their concentrations. They did mention the fact that the drug contains benzalkonium chloride, and the discussion implies that it does not contain polyethylene glycol. Rather than being reassured by the lack of adverse effects of the intrathecal injection of low doses of this preparation, I am concerned about the apparent toxic effect of modestly higher doses. I do not think this drug is the answer to the epidural steroid safety issue. The responsible method of solving this problem is the intentional development of a safe, single-use preparation formulated specifically for epidural use. Given the legal risks, the controversy regarding the efficacy of the technique, and the irrational public debate over the issue in Australia, I doubt that any pharmaceutical company will want to take on this project.

S.E. Abram, M.D.

Antinociception Induced by Civamide, an Orally Active Capsaicin Analogue

Hua X-Y, Chen P, Hwang J-h, et al (Univ of California, La Jolla)
Pain 71:313–322, 1997 8–40

Background.—Capsaicin's antinociceptive effects are believed to result from its binding with a specific membrane receptor that then desensitizes the associated nerve terminal. These investigators used a new capsaicin analogue, civamide, to characterize capsaicinoid receptor pharmacology and to determine the nociceptive effects of civamide in a rat model of pain.

Methods.—Male Sprague-Dawley rats given either vehicle or civamide (20, 60, or 200 mg/kg) by gavage were used in 3 different models of pain. In the formalin test, rats were briefly anesthetized, and 50 µL of 5% formalin solution was injected into the right hind paw. The flinching responses to vehicle or civamide were assessed in phase I (first 6 minutes) and phase 2 (after 10 minutes). In the thermal paw withdrawal test, a glass surface was maintained at 30°C, and the time it took for the rat to remove the hind paws (averaged) was measured. Rats were studied at 60 minutes and on days 1–4 after vehicle or civamide dosing. In the Chung model, surgery was performed to induce an allodynic state, to select rats that developed tactile allodynia with a 50% threshold for a hair ≤4 g. These animals recovered for 7 days, and positive responses (paw withdrawal) were measured at 60 minutes and on days 1–4 after vehicle or civamide dosing. Tissues were examined by radioimmunoassay for the presence of calcitonin gene-related peptide (CGRP) and substance P in dorsal and ventral spinal cords to determine the mechanism of drug action.

Findings.—In the formalin test, 200 mg/kg civamide significantly reduced the number of flinches in both phases I and II at 60 minutes and at 2 days after dosing (Fig 1). This inhibitory effect was evident for phase II responses even 7 days after dosing, and the effect was dose dependent. In the thermal test, civamide increased the paw withdrawal latency 1 and 2

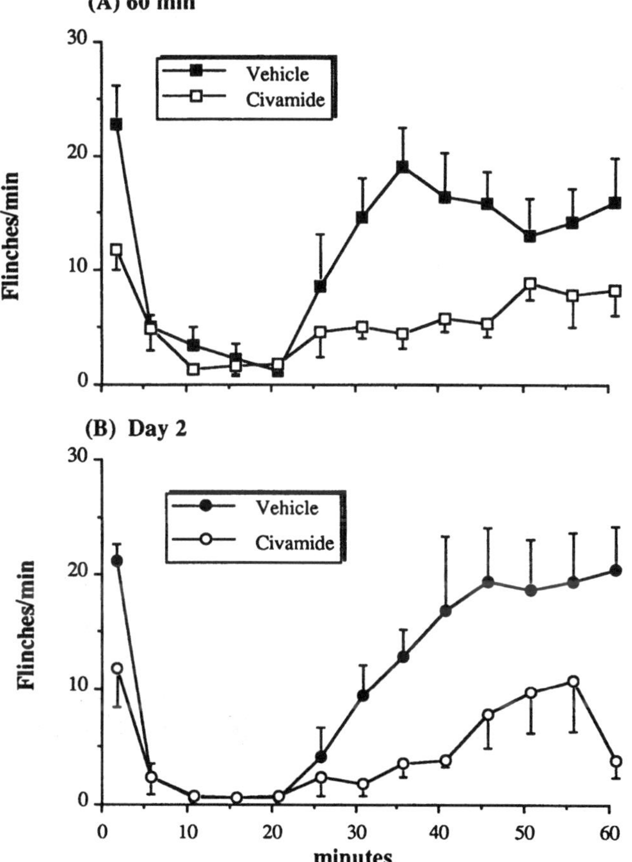

FIGURE 1.—The time-course effect of civamide, 200 mg/kg p.o., on the flinch response (flinches per min) evoked by injection of 50 μL of 5% formalin into the paw at 60 minutes (**A**) and at the third day (day 2) (**B**) after civamide/vehicle delivery. The data are presented as mean ± SEM of 5–6 animals in each group. (Courtesy of Hua X-Y, Chen P, Hwang J-h, et al: Antinociception induced by civamide, an orally active capsaicin analogue. *Pain* 71:313–322, 1997.)

days after dosing, compared with controls. This effect declined to predrug levels by day 3, but the effect also was dose dependent on day 2. In the Chung model, civamide had a significant antiallodynic effect on the tactile threshold on day 2. This effect, too, was dose dependent, and the effect returned to baseline levels in 4–5 days (Fig 7). The only change in peptide levels after civamide dosing was a decrease in the dorsal root ganglia and sciatic nerve concentrations of CGRP.

Conclusions.—Civamide showed significant antinociceptive activity in both phases of the formalin test. That this effect lasted for up to 7 days

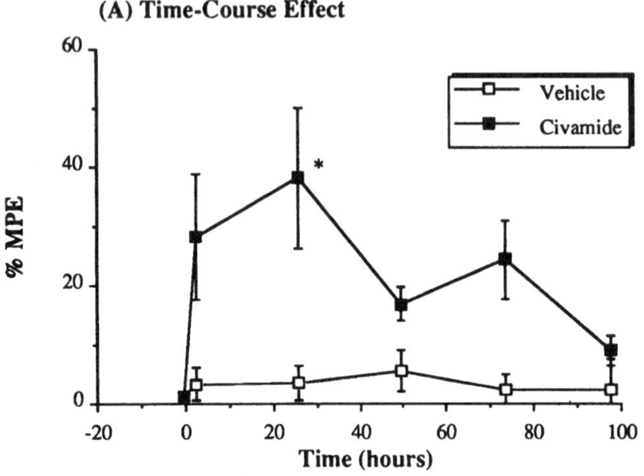

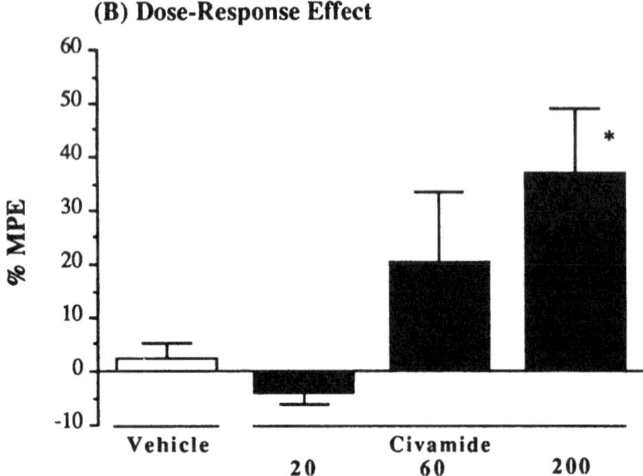

FIGURE 7.—Summary of (A) the time-course effect of civamide 200 mg/kg, and (B) the dose–response effect of civamide (20, 60, and 200 mg/kg, p.o.) measured on the second day after drug application on the Chung model. The data are presented as mean ± SEM of 5–11 animals in each group. *$P < 0.05$, 1-way analysis of variance. (Courtesy of Hua X-Y, Chen P, Hwang J-h, et al: Antinociception induced by civamide, an orally active capsaicin analogue. *Pain* 71:313–322, 1997.)

after dosing in phase II suggests that civamide acts by interrupting small afferent transmission with C-polymodal nociceptors. Nociceptive effects also were evident at 2 days after oral civamide in the thermal and Chung models, again in a dose-dependent manner. Because only CGRP activity in the dorsal spinal cord was altered, this further supports the hypothesis that civamide's analgesic effect occurs through desensitization of afferent terminals.

► It is interesting that with this capsaicin analogue there is a dissociation between the C-fiber stimulating effect and the ability of the drug to desensitize nociceptive afferent terminals. Thus, with oral administration, there is a substantial and prolonged antinociceptive and antihyperanalgesic effect without initially producing pain. For individuals who can tolerate high concentrations of capsaicin on the palate, however, the answer may lie in a visit to their favorite Thai or Mexican restaurant.

S.E. Abram, M.D.

Intraarticular Morphine Analgesia in Chronic Pain Patients With Osteoarthritis

Likar R, Schäfer M, Paulak F, et al (Abteilung für Innere Medizin, Klagenfurt, Austria; Johns Hopkins Univ, Baltimore, Md; NIH, Baltimore, Md; et al)

Anesth Analg 84:1313–1317, 1997 8–41

Objective.—In patients undergoing arthroscopic knee surgery, intraarticular (IA) injections of very small doses of morphine produces effective postoperative analgesia that is mediated by opioid receptors on the peripheral nerve terminals of primary afferent neurons. A double-blind, randomized, 2-period, crossover study compared the efficacy of IA morphine and saline treatment between different groups of osteoarthritis patients with chronic pain, as well as in the same patient.

Methods.—The study consisted of a first injection, a 48-hour assessment phase (phase 1) and a washout phase, followed by a second injection 7 days later with a 48-hour assessment phase (phase 2). Group A patients (n = 13) received simultaneous injections of 1 mg of morphine hydrochloride IA and 5 mL of saline intravenously; 7 days later they were crossed over to the opposite treatment of 5 mL of saline IA and 1 mg of morphine intravenously. Group B patients (n = 10) received the same treatments in the opposite order. Pain intensity was scored on a numerical rating scale (NRS) from 0 (no pain) to 100 (unbearable pain), a visual analogue scale (VAS)(0–100), and a German adaptation of the McGill Pain Questionnaire (MPQ) before, and at 6, 24, and 48 hours after the first and second injections. Knee pain intensity was compared at rest and during movement. Side effects were rated as none, moderate, or severe. Data were compared statistically using repeated measures analysis of variance.

Results.—Because pain intensity scores showed a carry-over for group A, mean pain intensity data for phase 1 alone were used. The group NRS and VAS scores of group A were significantly lower than baseline values at all time points. There were no changes in NRS scores from baseline values for group B before the second morphine injection. Phase I MPQ ratings were similar for groups A and B during phase 1.

Conclusions.—Single IA injections of small doses of morphine can relieve chronic knee pain for as long as 7 days in patients with osteoarthritis.

► The analgesic effect of articular morphine with chronic knee arthropathy was moderately effective and surprisingly long lasting. We are occasionally confronted with patients who have received a diagnosis of "RSD of the knee," a condition characterized by chronic burning pain, allodynia around the joint, joint swelling, and occasionally skin discoloration. Such patients usually experience minimal pain relief with sympathetic blocks, and the condition is probably the result of a chronic synovitis. It would be interesting to determine whether IA morphine would be helpful in such patients.

S.E. Abram, M.D.

Methylnaltrexone Prevents Morphine-induced Delay in Oral-Cecal Transit Time Without Affecting Analgesia: A Double-blind Randomized Placebo-controlled Trial

Yuan C-S, Foss JF, O'Connor M, et al (Univ of Chicago)

Clin Pharmacol Ther 59:469–475, 1996 8–42

Background.—Opioids such as morphine are commonly used for analgesia. The most common side effect of long-term morphine use is constipation, as the result of direct opioid action on the gut. This side effect can limit the use of morphine. Maintenance of the analgesic effect of morphine while reducing its inhibition of gastrointestinal motility and transit would be clinically useful. Methylnaltrexone is a quaternary opioid receptor antagonist that does not cross the blood-brain barrier. It is possible that methylnaltrexone could reverse opioid side effects such as constipation without interfering with analgesia. The effects of methylnaltrexone on analgesia and morphine-induced changes in gastrointestinal motility were assessed in healthy volunteers.

Methods.—Seven healthy male and 7 nonpregnant healthy female volunteers participated in this double-blind, randomized, placebo-controlled study. The average age of the participants was 26 years. Patients received, in random order and in a double-blinded fashion, either an injection of placebo plus placebo, placebo plus 0.05 mg/kg morphine, or 0.45 mg/kg methylnaltrexone plus 0.05 mg/kg morphine. Each injection was separated from the others by at least 1 week. Venous blood and urine samples were collected to assess drug levels. Gastrointestinal transit time was measured by pulmonary hydrogen. Perception of tonic pain was monitored by the cold-pressor test.

Results.—Morphine significantly increased oral-cecal transit time. Methylnaltrexone prevented the morphine-induced increase in oral-cecal transit time. Methylnaltrexone did not affect morphine's analgesic effects. Preliminary results with a higher dose of morphine, (0.1 mg/kg) indicates that at this dose also, methylnaltrexone interfered with the delay in oral-cecal transit time, but not with the analgesia of morphine.

Conclusion.—Methylnaltrexone can be used to reverse the morphine-induced increase in oral-cecal time without interfering with morphine's analgesic activity. Methylnaltrexone may be an important therapeutic adjuvant for the treatment of opioid-induced constipation.

► Constipation is a major problem for patients with chronic or cancer pain who take opioids for long intervals. Apparently, less tolerance develops to the constipating effect than to the analgesic, respiratory depressant, or sedative effects of opioids. Prolonged gastrointestinal transit time associated with opioids creates major problems for postoperative patients as well, delaying initiation of oral feeding, and thus, causing nutritional deficits that retard healing and prolong catabolic conditions. One of the major advantages of postoperative regional analgesic techniques is the reductions of systemic opioid effects of gastrointestinal mobility. If methylnaltrexone is, indeed, effective in maintaining normal mobility, it will be a real benefit in terms of function improvement as well as patient comfort.

S.E. Abram, M.D.

Benzodiazepine Mediated Antagonism of Opioid Analgesia

Gear RW, Miaskowski C, Heller PH, et al (Univ of California, San Francisco; Kaiser Found Hosp, Haywood, Calif)

Pain 71:25–29, 1997 8–43

Purpose.—Opioid analgesia is antagonized by activation of supraspinal γ-aminobutyric acid-A ($GABA_A$) receptors. Benzodiazepines, widely used as adjuncts to anesthesia during surgery, enhance the action of GABA at $GABA_A$ receptors. If using benzodiazepines for preoperative sedation antagonizes postoperative opioid analgesia, giving a benzodiazepine antagonist—flumazenil—should provide better-quality postoperative analgesia. Patients undergoing dental surgery were studied to see whether flumazenil would enhance postoperative morphine analgesia after preoperative sedation with a benzodiazepine.

Methods.—The double-blind, placebo-controlled trial included 71 patients undergoing surgical removal of 1 or more impacted mandibular third molars. The patients received routine IV sedation with the benzodiazepine diazepam. The operation was performed with nitrous oxide and mepivacine for local anesthesia. Postoperatively, each patient received a 6-mg IV injection of morphine sulfate. Forty minutes later, patients also received either flumazenil, 0.75 mg IV, or placebo. Pain intensity before and after morphine injection was assessed by visual analogue scale. Vital signs were assessed as well. For the 2 days after surgery, the patients' pain was assessed by diary and analgesic use.

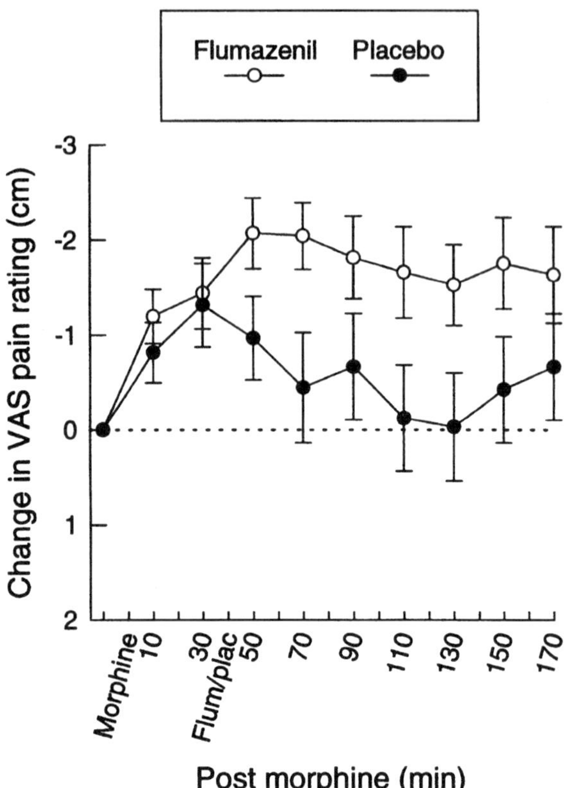

FIGURE 1.—The effect of flumazenil (0.75 mg IV) on morphine (6 mg IV) analgesia. Change in visual analogue scale (*VAS*) pain rating (ordinate), recorded on a 10-cm VAS represents changes from the baseline level (*dotted line*) after various times. Data points are plotted as mean ± SEM. (Reprinted from *Pain* courtesy of Gear RW, Miaskowski C, Heller PH, et al: Benzodiazepine mediated antagonism of opioid analgesia. *Pain* 71:25–29, 1997.)

Results.—Morphine analgesia was significantly enhanced in the patients who received flumazenil (Fig 1). Vital signs were not significantly different between groups. The flumazenil group also had significantly less nausea after discharge and used significantly less ibuprofen. There was no significant difference in postdischarge pain levels, suggesting that patients in the placebo group required more ibuprofen to achieve a comparable level of pain control (Fig 2).

Conclusion.—For surgical patients receiving preoperative benzodiazepine sedation, flumazenil significantly enhances postoperative morphine analgesia. The findings indicate that benzodiazepines cause clinically important antagonism of opioid analgesia. Postoperative analgesia may be improved by using short-acting benzodiazepines or giving flumazenil postoperatively. More study is needed to see whether patients with chronic pain—many of whom receive benzodiazepines for their anxiolytic ef-

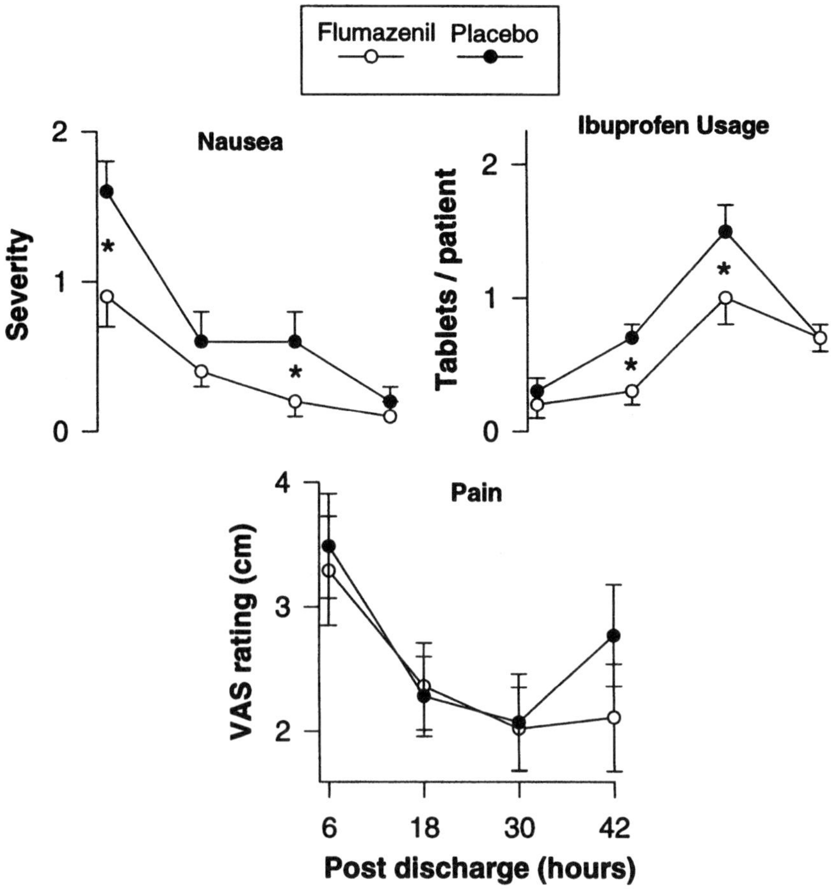

FIGURE 2.—The effect of flumazenil on postdischarge nausea (**top panel**), ibuprofen usage (**middle panel**), and pain (**bottom panel**). *Asterisks* denote statistically significant differences. (*P* less than 0.05). Data points are plotted as mean ±SEM. *Abbreviation*: *VAS*, visual analogue scale. (Reprinted from *Pain* courtesy of Gear RW, Miaskowski C, Heller PH, et al: Benzodiazepine mediated antagonism of opioid analgesia. *Pain* 71:25–29, 1997.)

fects—have a similar negative interaction between benzodiazepines and opioids.

▶ Although benzodiazepines are analgesic when injected spinally, their systemic administration produces predominantly supraspinal effects, 1 of which is interference with descending pain control mechanisms. Barbiturates probably exert their antanalgesic effect through activation of supraspinal GABA receptors as well. The implications of this finding, as the authors suggest, may be profound for the large numbers of patients with chronic pain who use benzodiazepines for sleep, anxiolysis, and muscle relaxation. Many of us discontinue these drugs in chronic pain patients in an effort to reduce depression and improve cognitive and coping abilities. As this study indicates, there may be even more compelling reasons for stopping their use.

S.E. Abram, M.D.

Extradural Sensory Rhizotomy in the Management of Chronic Lumbar Radiculopathy: A Minimum 2-Year Follow-up Study

Wetzel FT, Phillips FM, Aprill CN, et al (Univ of Chicago; Diagnostic Conservative Management, New Orleans, La; Spine Associates of Columbus, PC, Ga)

Spine 22:2283–2292, 1997 8–44

Introduction.—It can be very difficult to manage chronic radicular pain in a patient with failed lumbar surgery. Central ablative procedures—rhizotomy and ganglionectomy—have been variably effective in relieving pain. Extradural sensory rhizotomy was performed in carefully selected patients with chronic intractable lumbar radiculopathy.

Methods.—The retrospective analysis included 51 consecutive patients undergoing extradural sensory rhizotomy over a 15-month period. All patients had persistent, intractable lower extremity pain after failed lumbar spine surgery. Before surgery, each patient had extensive evaluations to rule out reversible structural lesions, as well as clinical and electrophysiologic assessments to confirm the presence of chronic radiculopathy. Selective nerve blocks were performed and repeated to confirm the symptomatic nature of the segments. Selective sensory rhizotomy or, in some cases, complete rhizotomy was performed. At least 2 years' postoperative follow-up was available in 37 patients. A visual analogue scale was used to assess pain relief. Other outcomes included sensory and motor deficits, use of narcotic analgesics, and patient ratings of the effectiveness of surgery.

Results.—At 6 months, outcomes were rated as excellent in 10% of patients, good in 45%, poor in 12%, and treatment failure in 33% (Table 2). Thirteen patients underwent secondary rhizotomies, and 5 had tran-

TABLE 2.—Clinical Results After Lumbar Extradural Sensory Rhizotomy at 6 Months' Follow-Up or Less (n = 51)

Rating Category	No. (%) of Patients	m VAS, Preoperative	m VAS, ≤6 mo
Excellent	5 (9.8)	8.6 (8.1–9.1)	2.6 (1–4)
Good	23 (45.1)	8.7 (7.7–9.6)	3.9 (3.0–4.6)
Poor	6 (11.7)	9.0 (7.9–9.8)	8.1 (7.0–8.7)
Failure	17 (33.3)	8.5 (7.9–9.5)	8.9 (7.7–9.9)

Note: There was no significant difference in visual analogue scale (*VAS*) scores between Excellent and Good categories (P = 0.1), or Poor vs. Failure (P = 0.2). However, VAS data were significantly different between the Excellent and Poor (P = 0.02), and Excellent vs. Failure Groups (P = 0.0002). Likewise, VAS data were significantly different between Good and Poor groups (P = 0.0001), and Good vs. Failure groups (P = 0.001). All P values, by the paired t test, 95% confidence interval.

(Courtesy of Wetzel FT, Phillips FM, Aprill CN, et al: Extradural sensory rhizotomy in the management of chronic lumbar radiculopathy: A minimum 2-year follow-up study. *Spine* 22:2283–2292, 1997.)

TABLE 3.—Clinical Results After Lumbar Extradural Sensory Rhizotomy at 2 Years' Follow-Up or Greater (n = 37)

Rating Category	No. (%) of Patients	m VAS, Preoperative	m VAS, ≤6 month Follow-up	No. (%) of Patients	m VAS, Preoperative	m VAS ≤2 yr Follow-up
Excellent	4 (12.1)	8.6 (8.1–9.1)	2.6 (1–4)	2 (5.4)	8 (7.9–8.1)	1.6 (1.2–2.0)
Good	18 (48.7)	8.6 (7.7–9.6)	3.6 (3.1–4.6)	5 (13.5)	8.5 (7.9–9.1)	3.8 (3.2–4.1)
Poor	4 (10.8)	9.0 (7.9–9.8)	8.0 (7.0–8.7)	13 (35.1)	8.8 (7.7–9.5)	8.8 (7.8–9.7)
Failure	10 (27.1)	9.0 (7.9–9.5)	8.8 (7.7–9.9)	17 (46.1)	8.3 (7.9–9.6)	8.8 (5.1–9.8)

Note: No significant difference in visual analogue scale (*VAS*) was apparent in Excellent vs. Good (P = 0.07), or Poor vs. Failure groups (P = 0.6). However, VAS scores were significantly different between Excellent and Poor (P = 0.04), Excellent vs. Failure (P = 0.05), Good vs. Poor (P = 0.0001), and Good vs. Failure (P = 0.0001). Paired t test, 95% confidence interval.

(Courtesy of Wetzel FT, Phillips FM, Aprill CN, et al: Extradural sensory rhizotomy in the management of chronic lumbar radiculopathy: A minimum 2-year follow-up study. Spine 22:2283–2292, 1997.)

sient improvement. At an average follow-up of 3.5 years, outcomes were excellent in 5% of patients, good in 14%, poor in 35%, and treatment failure in 46% (Table 3). Thus, the overall clinical success rate was only 19%. None of the patients believed that the rhizotomy significantly improved any aspect of their back pain.

Conclusion.—Even when rhizotomy provides good results in patients with chronic lumbar radiculopathy, the results deteriorate over time. The failure of this procedure may be related to anatomical factors and the lack of specific diagnostic techniques. Rhizotomy is not recommended for use in the treatment of chronic lumbar radiculopathy after lumbar surgery.

▶ Despite previous publication of disappointing results from rhizotomy, the authors proceeded with this project. The rationale for yet another look at this procedure was their meticulous selection and follow-up process. Their selection criteria included electromyographic evidence of radiculopathy without signs of active denervation; reproduction of pain during, and relief of pain after, selective root block; and lack of evidence for facet joint–related pain. Despite these measures, long-term benefit was extremely unlikely. Hopefully, this study will convince the most ardent proponents of this procedure to cease and desist.

S.E. Abram, M.D.

Effect of Racemic Mixture and the (S+)-Isomer of Ketamine on Temporal and Spatial Summation of Pain

Arendt-Nielsen L, Nielsen J, Petersen-Felix S, et al (Aalborg Univ, Denmark; Inselspital Bern, Switzerland)

Br J Anaesth 77:625–631, 1996 8–45

Background.—Few *N*-methyl-D-aspartate (NMDA) antagonists are available for use in humans, and the existing agents have severe psychomimetic effects. Ketamine is available commercially. The analgesic efficacy of a racemic mixture and the stereoisomer (S+)-isomer of ketamine on temporal and spatial summation of pain was reported.

Methods.—Twelve healthy subjects participated in the double-blind, 3-way crossover, placebo-controlled study. Reaction times of the following were assesed: pain evoked by small and large area pressure stimuli, pain detection threshold and pain ratings to small and large areas of heat stimuli, pain detection threshold and pain rating to heat stimuli of brief and long duration, summation pain threshold and pain ratings to repeated heat and electrical stimuli, adverse effects, and reaction times were assessed. Ketamine (racemic) and ketamine (S+) were assessed at plasma levels of 350 and 180 ng mL^{-1}, respectively.

Findings.—Ketamine (racemic) prolonged reaction time more than ketamine (S+). Both agents affected pain resulting from repeated stimuli or stimuli of long duration equally or more than a single stimulus of short duration. In addition, both agents affected pain evoked from large areas equally or more than pain evoked from small areas. The (S+)-isomer was about twice as potent as the racemic mixture in inhibiting central summation.

Conclusions.—Ketamine (racemic) and ketamine (S+) both had a general analgesic effect as well as an effect on repeated stimuli, long-duration stimuli, and stimuli covering large areas. The doses tested had the same number of adverse effects, which were minimal.

▶ Many drugs are administered as racemates. Pharmaceutical companies are showing an increased interest in developing drugs as single isomers. Ketamine is commercially available as a racemic mixture, but the (S+) ketamine is more potent than the (R-) isomer and may have fewer psychoactive side effects.

M. Wood, M.D.

The Twelfth Rib Syndrome

Cranfield KAW, Buist RJ, Nandi PR, et al (Univ College London; Natl Hosp for Neurology and Neurosurgery, London; Medway Hosp, Gillingham, Kent, England)

J Pain Symptom Manage 13:172–175, 1997 8–46

Background.—The twelfth rib syndrome, presumed to result from irritation of the twelfth intercostal nerve by the highly mobile twelfth rib, appears to be a fairly common, underdiagnosed chronic pain syndrome. It occurs in more women than men, at a ratio of 3:1. Usually patients describe a constant dull ache or sharp stabbing pain that may last for several hours to many weeks, but the presentation and course of this syndrome vary. Six patients are presented to illustrate the varied presentation of this syndrome.

Case Reports.—The first patient, a 66-year-old man, had a classic presentation. The pain was constant, radiated into the abdomen, and was exacerbated by sitting or other activities involving spinal extension. Clinical findings suggested the diagnosis, which was confirmed by pain production on movement of the twelfth rib with radiographic guidance. The pain was relieved by an intercostal nerve block with local anesthetic, and permanent symptomatic relief was achieved after twelfth rib resection.

The second patient was a 48-year-old woman with long-standing back pain, the nature of which had changed 2 years before her referral. She experienced a dull constant pain in the right loin and right costal margin that varied in severity, with no associated paresthesia or allodynia. Spinal extension and pressure over the midlumbar region exacerbated the pain, as had manipulations by physiotherapists and osteopaths. Tenderness over the twelfth rib, elicited during examination, was confirmed to be the source of pain under an image intensifier. This pain was relieved by 2 intercostal injections of local anesthetic and steroid, but chronic low back pain continued.

The third patient, a 22-year-old woman referred for right costovertebral angle tenderness, reported a 4.5-year history of an intermittent, sharp pain in the right loin that had begun during pregnancy. Exacerbations of the pain occurred every few months, resulting in pain of 2 weeks' duration. She had no paresthesia or allodynia. Lying flat, the use of a hot water bottle, and various simple analgesics alleviated the pain. The only abnormal finding was extreme tenderness inferior to the twelfth rib on the right side, associated with paravertebral muscle spasm. Transcutaneous electrical nerve stimulation was moderately successful. A twelfth intercostal nerve block markedly improved her symptoms, although maximum improvement was not apparent until 2 weeks after injection.

Patient 4 was a 39-year-old woman with a presumptive diagnosis of left-sided sciatica thought to be caused by arachnoiditis. The pain was deep, boring, and constant, in the region of the left loin. Acute exacerbations occurred on sitting, leaning forward, and lying on soft surfaces. Although diclofenac and coydramol decreased symptoms, she had to spend 9 hours a day lying down. Examination showed a mild right hemiparesis, dysphasia, and tenderness over the course of the left twelfth rib. Under an image intensifier, the loin pain was reproduced when pressure was applied to the twelfth rib. A twelfth intercostal nerve block relieved the loin pain for the duration of the anesthetic. Cryotherapy of the twelfth intercostal nerve was then performed. At the 6-month follow-up assessment, the patient was pain free.

Patient 5 had right loin pain thought to be caused by arachnoiditis after spinal surgery in 1970. Lower limb pain developed in 1980, which was initially treated successfully by insertion of a dorsal column stimulator. However, this treatment progressively failed. In addition, the patient experienced a new right loin pain, which she described as a deep ache with sudden exacerbations, especially on right lateral flexion of the lumbar spine. She had no associated sensory deficit. Examination revealed right loin tenderness. Direct pressure on the twelfth rib reproduced the pain under the image intensifier. An intercostal block with 2% lidocaine alleviated the pain. A subsequent course of intercostal blocks using bupivacaine and methylprednisolone decreased the loin pain. At her 6-month assessment, the loin pain had resolved, but the lower limb pain continued to be refractory to treatment.

The sixth patient, a 41-year-old man with Peutz-Jeghers syndrome, reported a 17-month history of right-sided subcostal pain, which developed after a laparotomy. The pain seemed to be related to posture. Pressure over the anterior region of the twelfth rib produced pain. A chest radiograph showed excessively long lower ribs. The pain was localized mainly to the twelfth rib under an image intensifier. His symptoms were relieved by local anesthetic and steroid injection into the costovertebral complex as an intercostal nerve block for the duration of the local anesthetic. Although a subsequent intercostal nerve block was unsuccessful, the use of a transcutaneous nerve stimulator provided this patient with considerable relief.

Conclusions.—The twelfth rib syndrome varies in presentation and course. Diagnosis of this syndome requires exclusion of specific causes. The diagnosis should only be made when the symptoms can be reproduced exactly by manipulation of the affected rib.

► Although 2 patients in this series obtained relief from neurodestructive procedures (rib resection, cryotherapy), such techniques may be associated with aggravation of pain and should be reserved for the most desperate, intractable cases. The most common presentation of this syndrome that I have seen is point tenderness over the tip of the twelfth rib. In these cases, pain is likely to resolve with local infiltration of the site with long-acting steroid plus local anesthetic.

S.E. Abram, M.D.

9 Anesthesia Mechanisms and Other Basic Science Studies

Mechanisms of Toxicity/Pathophysiology

Biotransformation of Halothane, Enflurane, Isoflurane, and Desflurane to Trifluoroacetylated Liver Proteins: Association Between Protein Acylation and Hepatic Injury

Njoku D, Laster MJ, Gong DH, et al (Johns Hopkins Med Insts, Baltimore, Md; Univ of California, San Francisco; NIH, Bethesda, Md)

Anesth Analg 84:173–178, 1997 9–1

Objective.—Halothane hepatitis is a fulminant hepatic necrosis associated with markedly increased serum alanine and aspartate transferase and bilirubin levels, with jaundice, hepatic encephalopathy, and frequently death. This condition, which can also occur in susceptible individuals after enflurane, isoflurane, and desflurane administration, is caused by an immune response against reactive anesthetic metabolites covalently bound to hepatic proteins. The hepatotoxicity has been directly correlated to anesthetic metabolism catalyzed by cytochrome P450-2E1 to trifluoroacetylated hepatic proteins. The relationship between acylation of hepatic proteins by anesthetics and reported relative rates of metabolism was studied in rats.

Methods.—Rats were pretreated with isoniazid to induce P450-2E1. They were then assigned to breathe oxygen alone or halothane, enflurane, isoflurane, or desflurane in oxygen at a minimum alveolar concentration (MAC) of 1.25 for 8 hours. The livers were taken for examination 18 hours after anesthetic exposure. Additional studies were performed using sera from patients with clinical halothane hepatitis.

Results.—Tissue acylation was greatest after exposure to halothane, followed by enflurane or isoflurane. Reactivity to isoflurane was compared with that for desflurane or oxygen. Halothane reactivity was greater than in any of the other 4 groups on enzyme-linked immunosorbent assay. The same assay found that enflurane reactivity was significantly greater than desflurane or oxygen reactivity. The sera of patients with halothane hepatitis demonstrated antibody reactivity against hepatic proteins from halothane- or enflurane-exposed rats. Rats exposed to anesthetics or oxygen alone showed no reactivity.

Conclusions.—Hepatotoxicity related to halothane or other anesthetics may be mediated by production of acylated proteins. The toxic potential of fluorinated inhaled anesthetics may be related to the degree of metabolism reflected by relative liver protein acylation. Thus drugs that are minimally metabolized may be better anesthetic choices.

▶ The idea that the less metabolism the better may or may not be true if mechanisms of hepatic injury are related to the immune system (i.e., the acylation of proteins and subsequent reaction of the immune system to those now-foreign proteins). We are beginning to discover greater incidences of liver "injury" after routine anesthetics than we formerly believed exists. Whether this "injury" is clinically significant is not so obvious. Njoku et al. would like to establish the idea that less metabolism correlates closely with less potential for the above mechanism—the immune mechanism. I doubt that the correlation is that close, but this is an interesting article and will bring the reader up to "snuff" in this important area of toxicology.

J.H. Tinker, M.D.

Inorganic Fluoride: Divergent Effects on Human Proximal Tubular Cell Viability

Zager RA, Iwata M (Fred Hutchinson Cancer Research Ctr, Seattle)
Am J Pathol 150:735–745, 1997 9–2

Purpose.—Fluoride is a widely distributed, nephrotoxic element. Fluoride nephrotoxicity can occur with the use of fluorinated anesthetics such as methoxyflurane. Inorganic fluoride is produced by the metabolism of fluorinated anesthetics by the cytochrome p450 system. Although recognition of methoxyflurane's nephrotoxicity has resulted in cutbacks in its use, other defluorinated anesthetics such as enflurane, isoflurane, sevoflurane, and halothane are still used. The subcellular determinants of fluoride cytotoxicity were examined, including an assessment of the effects of subtoxic fluoride exposure on tubular cell vulnerability to adenosine triphosphate (ATP) depletion and nephrotoxicity.

Methods.—HK-2 human proximal tubular cells were cultured in the presence of NaF concentrations of 0–20 mmol/L. This range included the clinically relevant intrarenal and urinary fluoride levels associated with the use of fluorinated anesthetics. Cell injury was assessed by vital dye uptake at the end of a 24-hour exposure period. Tests of fluoride's effects on cell deacylation and plasma leukocyte activation $(PLA)_2$ activity were performed as well. In further experiments, HK-2 cells were exposed to subtoxic levels of NaF for 0–24 hours. The cells were then challenged with ATP depletion plus Ca^{2+} overload to simulate ischemia, or with myoglobin exposure, a clinically relevant nephrotoxic insult.

Results.—Cytotoxicity increased together with NaF concentration. The nephrotoxic effects of NaF exposure were significantly lessened by extracellular CA^{2+} chelation and PLA_2 inhibitor therapy. Partial cytosolic PLA_2 depletion occurred rapidly in the face of subtoxic doses of NaF. Cells with partial PLA_2 depletion showed considerable resistance to ATP depletion/Ca^{2+} ionophore injury and to myoglobin-induced attack.

Conclusion.—This study demonstrates dose-dependent fluoride-induced cytotoxicity in human proximal tubular cells in vitro. The toxic effects of fluoride occur at least partly through Ca^{2+}- and PLA_2-dependent mechanisms and lead to partial cytosolic PLA_2 depletion. Acute cell resistance to fluoride exposure can be significantly increased by subtoxic fluoride exposure, possibly through reductions in cytosolic PLA_2 activity. The clinical applications of these findings to the use of fluorinated anesthetics remain to be determined.

► I include this paper so that we all understand that fluoride, at least at some concentration, is, in fact, a known nephrotoxin. This elegant paper discusses mechanisms and also reveals the surprising finding that subtoxic fluoride exposure may actually *increase resistance* to further attack by fluoride. I don't think the authors understand why that is true and I know I don't, despite careful reading of this paper. Nonetheless, as is the case with most things, we are simply talking about "how much."

J.H. Tinker, M.D.

Activin A and Inhibin A as Possible Endocrine Markers for Pre-Eclampsia

Muttukrishna S, Knight PG, Groome NP, et al (Univ of Oxford, England; Univ of Reading, England; Oxford Brookes Univ, England)

Lancet 349:1285–1288, 1997 9–3

Introduction.—The finding of inhibin A and activin A in term placental extracts suggests a placental origin for these proteins. Detection of varying concentrations of inhibin A and activin A in normal pregnancies and pregnancies complicated by pre-eclampsia might help in the diagnosis of pre-eclampsia, a placental disease of unknown cause. A retrospective cross-sectional study examined serum concentrations of these proteins in women with established pre-eclampsia and in controls.

Methods.—Blood samples were taken from 20 women hospitalized with pre-eclampsia and from 20 control pregnant women who were matched for duration of gestation, parity, and maternal age. Highly specific 2-site enzyme immunoassays were used to measure concentrations of inhibin A, inhibin B, proαC, and activin A. Pooled samples of controls and pre-

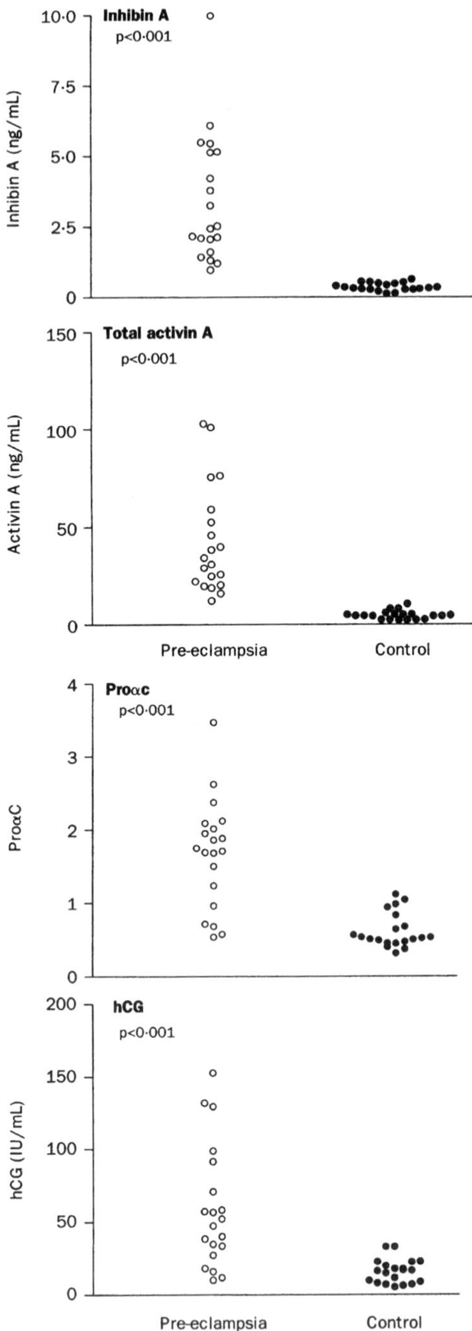

FIGURE 1.—Individual concentrations of inhibin A, total activin A, proαC, and human chorionic gonadotropin (*h*CG) in pre-eclamptic and control women. (Courtesy of Muttukrishna S, Knight PG, Groome NP, et al: Activin A and inhibin A as possible endocrine markers for pre-eclampsia. *Lancet* 349:1285–1288. Copyright by the Lancet Ltd., 1997.)

eclampsia serum subsequently underwent fast protein liquid chromatographic analysis to establish the molecular weight forms of circulating inhibin A and activin A. Correlation analyses were used to investigate the relation between hormones, platelet counts, and blood pressure in pre-eclampsia.

Results.—Women with pre-eclampsia had mean serum concentrations of inhibin A and of activin A that were significantly higher (Fig 1) than those in control pregnant women. Mean concentrations were approximately 8 times higher for inhibin A and 9 times higher for activin A. Women with pre-eclampsia also had significantly higher peripheral concentrations of proαC and of human chorionic gonadotropin (hCG). The control and pre-eclampsia groups had similar inhibin B concentrations. Molecular-weight forms of inhibin A (32 kd) and activin A (greater than 100 kd) were similar in the 2 groups. Chromatographic profiles of pooled serum samples showed only 1 major peak of inhibin A (32 kd) and 1 major peak of activin A (greater than 100 kd). The elution positions of each peak were identical in the 2 groups.

Conclusions.—Maternal serum concentrations of inhibin A and activin A are significantly higher in women with pre-eclampsia than in control women matched for duration of gestation. The magnitude of the difference suggests that these hormones could act as sensitive endocrine markers for pre-eclampsia and provides further evidence for trophoblast dysfunction in this disease.

► I selected this article to illustrate the continuing search for markers for pre-eclampsia in obstetric practice. This study demonstrated that the maternal serum concentrations of activin A and inhibin A are increased in pre-eclampsia—it is thought that these 2 proteins are produced by the placenta during pregnancy and that increased concentrations are evidence of trophoblast dysfunction in pre-eclampsia. The next step is to perform large prospective studies to assess whether the routine measurement of these proteins are valid endocrine markers of pre-eclampsia; the ultimate aim would be to prevent development of the disease and/or improve management and thereby improve outcome.

M. Wood, M.D.

Antinociception

Characterization of Muscarinic Receptor Subtypes That Mediate Antinociception in the Rat Spinal Cord

Naguib M, Yaksh TL (King Saud Univ, Riyadh, Saudi Arabia; Univ of California—San Diego, La Jolla)

Anesth Analg 85:847–853, 1997 9–4

Background.—Although we know that cholinergic receptors in the spine help mediate antinociceptive effects, exactly which receptor subtypes are involved has yet to be elucidated. Subtypes of muscarinic receptors that have been identified include neuronal (M_1), cardiac (M_2), and functional smooth muscle or glandular (M_3) receptors. These authors used muscarinic agonists and a cholinesterase inhibitor to characterize the M1, M_2, and/or M_3 subtypes of muscarinic agonist receptors in the rat spinal cord.

Methods.—Three studies were performed in 80 male Sprague-Dawley rats with an intrathecal catheter implanted for drug delivery. A washout period of at least 5 days was allowed between studies. In the agonist study, various doses of the muscarinic agonists carbachol and McN-A-343 and the cholinesterase inhibitor neostigmine were administered. Blood levels were measured regularly for up to 35 minutes after injection to determine the time to peak agonist effect. The just maximally effective (JME) dose was calculated as the smallest dose that still produced the maximum effect. In the antagonist study, administration of the various antagonists (atropine, pirenzepine, methoctramine, and 4-DAMP) was timed (based on the JME dose of agonist) so that the maximum antagonist effect occurred at the same time as the maximum agonist effect. Response latencies were measured for up to 20 minutes after the antagonist injection. In the choline uptake blocker study, hemicholinium was injected, and then 4 hours later the JME dose of neostigmine or carbachol was injected, with response latencies measured 5 minutes later.

Findings.—In the agonist study, McN-A-343 reached its peak antinociceptive effect at 5 minutes, and neostigmine and carbachol reached theirs at 15 minutes. The JME doses were, respectively, 630, 14.3, and 110 nmol. When antagonists were added, all 3 of the agonists showed a dose-dependent reversal of effect. Atropine (a nonspecific muscarinic blocker) and 4-DAMP (affinity for M_3 receptors) were most potent for neostigmine, and pirenzepine (affinity for M_1 receptors) and atropine were most potent for carbachol and McN-A-343. Methoctramine (affinity for M_2 receptors) never produced more than a 50% reduction in response for any of the agonists. In the choline uptake blocker study, hemicholinium antagonized the effects of neostigmine but not those of carbachol.

Conclusions.—Neostigmine, McN-A-343, and carbachol all induced a potent analgesic effect. The nociceptive responses to 4-DAMP, atropine, methoctramine, and pirenzepine indicate that the receptor subtypes involved are M1 and M3. Further research should focus on discriminating between M1 and M3 muscarinic receptors for the targeting of specific binding between drug and receptor subtype.

► The multiplicity of receptor subtypes increases not only the complexity of receptor agonist and antagonist effects but also the possibilities for finding receptor subtype-specific drugs that maximize beneficial effects and minimize side effects. We recently assessed the analgesic potential for 2 clinically available muscarinic agonists, methacholine and bethanechol, in rats.[1] Both of these drugs are available without preservatives, making them tempting candidates for future human trials. Unfortunately, both preparations produced substantial adverse effects and minimal analgesia, presumably because they did not affect the right receptor subtypes.

S.E. Abram, M.D.

Reference

1. Abram SE, Fouch RA: Comparison of the antinociceptive properties of intrathecal and systemic tramadol in rats. *Reg Anesth* 22:S27, 1997.

Distinct Electrophysiological Effects of Two Spinally Administered Membrane Stabilising Drugs, Bupivacaine and Lamotrigine

Chapman V, Wildman MA, Dickenson AH (Univ College London)

Pain 71:285–295, 1997 9–5

Background.—In the spinal cord, blocking C fibers should prevent nociceptive transmission into the central nervous system and thus block pain. Various drugs have such blocking effects, including the sodium channel blocker bupivacaine. Would another sodium channel blocker, such as the antiepileptic lamotrigine, have similar effects? These researchers examined the responses to these drugs in single dorsal horn neurons receiving stimulation from Aβ or C fibers.

Methods.—Laminectomy was performed on male Sprague-Dawley rats to expose segments L4–L5. Transcutaneous electrical stimulation administered 16 times was used to differentiate Aβ fiber responses (0–20 msec after stimulation) from C fiber responses (90–300 msec after stimulation). Responses occurring more than 300 msec after the stimulus represented the neuron's postdischarge. Windup (i.e., the enhanced response) was measured as the difference between the number of C fiber potentials at baseline and after induction by 16 stimuli. The baseline potential was measured as the initial baseline response to the first stimulation multiplied by 16. Once C fiber responses were established, various doses of bupivacaine or lamotrigine were applied to dorsal horn neurons and the electrically evoked responses were measured 5 minutes later and thereafter at 10-minute intervals.

Findings.—Compared with control values, bupivacaine at doses between 25 and 1,000 μg significantly reduced C fiber activity. The effect was dose dependent; at the highest dose, bupivacaine significantly reduced the Aβ fiber, windup, and postdischarge responses, too. In contrast, lamotrigine at doses from 50 to 100 μg/μL had no overall significant effect on Aβ fiber, C fiber, windup, or postdischarge responses. However, individual neuron responses to lamotrigine varied greatly (Fig 8), in that sometimes this drug enhanced windup and sometimes it reduced windup. Overall, lamotrigine tended to increase responses.

Conclusions.—While both bupivacaine and lamotrigine are sodium channel blockers, their effects on nerve transmission in the spinal cord are very different. Bupivacaine uniformly blocked Aβ and C fiber responses, whereas lamotrigine had vastly different effects in individual neurons. These results do not support the use of lamotrigine as a spinal analgesic.

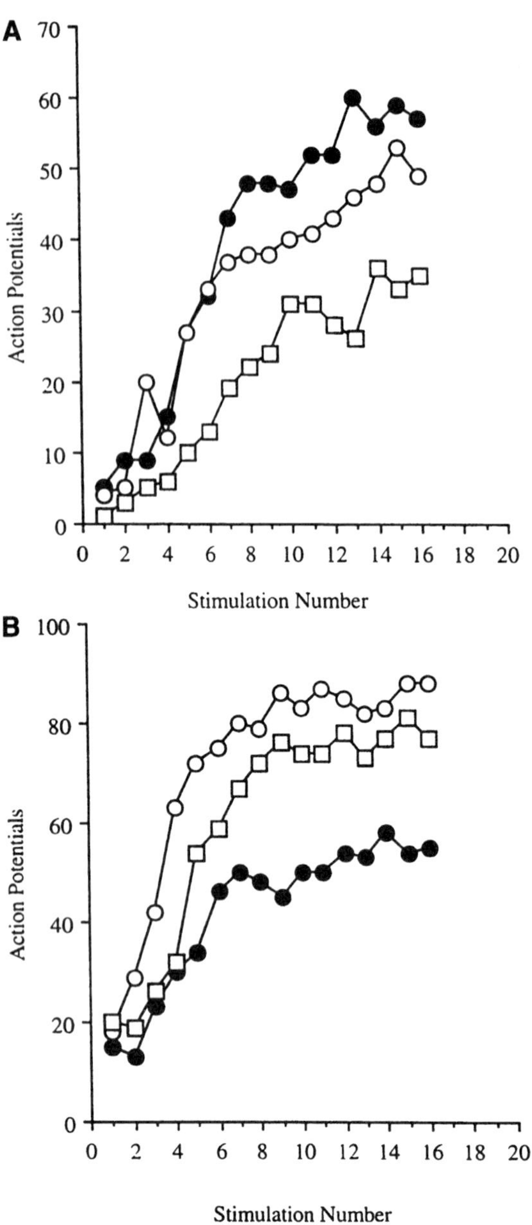

FIGURE 8.—Examples of individual neurons displaying windup and the effect of varying concentrations of lamotrigine on the windup of these individual neurons. A, in this case, lamotrigine 250 µg (*open circle*) and 100 µg (*open square*) reduced the windup of this individual neuron as compared to control (*filled circle*). B, in this case, lamotrigine 250 µg (*open circle*) and 100 µg (*open square*) facilitated the windup of this individual neuron as compared to control (*filled circle*). (Reprinted from *Pain* Chapman V, Wildman MA, Dickenson AH: Distinct electrophysiological effects of two spinally administered membrane stabilising drugs, bupivacaine and lamotrigine. *Pain* 71:285–295, 1997.)

► Lamotrigine is thought to have potential benefits for patients with neuropathic pain because of a unique combination of pharmacologic properties: sodium channel blockade and interference with release of glutamate spinally. The lack of suppression of windup and, indeed, the facilitation of that response, suggests that optimism regarding the antihyperalgesic effect of this drug may be premature.

S.E. Abram, M.D.

Selective N-Type Neuronal Voltage-sensitive Calcium Channel Blocker, SNX-111, Produces Spinal Antinociception in Rat Models of Acute, Persistent and Neuropathic Pain

Bowersox SS, Gadbois T, Singh T, et al (Neurex Corp, Menlo Park, Calif)

J Pharmacol Exp Ther 279:1243–1249, 1996 9–6

Background.—Previous research suggests that N-type voltage-sensitive calcium channels (VSCCs) play a fundamental role in transmitting noxious somatosensory stimuli and endogenous neuropathic pain signals. The effects of intrathecally administered SNX-111, a VSCC blocker, on nociceptive behavior induced in rats by subcutaneous injection of dilute formalin into the dorsal hindpaw and on tactile allodynia in a spinal nerve ligation model of painful peripheral neuropathy were studied.

Methods and Findings.—Male Sprague-Dawley rats were used. SNX-111 suppressed both the acute and tonic phases of the formalin test when infused for 72 hours immediately before testing, resulting in significant, dose-dependent antinociceptive effects. Bolus injections of 100 ng SNX-111 suppressed phase 2 nociceptive responses. SNX-111 was about 1000-fold more potent than morphine in blocking phase 2 responses when the compounds were given by intrathecal bolus injection. Intrathecal bolus injections of 30–300 ng SNX-111 blocked mechanical allodynia in a dose-dependent fashion in rats with experimentally induced painful peripheral neuropathy. Subacute SNX-111 administration by continuous intrathecal infusion produced a reversible blockade of mechanical allodynia with no apparent development of tolerance.

Conclusions.—Selective N-type VSCC blockers are potent, effective antinociceptive agents when given by the spinal route. Selective N-type VSCC blockers are effective in rat models of acute, persistent and neuropathic pain. N-type VSCCs play an important role in the spinal processing of noxious somatosensory input.

► Neuropathic pain is generally more difficult to control than either somatic nociceptive pain or visceral pain using conventional analgesic techniques. Spinal and epidural administration of combinations of opioids and dilute local anesthetics may be effective, but often produce unacceptable degrees of sensory or motor blockade. Spinal administration of N-type calcium channel blockers, such as the conopeptide SNX-111, provide analgesia in neuropathic as well as somatic nociceptive pain models. Initial trials of intrathecal infusions of this drug in patients with cancer pain have demonstrated benefits for patients resistant to intrathecal morphine. It is likely that side effects will limit the systemic use of this compound.

S.E. Abram, M.D.

Synergistic Antinociceptive Interactions of Morphine and Clonidine in Rats With Nerve-Ligation Injury

Ossipov MH, Lopez Y, Bian D, et al (Univ of Arizona, Tucson)

Anesthesiology 86:196–204, 1997 9–7

Background.—In a rat model, ligation injury of the L5/L6 nerve roots results in behavioral signs representing the clinical conditions of neuropathic pain, including tactile allodynia and thermal and mechanical hyperalgesia. Intrathecal morphine has no antiallodynic activity in such models. Antinociceptive potency and efficacy are reduced. The antinociceptive activity of intrathecal clonidine alone or combined with intrathecal morphine in nerve-injured rats is presented.

Methods.—Male Sprague-Dawley rats were used. Unilateral nerve injury was produced by ligation of the L5 and L6 spinal roots. A group of sham-operated rats was subjected to similar surgery without nerve ligation. Morphine and clonidine were administered intrathecally through implanted catheters alone or in a 1:3 fixed ratio.

Findings.—In both groups, morphine produced a dose-dependent antinociceptive effect. The doses calculated to produce a 50% maximal possible effect (MPE) were a mean 15 and 30 µg in the experimental and control groups, respectively. Although morphine produced a 100% MPE in the control group, the MPE in the nerve-injured rats was only 69%. Clonidine had a dose-dependent effect, with an A_{50} of 120 µg in sham-operated rats. The maximal effect of clonidine plateaued at 55% and 49% MPE at 100 and 200 µg, respectively, in the nerve-injured rats, which prevented the calculation of an A_{50}. In the control group, a morphine-clonidine mixture produced maximal efficacy, with an A_{50} of 15 µg, which was significantly less than the theoretical additive A_{50} of 44 µg. Morphine and clonidine combined produced a maximal efficacy in nerve-ligated rats, with an A_{50} of 11 µg, significantly less than the theoretical additive A_{50} of 118 µg, indicating a synergistic antinociceptive interaction.

Conclusions.—Clonidine, like morphine, loses antinociceptive potency and efficacy after nerve ligation injury. A spinal combination of morphine and clonidine appears to synergize under conditions of nerve injury to elicit a significant antinociceptive action when either drug alone may be ineffective.

▶ In both animal models and clinical experience, chronic neuropathic pain is relatively unresponsive to spinal and epidural opioids. The pharmacologic basis for this phenomenon is now fairly well understood: persistent barrages of afferent traffic produce activation of the NMDA receptor; calcium enters the cell, producing, among other actions, an increase in protein kinase C, which in turn interferes with the G-protein–coupled opening of potassium channels in response to opiate receptor occupation. This study confirms this resistance of neuropathic pain to suppression by opioids, but also shows clonidine to be fairly ineffective. Remarkably, however, the combination of an opiate and an alpha-2 adrenergic agonist have a synergistic effect in this model of neuropathy. Similarly, clonidine appears to be effective in models of opioid tolerance, and there is evidence from both animal and human studies that tolerance develops more slowly when morphine and clonidine are combined.

S.E. Abram, M.D.

Antinociceptive Interaction of Intrathecal α_2-Adrenergic Agonists, Tizanidine and Clonidine, With Lidocaine in Rats

Kawamata T, Omote K, Kawamata M, et al (Sapporo Med Univ, Japan)
Anesthesiology 87:436–448, 1997 9–8

Introduction.—In the control of acute and chronic pain, intrathecal-epidural clonidine, an α_2-adrenergic agonistic, produces potent analgesia. Hypotension and bradycardia are induced by intrathecal-epidural clonidine. Antinociception in a similar manner to clonidine has been provided by tizanidine without producing pronounced hemodynamic changes. Little is known, however, about the interaction between tizanidine and local anesthetics on antinociceptive and hemodynamic effects. Using isobolographic analysis, the antinociceptive interactions of intrathecal tizanidine and clonidine with lidocaine in rats on antinociception were evaluated.

Methods.—Lumbar intrathecal catheters were implanted into rats. To assess the thermal nociceptive threshold, the tail-flick test was used. The ability of intrathecal tizanidine, clonidine, lidocaine, or the combinations of α_2-adrenergic agonist and lidocaine to alter the tail-flick latency was examined. The isobolographic analysis was applied to characterize the antinociceptive interaction. After intrathecal administration of drugs and combinations, the motor function, blood pressure, and heart rate were monitored.

Results.—The tail-flick latency in dose- and time-dependent fashion was increased by intrathecal tizanidine, clonidine, or the combination without affecting motor function. The order potency of tizanidine was 1.8 and the order potency of clonidine was 0.75 (dose producing a 50% of peak effect, in micrograms). Significantly synergistic antinociceptive interaction was seen with tizanidine with lidocaine, and clonidine with lidocaine, according to isobolographic analysis. The synergistic interaction was also confirmed by potency ratio analysis and fractional analysis. Tizanidine with lidocaine did not affect motor function or blood pressure at the dose in the combinations showing comparable antinociception, unlike clonidine with lidocaine.

Conclusions.—The degree of antinociception to somatic noxious stimuli are enhanced when intrathecal tizanidine and clonidine synergistically interact with lidocaine. Without affecting blood pressure, heart rate, or motor function, the antinociceptive synergistic interaction between tizanidine and lidocaine may be useful in clinical practice.

▶ The relevance of this animal study to clinical anesthesia is that another new α_2-adrenergic agonist is undergoing investigation—tizanidine. Clonidine is a relatively selective α_2-adrenergic agonist, but even more selective α_2-agonists may become available in the future. Adverse side effects of clonidine include hypotension, bradycardia, and sedation. If new drugs could become available without such side effects, then clinical studies to determine optimum drug combinations (e.g., α_2-agonist and local anesthetic) for pain management would then become a real possibility.

M. Wood, M.D.

Opiate Receptor Knockout Mice Define μ Receptor Roles in Endogenous Nociceptive Responses and Morphine-induced Analgesia

Sora I, Takahashi N, Funada M, et al (NIH, Baltimore, Md; Johns Hopkins Univ, Baltimore, Md)

Proc Natl Acad Sci USA 94:1544–1549, 1997 9–9

Purpose.—Nociceptive circuits express opiate receptors that are the site of action of morphine. The μ, δ, and κ receptor subtypes are expressed in circuits capable of modulating nociception and receiving inputs from endogenous opioid neuropeptide ligands. However, it is uncertain how each receptor subtype influences nociceptive processing, whether in the drug-free or morphine-treated state. Homologous, recombinant, and μ receptor knockout mice were used to determine the role of morphine-preferring opiate receptors in nociceptive drug responses.

Methods.—Both heterozygous and homozygous μ receptor knockout mice were produced. Compared with wild-type animals, these mice had 54% and 0% expression of μ receptors. Both μ knockout mice expressed κ and δ receptors at near wild-type levels. Knockout and wild-type mice were compared for their spinal and supraspinal nociception to tail flick and hot plate tests in the untreated and morphine-treated states.

Results.—Latencies to response to both tests were significantly shorter for untreated knockout mice than for wild-type mice (Fig 2). This suggested that normal nociceptive processing was influenced by endogenous opioid-peptide interactions with μ opiate receptors. In homozygous knockout mice, morphine treatment did not significantly reduce the nociceptive responses to either test. In the heterozygous knockout mice, treatment produced a rightward and downward shift in the morphine analgesia dose-effect relationships (Fig 3).

Conclusions.—Endogenous opioid-peptide actions are evident at μ opiate receptors in tests of nociceptive responsiveness in mice. The findings

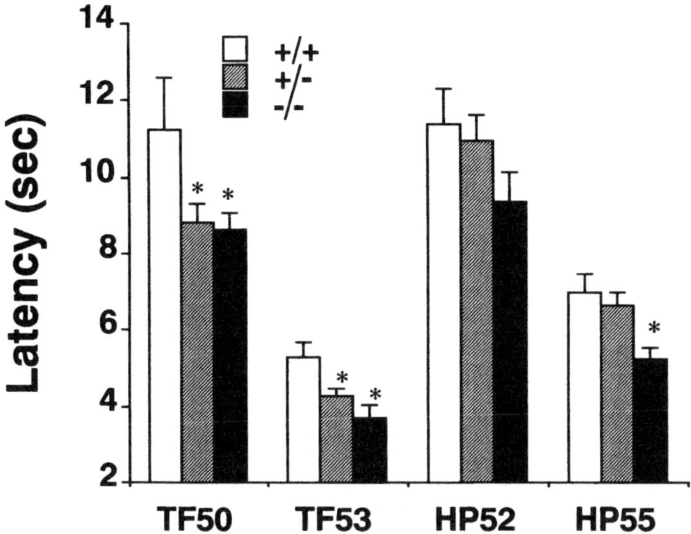

FIGURE 2.—Latencies for nociceptive responses in tail flick (*TF*) and hot plate (*HP*) tests in unpretreated mice. Mice of +/+ (n = 14), +/− (n = 24), and −/− (n = 15) μ receptor genotypes underwent tail flick testing in 50° or 53° C water and hot plate testing at 52°or 55° C, as indicated. *$P < 0.05$ compared with wild-type control values. (Courtesy of Sora I, Takahashi N, Funada M, et al: Opiate receptor knockout mice define μ receptor roles in endogenous nociceptive responses and morphine-induced analgesia. *Proc Natl Acad Sci USA* 94:1544–1549. Copyright 1997, National Academy of Sciences, USA.)

suggest that the μ receptor mediates morphine-induced analgesia in tests of spinal and supraspinal analgesia. Further study of these processes should contribute to the ongoing efforts to improve treatment for pain, so as to maximize the effects of exogenous drugs while minimizing suppression of the body's endogenous pain suppression mechanisms.

► Transgenic technology, which allows the transfer of genes between species, has provided powerful methods for exploring the mechanisms of drug actions. A relatively new technique called "gene targeting" has made it possible to delete a single gene without affecting the rest of the genome. Mice that are missing both copies of a given gene (abbreviated as −/−) are called "knockouts," and can be compared with wild type (+/+) and heterozygous (+/−) mice to conclusively determine the site(s) of action of pharmacologic agents. It is no understatement to say that knockout technology is revolutionizing the field of vertebrate biology.

This article provides a nice example of the powerful ability of knockout strategies to address pharmacologic and physiologic questions. The authors used gene targeting to generate a line of mice that are lacking the gene encoding the μ opioid receptor. By comparing the μ receptor knockouts with wild-type and heterozygous mice, the authors were able to discriminate the activities of μ opioid receptors from δ and κ opioid receptor functions.

The findings are striking. Most importantly, morphine is almost totally devoid of analgesic activity in the −/− mice; the +/− mice demonstrate an intermediate sensitivity to morphine, consistent with their intermediate lev-

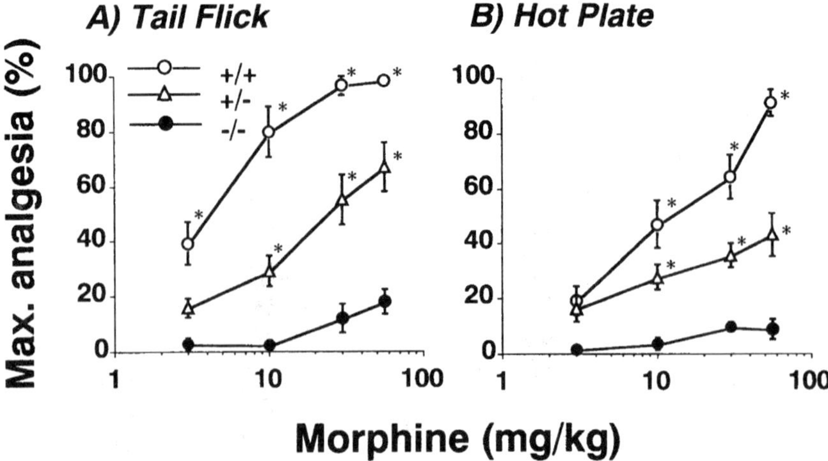

FIGURE 3.—Latencies for nociceptive responses in 53°C tail flick and 55°C hot plate tests in pretreated mice. **A,** dose-response relationships for morphine-induced alterations in latencies on 53°C tail flick testing in mice with mild-type (+/+), heterozygote (+/−), and homozygote (−/−) μ opiate receptor genotypes using a cumulative dose-response paradigm as described. Percentage of maximal analgesia was calculated for each mouse as: 100 × {[(latency to tail flick after morphine) − (latency to tail flick at baseline)]/[(15-sec cutoff time) − (baseline latency)]}. *, $P < 0.05$ compared with preinjection control values for the appropriate genotype. Dose-effect relationships were significant for +/+ and +/− mice but not for −/− mice. Among genotype differences, dose-response relationships also were significant for animals of each genotype [$P < 0.001$, df(2, 120), $F = 66$ by repeated measures ANOVA]. **B,** dose-response relationships for morphine-induced alterations in latencies on 55°C hot plate testing in mice with wild-type (+/+), heterozygote (+/−), and homozygote (+/+) μ opiate receptor genotypes using a cumulative dose-response paradigm as described. Percentage of maximal analgesia was calculated for each mouse using a 30–sec cutoff time. *, $P < 0.05$ compared with preinjection control values for the appropriate genotype. Dose-effect relationships were significant for +/+ and +/+ mice but not for −/− mice. Among genotype differences, between dose-response relationships also were significant for animals of each genotype [$P < 0.001$, df(2, 124), $F = 27$ by repeated measures ANOVA]. Max., maximum. (Courtesy of Sora I, Takahashi N, Funada M, et al: Opiate receptor knockout mice define μ receptor roles in endogenous nociceptive responses and morphine-induced analgesia. *Proc Natl Acad Sci USA* 94:1544–1549. Copyright 1997, National Academy of Sciences, USA.)

els of μ opioid receptor expression. This convincingly demonstrates that the μ opioid receptor is the sole molecular target for the analgesic activity of morphine.

Second, the −/− mice display decreased latencies on tail flick and hot plate tests, meaning that they respond more rapidly to noxious stimuli. This finding indicates that μ opioid receptors play a role in the modulation of acute nociceptive processing.

Expect to see a large number of studies using knockout technology to explore anesthetic targets. A related article[1] uses gene targeting to study the role of the μ opioid receptor in the response of reward pathways to morphine.

M.J.S. Heath, M.D.

Reference

1. Matthes HWD, Maldonado R, Simonin F, et al: Loss of morphine-induced analgesia, reward effects and withdrawal symptoms in mice lacking the μ-opioid-receptor gene. *Nature* 383:819–823, 1996.

Enhancement of Analgesia From Systemic Opioid in Humans by Spinal Cholinesterase Inhibition

Hood DD, Mallak KA, James RL, et al (Wake Forest Univ, Winston-Salem, NC)

J Pharmacol Exp Ther 282:86–92, 1997 9–10

Background.—Intravenous opioids produce analgesia and have been shown to increase the release of acetylcholine (ACh) in spinal cord dorsal horn in animal studies. These effects can be enhanced by intrathecal neostigmine. The capability of intrathecal neostigmine to enhance analgesia and increase CSF concentrations of ACh more than IV was tested, as well as the effect of neostigmine on side effects induced by alfentanil.

Methods.—There were 40 healthy volunteers; 17 were men, and the mean age was 31 years. Participants were given 50, 100, or 200 μg intra-

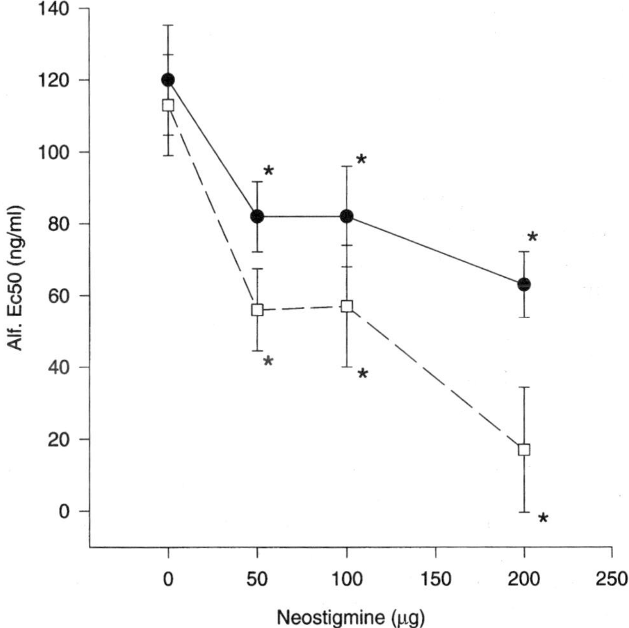

FIGURE 3.—Median effective concentration EC_{50} value for alfentanil in the foot *open squares* and hand *closed circles* in the absence or presence of 50, 100, or 200 μg intrathecal neostigmine. $*P < 0.05$ vs. IV alfentanil without intrathecal neostigmine. (Courtesy of Hood DD, Mallak KA, James RL, et al: Enhancement of analgesia from systemic opioid in humans by spinal cholinesterase inhibition. *J Pharmacol Exp Ther* 282:86–92, 1997.)

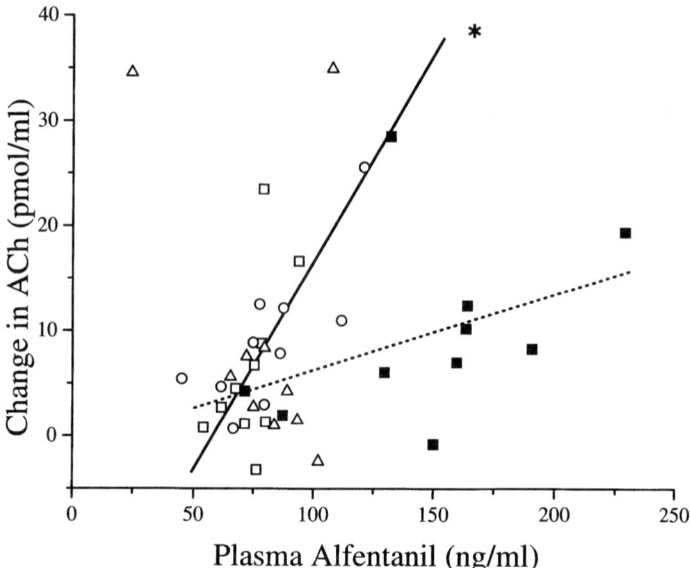

FIGURE 7.—Effect of alfentanil and neostigmine on change in acetylcholine (ACh) concentrations in CSF. For each volunteer, the effect of alfentanil was determined as the difference between the CSF ACh concentration after the IV alfentanil infusion and the CSF ACh concentration before infusion. Alfentanil in the absence of intrathecal neostigmine produced a significant ($P < 0.01$) plasma alfentanil concentration-independent increase in CSF ACh (*closed squares*, dotted regression line). Intrathecal neostigmine produced a dose-dependent increase in the effect of alfentanil ($P < 0.01$ for interaction) and resulted in an alfentanil concentration-dependent increase in CSF ACh (*open circles*, 50 µg; *open squares*, 100 µg; *open triangles*, 200 µg, solid regression line for entire neostigmine–alfentanil data set). *$P < 0.05$ compared with alfentanil alone. (Courtesy of Hood DD, Mallak KA, James RL, et al: Enhancement of analgesia from systemic opioid in humans by spinal cholinesterase inhibition. *J Pharmacol Exp Ther* 282:86–92, 1997.)

thecal neostigmine or saline. After 60 minutes, participants were given a computer-controlled, stepped IV infusion of alfentanil in increasing targeted plasma concentrations. Sixty minutes after spinal injection and after each 20-minute alfentanil infusion, pain scores from hand and foot immersion in ice water, as well as sedation, nausea, weakness, vital signs, end tidal CO_2, and oxyhemoglobin saturation were measured. Samples of CSF fluid were analyzed once after drug administration.

Results.—Measurements showed that neostigmine alone produced analgesia in the foot but not in the hand (Fig 3), and caused leg weakness. Alfentanil alone produced a similar level of analgesia in the foot and the hand and caused nausea, sedation, increased end-tidal CO_2, and decreased oxyhemoglobin saturation. Neostigmine enhanced analgesia but not respiratory effects induced by alfentanil, and it enhanced nausea and sedation. An increased CSF ACh concentration was seen with alfentanil; this was enhanced by neostigmine (Fig 7).

Discussion.—These findings support a spinal cholinergic mechanism of IV opioid analgesia. Neostigmine enhanced analgesia and side effects from IV alfentanil in these participants. Neostigmine did not enhance respiratory depression induced by alfentanil. The clinical value of neostigmine and alfentanil combined will depend on the strength of their interactions.

► Neostigmine has recently been introduced into clinical trials to test whether intrathecal neostigmine is useful in producing analgesia in a clinical setting. This is 1 of the first reports in human volunteers—the next step is to extend the study to patients with pain symptoms.

M. Wood, M.D.

Cardiac Physiology and Pharmacology

Stereospecific Effect of Bupivacaine Isomers on Atrioventricular Conduction in the Isolated Perfused Guinea Pig Heart

Graf BM, Martin E, Bosnjak ZJ, et al (Med College of Wisconsin, Milwaukee; Univ of Heidelberg, Germany)

Anesthesiology 86:410–419, 1997 9–11

Background.—Local anesthetics are known to be cardiotoxic, yet some drug isomers have been found to exert less cardiotoxicity than their racemates. This study evaluated the effects of (±) racemic bupivacaine and its (+) and (−) isomers on cardiac function.

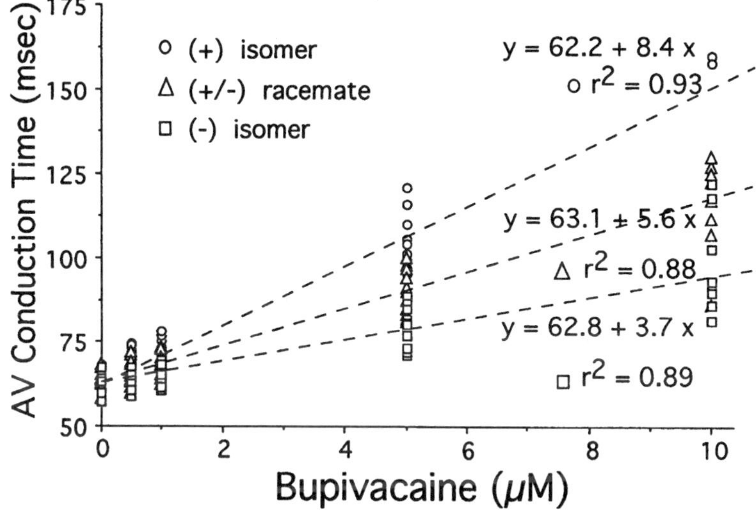

FIGURE 2.—Concentration-response curves (*dashed lines*) for the optical isomers and the racemate of bupivacaine on atrioventricular conduction time in 12 isolated perfused guinea pig hearts beating spontaneously. Data were analyzed using best-fit linear regression. Y intercepts are nearly identical in the 3 groups for an average of 62.7 msec; however, the average slope of the (+) bupivacaine group is more than double that of the (−) bupivacaine group, and the slope of the racemate lays between that of the isomers. Control values between the individual concentrations are not displayed. At 10 μm only 2, 8, and 11 of 12 hearts treated with (+), (±), and (−) bupivacaine, respectively, remained in sinus rhythm and are displayed in this graph (see Fig 3). (Courtesy of Graf BM, Martin E, Bosnjak ZJ, et al: Stereospecific effect of bupivacaine isomers on atrioventricular conduction in the isolated perfused guinea pig heart. *Anesthesiology* 86:410–419, 1997. Copyright American Society of Anesthesiologists, Inc. Used with permission of Lippincott-Raven Publishers.)

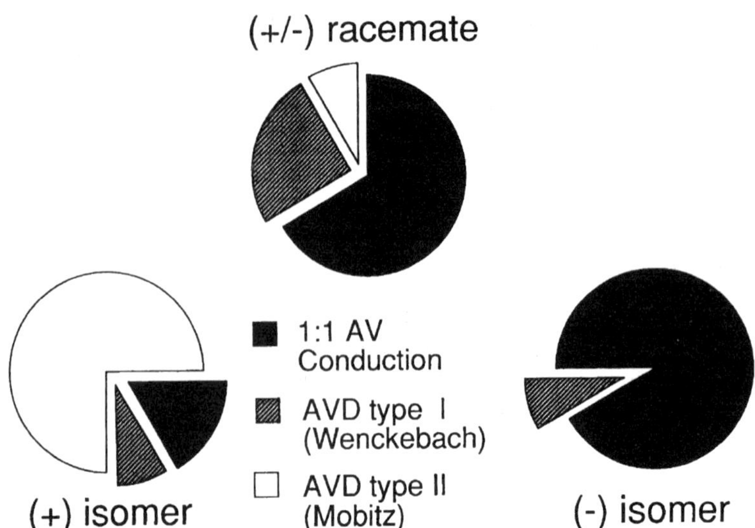

FIGURE 3.—Effect of 10 μm (+), (−), and (±) bupivacaine on second-degree atrioventricular dissociation of the Wenckebach (type I) and Mobitz (type II) classification in 12 isolated guinea pig hearts. Each pie chart comprises 12 hearts. Significance of atrioventricular dissociation is indicated in the text. Third-degree atrioventricular dissociation and dysrhythmias other than atrioventricular dissociation were not observed. Atrioventricular dissociation reverted to sinus rhythm without atrioventricular prolongation during the drug-free washout periods. (Courtesy of Graf BM, Martin E, Bosnjak ZJ, et al: Stereospecific effect of bupivacaine isomers on atrioventricular conduction in the isolated perfused guinea pig heart. *Anesthesiology* 86:410–419, 1997. Copyright American Society of Anesthesiologists, Inc. Used with permission of Lippincott-Raven Publishers.)

Methods.—The hearts of 12 ketamine-anesthetized guinea pigs were excised during continuous perfusion with Krebs-Ringer's solution via the Langendorff technique. Atrioventricular (AV) conduction time, heart rate, left ventricular pressure, coronary perfusion pressure, and inflow and outflow oxygen tensions were measured. Oxygen delivery, oxygen tension, percentage oxygen extraction, and myocardial oxygen consumption were calculated. After stabilization of the heart, random concentrations (0.5, 1, 5, and 10 μm) of bupivacaine and its isomers were injected into the perfusate. Hearts were perfused for 15 minutes with each of the 3 racemates at each concentration, with a washout period between different concentrations and different racemates.

Findings.—All 3 racemates showed dose-dependent decreases in atrial heart rate (mean [± SEM], −17% ± 1% at 10 μm dose) and left ventricular pressure (−50% ± 3% at 10 μm dose). All 3 also decreased coronary flow (−20% ± 4% at 10 μm dose) and myocardial oxygen consumption (−46% ± 4% at 10 μm dose). However, no significantly different effects were noted among these parameters at equimolar concentrations of racemic or isomeric bupivacaine.

However, AV conduction increased significantly in a dose-dependent manner with increasing concentrations of (+), (−), and (±) bupivacaine (Fig 2). Differences in AV conduction were more pronounced at higher concentrations, with the (+) isomer producing significantly more AV delay than the (−) isomer or racemic drug. The racemates also exhibited very different effects on second-degree type I (Wenckebach) and type II (Mobitz) AV dissociation (Fig 3). At the 10 μm dose, the (+) isomer was associated with type II AV dissociation in 9 of 12 hearts, compared with only 1 of 12 hearts for the racemic mixture and 0 of 12 hearts for the (−) isomer. The incidence of type I AV dissociation for either isomer was 1 of 12 hearts, whereas with (±) bupivacaine, this effect was seen in 3 of 12 hearts.

Conclusions.—Equimolar concentrations of (+), (−), and (±) bupivacaine showed no inter-racemate differences in any variable measured except AV conduction. The (+) isomer produced the greatest prolongation in AV conduction and the greatest amount of second-degree AV dissociation. Likewise, the (−) isomer produced the least prolongation in AV conduction and the least amount of second-degree AV dissociation. These findings suggest the presence of a specific receptor site on or within the sodium channels on the AV node, which responds to the (+) isomer with greater conduction blockade (fast cardiac sodium channel stereospecificity).

► Many drugs in anesthesia are administered as racemates or mixtures of isomers: bupivacaine, ketamine, and thiopental to name just a few. Ropivacaine, a new long-acting local anesthetic is a pure S (−) enantiomer that is said, at equivalent local anesthetic potency with racemic bupivacaine, to have reduced cardiac toxicity. Thus, there is an increased interest in separating out the effects of the bupivacaine isomers to determine whether a single isomer of bupivacaine has the potential to be a safer local anesthetic than bupivacaine itself. At the present time, research has centered on levobupivacaine.

In the study that I have selected, the (+) isomer prolonged AV conduction more than racemic bupivacaine and the (−) isomer also known as levobupivacaine. This and other studies have led clinical investigators to believe that levobupivacaine may have advantages over the racemate and the (+) isomer in terms of cardiac side effects. The development of single isomers does not apply only to local anesthetics, and it is possible that over the next decade, we will witness the introduction of a large number of single isomer drugs with reduced or attenuated toxicity.

M. Wood, M.D.

Calcitonin Gene-related Peptide–induced Preconditioning Improves Preservation with Cardioplegia

Lu E-X, Peng C-F, Li Y-J, et al (Xiang Ya Hosp, China; Hunan Med Univ, China)

Ann Thorac Surg 62:1748–1751, 1996 9–12

Objective.—Calcitonin gene-related peptide (CGRP) appears to be an endogenous myocardial protective substance. The effect of ischemic or

CGRP-induced preconditioning on myocardial salvage after prolonged cardioplegic arrest was determined in the isolated rat heart.

Methods.—Hearts were rapidly removed from Male Wistar rats. Contractile function was measured. Hearts were treated with St. Thomas cardioplegic solution at 4°C for 4 or 8 hours, and then reperfused with a modified Krebs-Henseleit bicarbonate buffer for 60 minutes at 37°C. Control hearts were equilibrated for 45 minutes before treatment. Ischemic preconditioned hearts were equilibrated for 20 minutes and then treated for 2 cycles of 5 minutes of normothermic ischemia and 10 minutes of reperfusion before immersion in cardioplegia solution. CGRP-treated hearts were equilibrated for 20 minutes and then treated for 2 cycles of 5 minutes with CGRP and 10 minutes of CGRP-free Krebs-Henseleit solution before cardioplegic arrest.

Results.—After 4 hours in hypothermic storage and 30 minutes of reperfusion, left ventricular pressure (LVP) and its first derivative were 65 mm Hg and 1,170 for control hearts, 94 mm Hg and 1,928 for preconditioned hearts, and 85 mm Hg and 1,900 for CGRP-treated hearts. After 8 hours in hypothermic storage and 30 minutes of reperfusion, LVP and its first derivative were 51 mm Hg and 815 for control hearts, 83 mm Hg and 1,480 for preconditioned hearts, and 85 mm Hg and 1,396 for CGRP-treated hearts. Coronary flow decreased and release of myocardial enzymes was increased during reperfusion. Decreases in coronary flow of hearts in hypothermic storage for 8 hours were significantly greater than for hearts in hypothermic storage for 4 hours.

Conclusion.—CGRP provides ischemic preconditioning cardioprotection against myocardial damage in isolated rat hearts even after 8 hours of cardioplegic arrest.

► CGRP has been found to play increasingly important roles as a neuromodulator. This article highlights one of its direct effects, that CGRP exerts preconditioning-like cardioprotection. That is, it enhances the recovery of cardiac function and reduced release of myocardial enzymes signifying cell damage. This might indicate a role for protein kinase and cardioprotection because CGRP activates it and protein kinase has been thought to be involved in the cardioprotective pathway. However, this hypothesis would not fit for its mechanism in the brain, and one hates to think that there is a different mechanism whereby ischemic preconditioning protects for brain and heart. Thus, this is an important study trying to elucidate the mechanism of ischemic preconditioning, a field that, I think, will probably have increasing importance as we understand its role.

M.F. Roizen, M.D.

Reduction of Neutrophil Margination by L-Arginine During Hypothermic Cardiopulmonary Bypass in a Pig Model

Dewanjee MK, Wu SM, De D, et al (Univ of Miami, Fla; Bentley Labs, Irvine, Calif)

ASAIO J 42:M661–M666, 1996 9–13

Purpose.—Cardiopulmonary bypass (CPB) and hemodialysis are associated with transient neutropenia in animals and human beings. Infusion of L-arginine, 2 mg/kg/min, during CPB generates nitric oxide, leading to increased blood flow to all organs. L-Arginine also reduces the level of marginated neutrophils (Ns), thus reducing cytokine-induced organ damage. A pig model of CPB was used to determine whether L-arginine infusion helps to increase blood flow to organs by counteracting regional and global ischemia, platelet thrombi, and decreasing N-endothelial cell adhesion.

Methods.—Yorkshire pigs were placed on CPB for 180 minutes or 90 minutes with 90 minutes of reperfusion. CPB was performed at a rate of 2.5–3.5 L/min and a temperature of 18° or 28° C. L-Arginine was infused at a rate of 2 to 15 mg/kg/min. Fifteen minutes before CPB, the pigs were administered indium-111–labeled autologous neutrophils (INN), 650 to 780 μCi. All animals received systemic heparin to achieve an activated coagulation time of greater than 400 seconds. A roller pump (Univox 1.8 m^2 membrane oxygenator, 0.25 m^2 arterial filter, and BCR-3500 cardiotomy reservoir were used for CPB. A gamma camera was used to image the distribution of INN in the CPB machine and organs. Measurements of INN were performed with an ion chamber and gamma counter.

Results.—Treatment with L-arginine significantly reduced N-trapping. Expressed as a percent of injected INN, N-trapping in the oxygenator decreased from 2.7% in control animals to 0.94% in those receiving L-arginine infusion. In the lung, N-margination was reduced from 48% to 23%. In animals undergoing CPB and reperfusion, the low dose of L-arginine had a beneficial effect. In those receiving the 15 mg/kg/min infusion rate, toxic effects of higher N-margination were noted. Neutrophil margination was not significantly affected by CPB temperature or Leumedin administration.

Conclusions.—This pig model of CPB shows that L-arginine infusion can reduce neutrophil margination. An infusion rate of 2 mg/kg/min may offer optimal reduction of thrombi, emboli, and marginated Ns in such sensitive organs as the brain, lungs, heart, and kidneys. The authors' experiments clearly show that nitric oxide generation through low-dose L-arginine infusion will benefit patients undergoing CPB.

► This article highlights the importance of doing studies with things as transient as nitric oxide stimulators and inhibitors. The study shows the effect of low dose being the opposite of high dose, and once again, demonstrating that with vasoactive compounds or compounds that appear to have vasoactive effects, even if they have principle effects on the immune and inflammatory systems, more is not necessarily better.

M.F. Roizen, M.D.

Comparative Pharmacology

Comparative Pharmacokinetics of Ropivacaine and Bupivacaine in Nonpregnant and Pregnant Ewes

Santos AC, Arthur GR, Lehning EJ, et al (Albert Einstein College of Medicine/Montefiore Med Ctr, New York; State Univ of New York, Stony Brook; Harvard Med School, Boston; et al)

Anesth Analg 85:87–93, 1997 9–14

Background.—The changes in body fluid volume, body composition, and hemodynamics during pregnancy may affect the pharmacokinetics of local anesthetics. Little is known about the effects of pregnancy on the disposition of bupivacaine, currently the local anesthetic most commonly used in obstetrics. The pharmacokinetics and protein binding of bupivacaine and ropivacaine administered intravenously to pregnant and nonpregnant sheep were investigated.

Methods and Findings.—Twelve pregnant ewes near term and 12 nonpregnant ewes were studied. All were in good condition during the study. The greatest mean total serum drug concentrations occurred at the end of IV infusion. Pregnancy was associated with lower distribution volumes of both bupivacaine and ropivacaine in the terminal phase of drug elimination (V_{d_β}) and steady state ($V_{d_{ss}}$) and with lower total body clearance (CL). Analysis of the relationship between V_{d_β} and CL showed that elimination half-time was not changed. Compared with ropivacaine, however, bupivacaine was associated with a greater distribution half-life, elimination half-life, volume of central compartment, V_c, V_{d_β}, $V_{d_{ss}}$, and mean residence times and lower CL. Protein binding depended on concentration and was greater in the pregnant ewes for both drugs.

Conclusions.—Pregnancy in this ovine model altered the pharmacokinetics of ropivacaine and bupivacaine in a similar manner. If these findings can be extrapolated to humans, an unintended intravascular injection of either drug may be expected to result in greater total serum concentrations in pregnant than in nonpregnant women, with drug levels declining at similar rates in both groups. The differences documented between the drugs in this study may make ropivacaine preferable for obstetric anesthesia.

► The role of ropivacaine in obstetric anesthesia remains to be defined. In my judgment, the purported advantages of ropivacaine (e.g., decreased cardiotoxicity, decreased motor block) have little relevance during the administration of epidural analgesia for laboring women, given the fact that most anesthesiologists now administer dilute solutions of bupivacaine during labor. When providing epidural anesthesia for cesarean section, I have long preferred to administer 2% lidocaine with epinephrine rather than bupivacaine. When providing epidural anesthesia for cesarean section, ropivacaine may be safer than bupivacaine, but it is unclear that ropivacaine is preferable to lidocaine.

D.H. Chestnut, M.D.

Acute In Vitro Neuromuscular Effects of Carbamazepine and Carbamazepine-10,11-epoxide

Nguyen A, Ramzan I (Univ of Sydney, Australia)

Anesth Analg 84:886–890, 1997 9–15

Background.—A drug interaction is possible during surgery in patients given anticonvulsants before or during anesthesia using neuromuscular blocking drugs. One study reported that a short-term dose of phenytoin increased neuromuscular paralysis induced by vecuronium in patients undergoing neurosurgery. It was also reported that diazepam increased the magnitude and duration of neuromuscular block induced by gallamine and reversed the block induced by succinylcholine. In another study, a short-term dose of diazepam did not alter recovery from *d*-tubocurarine, gallamine, or decamethonium and did not alter the neuromuscular block induced by alcuronium, pancuronium, or fazadinium. There are no com-

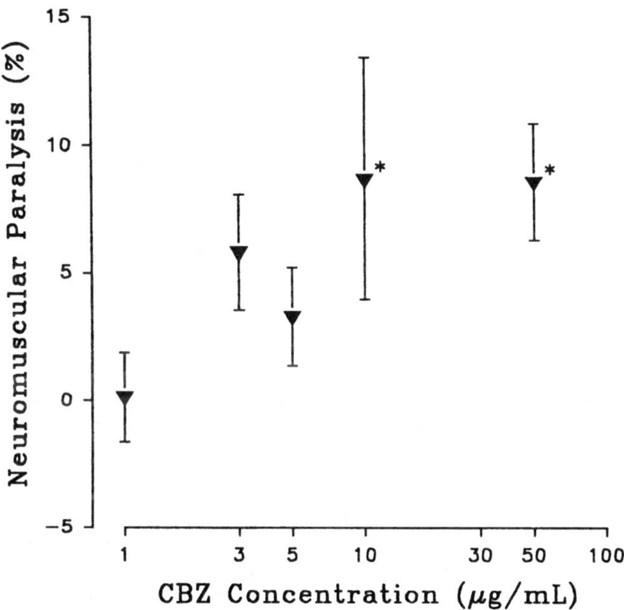

FIGURE 1.—Neuromuscular paralysis concentration profile for carbamazepine (CBZ). Values are expressed as mean plus or minus standard error of the mean from 12 phrenic nerve–hemidiaphragm preparations. *Asterisk*, significantly greater than 0, $P < 0.05$. (Courtesy of Nguyen A, Ramzan I: Acute in vitro neuromuscular effects of carbamazepine and carbamazepine-10,11-epoxide. *Anesth Analg* 84[4]:886–890, 1997.)

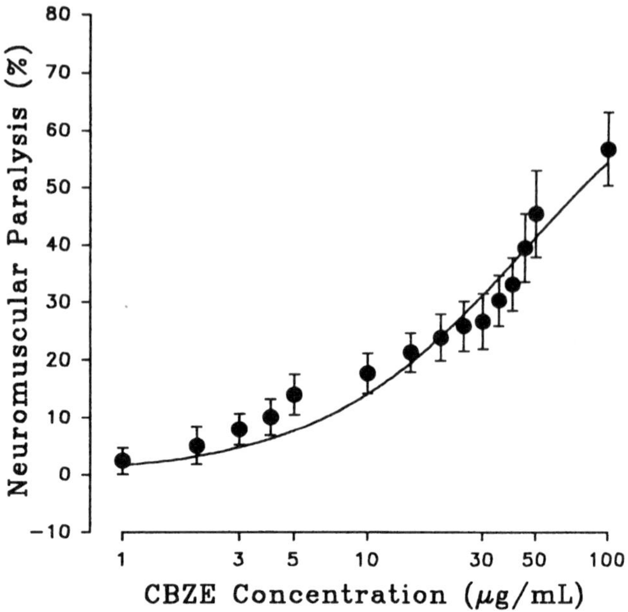

FIGURE 2.—Neuromuscular paralysis concentration profile for carbamazepine-10,11-epoxide (CBZE). Mean values plus or minus standard error of the mean from 10 phrenic nerve–hemidiaphragm preparations and the predicted relationship using a maximum paralysis (E_{max}) equation are presented. (Courtesy of Nguyen A, Ramzan I: Acute in vitro neuromuscular effects of carbamazepine and carbamazepine-10,11-epoxide. *Anesth Anal* 84[4]:886–890, 1997.)

parable data on the short-term neuromuscular effects of carbamazepine or on interactions between carbamazepine and neuromuscular blocking drugs.

Methods.—The short-term neuromuscular effects of the anticonvulsant carbamazepine and carbamazepine-10,11-epoxide, its major metabolite, were examined using an in vitro rat phrenic nerve–hemidiaphragm muscle preparation.

Results.—As the concentration of carbamazepine was increased from 1 μg/mL to 50 μg/mL, it produced 8.8% neuromuscular paralysis (Fig 1). A maximum paralysis of 65% was produced by carbamazepine-10,11-epoxide at concentrations of 1–100 μg/mL (Fig 2). The concentration needed to produce half this paralysis was 36 μg/mL. Carbamazepine (10 μg/mL) shifted the response concentration curve for the depolarizing neuromuscular blocker succinylcholine and the nondepolarizing neuromuscular blocker atracurium and also reduced the concentrations of these agents needed for half paralysis by 30%. Although carbamazepine-10,11-epoxide was a stronger neuromuscular blocker, it did not change the effect of succinylcholine or atracurium.

Discussion.—Carbamazepine and carbamazepine-10,11-epoxide produce partial neuromuscular paralysis. It may be possible to enhance, on a short-term basis, the block from neuromuscular blockers with carbamazepine or carbamazepine-10,11-epoxide. Long-term use of carbamazepine produces resistance to neuromuscular blockers. These findings confirm the results of other studies showing that anticonvulsants have reduced neuromuscular blocker dose requirements in the short term.

► The drug interaction between anticonvulsants and neuromuscular blocking agents is well recognized, and there are numerous clinical reports in the literature showing that short-term administration of anticonvulsants (e.g., phenytoin) reduces neuromuscular relaxant requirements (e.g., vecuronium).[1] This interesting short-term in vitro study demonstrated that the parent compound carbamazepine, which is not a potent neuromuscular blocker, enhanced the neuromuscular effect of succinylcholine and atracurium. In contrast, the carbamazepine metabolite, a potent blocker in its own right, failed to affect the activity of either muscle relaxant.

M. Wood, M.D.

Reference

1. Gray HStJ, Slater RM, Pollard BJ. The effect of acutely administered phenytoin on vecuronium-induced neuromuscular blockade. *Anaesthesia* 44:379–381, 1989.

Intraabdominal Carbon Dioxide Insufflation in the Pregnant Ewe: Uterine Blood Flow, Intraamniotic Pressure, and Cardiopulmonary Effects

Cruz AM, Southerland LC, Duke T, et al (Western College of Veterinary Medicine, Sask; Royal Univ, Sask)

Anesthesiology 85:1395–1402, 1996 9–16

Background.—Pregnant women are increasingly undergoing laparoscopic surgical procedures. However, maternal-fetal physiologic changes during intra-abdominal carbon dioxide insufflation are not well understood. Also, maternal and fetal safety is of concern during carbon dioxide pneumoperitoneum.

Methods.—Nine ewes received abdominal insufflation with carbon dioxide to an intra-abdominal pressure of 15 mm Hg or no insufflation in a prospective, randomized, crossover study. Thiopental was used to induce anesthesia and end-tidal halothane to maintain it. Partial pressure of carbon dioxide, arterial ($Paco_2$) was maintained between 35 and 40 mm Hg by serial maternal arterial blood gas analysis–guided mechanical ventilation.

Findings.—Maternal $Paco_2$ to $ETco_2$ gradient and minute ventilation was increased significantly during insufflation. Maternal $ETco_2$ and partial pressure of oxygen, arterial declined concomitantly. During insufflation, intra-amniotic pressure increased significantly. There were no significant changes in maternal hemodynamic variables, fetal variables, or uterine blood flow. No fetal deaths nor preterm labor occurred during the experiment.

Conclusions.—In this animal model, $PaCO_2$-to-$ETCO_2$ gradient increased markedly during the 1 hour of insufflation, suggesting that capnography may not be adequate to guide ventilation during carbon dioxide pneumoperitoneum in pregnant women. There were no other significant circulatory changes.

▶ The authors observed a significant increase in the $PaCO_2$-($ETCO_2$) gradient during insufflation, and they concluded that "a considerable underestimation of $PaCO_2$ can occur if $ETCO_2$ is used to monitor the adequacy of ventilation of pregnant patients undergoing $IACO_2$ insufflation." But it is unclear to me that this limitation of $ETCO_2$ monitoring is unique to pregnant patients. Instead, I suspect that $ETCO_2$ monitoring may underestimate $PaCO_2$ in all patients undergoing intra-abdominal carbon dioxide insufflation. Perhaps the potential consequences of unrecognized hypercarbia (i.e., maternal and fetal acidosis) are greater in pregnant than in nonpregnant patients. This is unclear, given that laparoscopic surgery is becoming increasingly popular in pregnant patients.

D.H. Chestnut, M.D.

Mechanisms of Action

Insensitivity to Anaesthetic Agents Conferred by a Class of $GABA_A$ Receptor Subunit

Davies PA, Hanna MC, Hales TG, et al (Inst for Genomic Research, Rockville, Md; Univ of California, Los Angeles)
Nature 385:820–823, 1997 9–17

Background.—One common feature of anesthetic agents is their potentiation of neuronal inhibition through γ-aminobutyric acid ($GABA_A$) receptors. In mammals, 13 subtypes of $GABA_A$ receptor subunits have been identified and categorized within 4 structural classes (α, β, γ, δ). A further structural category of $GABA_A$ receptor subunit with unique properties was identified.

Methods and Results.—Recombinant DNA techniques were utilized to identify a new class of $GABA_A$ receptor subunit class (ε). The expression of ε-subunit mRNA was analyzed in various tissues by Northern blotting. Two size lengths of mRNA were detected and were relatively abundant in amygdala and thalamus, especially the subthalamic nucleus. The biophysical and pharmacologic properties conferred on $GABA_A$ receptors by this novel subunit were examined by transient expression in HEK-293 cells. When these cells were transfected with only the ε-subunit cDNA, the cells did not express binding sites for GABA ligands or exhibit chloride currents in response to GABA administration. Therefore, this subunit does not appear able to assemble chloride channels on its own. When these cells were co-transfected with cDNAs for the ε-subunit and either α- or β-subunits, ligand-binding activity was not detected. When the cells were transfected with all 3 subunits, GABA-activated currents and ligand binding were detected. However, there was no binding of benzodiazepines. A comparison of current-voltage relationships demonstrated that inclusion of the ϵ-subunit confers novel biophysical properties. Inclusion of this subunit in transfection experiments abolishes normal outward rectification of $GABA_A$ receptors. Inclusion of this subunit also conferred insensitivity to the potentiating, but not the activating, effects of IV anesthetics.

Conclusions.—This report describes a novel class of human $GABA_A$ receptor subunit (ϵ) that can assemble to form heteromeric complexes with other receptor classes. The presence of this novel subunit in receptor complexes confers insensitivity to the potentiating, but not the activating, effects of IV anesthetics and abolishes outward rectification. This finding supports the idea that the 2 types of responses to anesthetic agents are mediated by different anesthetic-binding sites on the receptor complex. The ϵ-subunit may have other novel properties that have not yet been uncovered. Its abundant expression in the subthalamic nucleus suggests it may have a role to play in the treatment of movement disorders, such as Parkinson's disease.

► I selected this paper for our YEAR BOOK OF ANESTHESIOLOGY because it is published in what quite possibly is the world's most prestigious scientific journal. We have long understood that the phenomenon we call "anesthesia" must be a major yet at the same time minor physiologic or neurophysiologic change. By "major," I mean widespread removal of the defense against unconsciousness, yet not fatal. By "minor," I mean completely and rapidly reversible. Geneticists have been studying the genes that produce the various receptor subunits which respond to GABA. They believe that by understanding genetic alterations, which confer either sensitivity or insensitivity to anesthetics, and understanding the underlying nature of the involved genes, they can gain an understanding of how anesthetics work. Perhaps this is so, perhaps not, but just reading this complex paper and trying to understand it at least at some level, probably is a valuable exercise for clinicians, because basic science is racing along at an unprecedented clip these days, and we clinicians must do everything we can to make sure it doesn't race too far away from us. This is the very first paper published in *Nature* that I have ever included in the YEAR BOOK in my years as your Editor-in-Chief. I am not trying to say to you, dear reader, that I understand this, only that I am trying to gain an appreciation for it.

J.H. Tinker, M.D.

Increase of Glutamate Uptake in Astrocytes: A Possible Mechanism of Action of Volatile Anesthetics

Miyazaki H, Nakamura Y, Arai T, et al (Ehime Univ, Japan)
Anesthesiology 86:1359–1366, 1997 9–18

Background.—Glutamate is the most important excitatory neurotransmitter in the vertebrate CNS. Astrocytes are the most abundant cell type in the CNS and are involved in terminating glutamatergic neurotransmission by removing released glutamate from the synaptic cleft. The effects of various anesthetics on glutamate uptake activity of primary cultured astrocytes from rat hippocampus were examined.

Methods.—Cultured astrocytes from rat hippocampi were incubated in solution containing [^{3}H]glutamate pre-equilibrated with 0% to 4% halothane. Glutamate activity was measured as the amount of radioactivity per cell of protein.

Results.—Glutamate uptake increased to 165% of the control with 4% halothane. This increase was dose-dependent, and a significant increase of 30% to 50% in glutamate uptake was seen with a range of clinical use concentrations. Halothane, 1% to 4%, had little effect on the uptake of the inhibitory transmitter γ-aminobutyric acid. In neuron-rich cultures, a similar increase in glutamate uptake was seen, although to a lesser degree. A small increase in glutamate uptake was seen in biochemical subcellular fractions. Glutamate uptake was enhanced by enflurane, isoflurane, sevoflurane, and other volatile anesthetics but was not affected by the IV anesthetics ketamine or pentobarbital.

Discussion.—These findings show that the glutamate uptake activity of astrocytes increases in the presence of volatile anesthetics. This increase may lessen the excitatory synaptic transmission in the CNS. This increase of glutamate uptake may be the mechanisms of action of volatile anesthetics.

► Anesthetic action has been studied at the subcellular level with respect to various kinds of disruption of membrane function by either physical solution in membranes or in hydrophobic areas of proteins acting as channels. At the cellular level, volatile anesthetic action has been studied with respect to inhibition of excitatory synaptic transmission. It is well known that the brain's neurons are "played upon," each one by literally thousands of dendrites from surrounding cells. Glutamate is the most important fast-acting neurotransmitter and it is, in essence, a "positive" transmitter, i.e., excitatory. I selected this study because I believe anesthesiologists should keep themselves abreast of developments in our understanding of the mechanisms of action of the anesthetics we deliver. This paper is nicely written and well edited. It does, indeed, give the reader a reasonably painless update in this complex arena.

J.H. Tinker, M.D.

Sodium Channel in Human Malignant Hyperthermia

Fletcher JE, Wieland SJ, Karen SM, et al (Allegheny Univ, Philadelphia; Uniformed Services Univ, Bethesda, Md; Univ of Pennsylvania, Kennett Square, Penn)

Anesthesiology 86:1023–1032, 1997 9–19

Objective.—Malignant hyperthermia (MH) is associated with a ryanodine receptor defect. In cell cultures from MH-susceptible individuals, the function and expression of Na+ currents is altered. Results of a study examining if such alterations are artifacts of cell culture or are associated with MH are presented.

Methods.—mRNA was extracted from muscle fascicles of the vastus lateralis of 12 patients with MH susceptibility and 16 control subjects and amplified using PCR. β_1-subunit and SkM2 were identified and quantitated. The effects of added tetrodotoxin on directly elicited muscle twitch of human vastus lateralis (or equine semimembranosus) muscle strips was determined at increasing doses of tetrodotoxin as a means of estimating the functional SkM2 protein present.

Results.—The level of SkM2 was significantly depressed by 20-fold in muscle of the 7 MH-susceptible patients tested and by 115-fold in 6 of the 7 MH-susceptible patients. The functional expression of SkM2 protein was significantly decreased by at least a factor of 4 in muscle tissue of MH-susceptible patients compared with muscle tissue from controls.

Conclusion.—Muscle tissue from MH-susceptible patients contained altered mRNA and decreased functional expression of SkM2 when compared with muscle tissue from controls. Changes in sodium channels in the presence of anesthesia play a role in the development of the skeletal muscle rigidity that can lead to the severe acidosis characteristic of MH.

▶ I usually avoid extreme "basic science" types of studies in the YEAR BOOK because most clinicians are hard-pressed to apply that knowledge in the operating room. Nevertheless, when a basic science study comes along that materially adds to our knowledge of how something works, I attempt to include it, and that is the case here. The authors have shown a specific genetically determined alpha subunit of the sodium channel to be involved in human malignant hyperthermia. Although this paper is difficult to digest, I think the authors have made an important step forward in understanding how the genetically determined disorder is actually expressed at the subcellular level. This particular sodium channel dysfunctional unit, genetically determined, may help explain why MH seems to be somewhat heterogeneous, because two types of channels, calcium and now sodium, seem to be involved, each with apparently separate genetics. Since malignant hyperthermia is "our" disease, i.e., "anesthetic disease," I think we should take an interest when advances are made in the mechanistic understanding of it. This is such an article, in my opinion.

J.H. Tinker, M.D.

Anaesthetic Potency of Inhalation Agents Is Independent of Membrane Microviscosity

Norman RI, Hirst R, Appadu BL, et al (Univ of Leicester, England)

Br J Anaesth 78:290–295, 1997 9–20

Background.—Though inhalation anesthetics are widely used in clinical practice, their mechanism of action remains unknown. The reduction of membrane microviscosity of erythrocyte ghosts in the presence of clinically relevant levels of 7 inhalation anesthetics was investigated.

Methods.—The anesthetic agents used were desflurane, halothane, trichloroethylene, isoflurane, enflurane, methoxyflurane, and nitrous oxide. Fluorescence polarization anisotropy of the membrane incorporated fluorescent probes 1,6-diphenyl-1,3,5-hexatriene and 1-[-4-trimethylammoniumphenyl]-6-phenyl-1,3,5-hexatriene was used to study the decrease in membrane microviscosity of erythrocyte ghosts.

Findings.—All the anesthetic agents resulted in a dose-dependent reduction in anisotropy of both probes, demonstrating a decrease in membrane microviscosity. The decrease in anisotropy determined at the minimum alveolar concentration for anesthesia was inversely associated with the anesthetic potency of the agent. In addition, it was directly proportional to the hypothetical concentration of the agent in the membrane calculated from lipid-water partition coefficients.

Conclusions.—These data do not suggest a role for perturbation in membrane microviscosity in the mechanism of anesthesia of volatile agents. Though perturbation of the dynamic properties of the bulk phase of the membrane may not be important, the ability of anesthetic agents to dissolve in membrane bilayers may be important in their action.

▶ My long-cherished hypothesis of anesthetic action—that anesthetics insinuated themselves in more or less physical solution into lipophilic regions of membrane or hydrophobic regions of protein membrane channels, thus changing the configuration or swelling the membrane or protein, thus altering or depressing its function in a reversible fashion—is challenged in this paper. The authors used something called "fluorescence polarization anistropy." I wouldn't begin to try to understand what that is, but I do know that new "tools" become available from time to time, and this is one of those times in the long and checkered history of the study of the mechanism of volatile anesthetics. I still like the membrane swelling idea, if for no other reason but that I can understand it!

J.H. Tinker, M.D.

The Effects of Mexiletine, Desipramine and Fluoxetine in Rat Models Involving Central Sensitization

Jett M-F, McGuirk J, Waligora D, et al (Roche Bioscience, Palo Alto, Calif)
Pain 69:161–169, 1997 9–21

Background.—Peripheral nerve injury can result in chronic and disabling neuropathic pain. This type of pain does not always respond to conventional analgesics, such as opiates and nonsteroidal anti-inflammatory drugs. Any drug that is effective in the treatment of neuropathic pain must interfere with injury-induced sensitization of the dorsal horn neurons, also called central sensitization, which is part of the hyperalgesia and allodynia associated with this pain. Mexiletine, a class I_b antiarrhythmic drug, has been used to treat neuropathic pain. Desipramine, a selective, neuronal norepinephrine (NE) re-uptake inhibitor is effective in reducing the pain of diabetic neuropathy. The activity of selective 5-hydroxytryptamine (5-HT) uptake inhibitors, such as fluoxetine, in the treatment of neuropathic pain remains controversial. The efficacy of mexiletine, desipramine, and fluoxetine was evaluated in 2 rat models of neuropathic pain.

Methods.—In the formalin model of neuropathy, adult male Sprague-Dawley rats were administered formalin subcutaneously into the plantar surface of the hindpaw. Formalin treatment provoked a biphasic response, with a phasic response separated by an interphase from an enduring tonic response. In this model, the tonic phase reflects central sensitization. The agitation response of rats to formalin treatment was assessed by the dynamic force the rat places on a load cell with an automated detection system. The spinal nerve ligation (SNL) model was also used as a model of neuropathy. The spinal nerves L5 and L6 were tightly ligated to provoke central sensitization reflected by tactile allodynia and thermal hyperalgesia of the affected hindpaw. Mechanical hyperalgesia was monitored by the pin prick test. Tactile allodynia was monitored with a calibrated series of 8 von Frey filaments. Analgesic drugs were administered subcutaneously 1–3 hours before testing.

Results.—Mexiletine, 10–100 mg/kg administered subcutaneously, significantly decreased hyperalgesia in the formalin treated and SNL rats. It also reduced tactile allodynia in the SNL rats. Desipramine, 1–100 mg/kg administered subcutaneously, significantly reduced hyperalgesia in formalin-treated and SNL rats, but did not reduce tactile allodynia in SNL rats. Fluoxetine, 3–30 mg/kg administered subcutaneously, did not decrease hyperalgesia or allodynia in any of the tests or models used in this study.

Conclusion.—The 2 drugs that have proven effective in treating human neuropathic pain, mexiletine and desipramine, were also effective in reducing hyperalgesia in 2 rat models. Desipramine differentially affected mechanical hyperalgesia and tactile allodynia. This is consistent with the hypothesis that the neuronal mechanisms that underlie these manifestations of neuropathic pain are not identical. Fluoxetine, a selective 5-HT inhibitor, was not effective in reducing pain in either rat model of neuropathy. These 2 rat models may prove useful in understanding the mechanisms of central sensitization and in the evaluation of potential therapies.

▶ The analgesic properties of the serotonin-specific reuptake inhibitors such as fluoxetine and sertraline have been disappointing. Early studies of spinally administered serotonin agonists showed promising analgesic effects, and it was postulated that descending serotoninergic pathways from the medulla to the spinal cord were important mediators of endogenous antinociceptive mechanisms. More recent studies have shown less dramatic analgesic effect from serotonin agonists. There is also speculation that a portion of the analgesic effect of tricyclic antidepressants is related to mechanisms other than serotonin and norepinephrine re-uptake inhibition. *N*-methyl-D-aspartate antagonism is a possible candidate.

S.E. Abram, M.D.

Mechanisms Whereby Propofol Mediates Peripheral Vasodilation in Humans: Sympathoinhibition or Direct Vascular Relaxation?

Robinson BJ, Ebert TJ, O'Brien TJ, et al (Med College of Wisconsin, Milwaukee; VA Med Ctr, Milwaukee, Wis)

Anesthesiology 86:64–72, 1997 9–22

Introduction.—The induction and maintenance of anesthesia with propofol leads to decreased arterial blood pressure, caused in part by decreased peripheral resistance. Studies of propofol-associated hypotension have proposed several possible mechanisms, including a direct action of the drug on vascular smooth muscle, inhibition of sympathetic activity to the vasculature, or both. Two studies were designed to examine these possibilities.

Methods.—The 11 patients in study 1 had intralipid (time control) and propofol infused into the brachial artery at rates between 83 and 664 µg/min. Forearm vascular resistance (FVR) and forearm vein compliance (FVC) were determined by means of bilateral forearm venous occlusion plethysmography. Responses were compared to arterial infusions of sodium nitroprusside (SNP) at 0.3, 3.0, and 10 µ/min. In study 2, 6 healthy men underwent left stellate block and were anesthetized and maintained with propofol infusions of 125 and 200 $\mu g/kg^{-1}$ per min^{-1}. The time control in this study was blood flow dynamics in the unblocked right arm. Three additional conscious participants had intrabrachial artery infusions of SNP and nitroglycerin (both at 10 µg/min) before and after stellate blockade of the left forearm. Their arterial and venous responses were evaluated to determine whether the sympathetically denervated forearm vessels could dilate beyond the level produced by denervation alone.

Results.—Neither the intralipid or propofol infusions altered FVR, FVC, or skin blood flow. Infusion of SNP significantly decreased FVR in a dose-dependent manner but did not change FVC. Plasma propofol concentrations increased from 0.2 to 10.1 µg/mL during the incremental propofol infusions. In the second study, stellate ganglion blockade decreased FVR by a mean of 50% and increased FVC by a mean of 58%. The 2 infusion rates of propofol progressively reduced mean arterial pressure. No further changes in FVR and FVC occurred in the arm with sympathetic denervation after administration of propofol anesthesia. In the control arm, however, significant decreases in FVR and significant increases in FVC occurred at both infusion rates (Fig 3). Intra-arterial infusion of SNP and nitroglycerin after stellate blockade led to further decreases in FVR and further increases of FVC.

Conclusion.—The hypothesis that propofol acts directly on peripheral vessels was not supported, for no arterial or venous responses to the agent were observed in the forearm. But effects of propofol anesthesia on FVR and FVC were similar to the effects of sympathetic denervation by stellate ganglion blockade, indicating that the peripheral vascular actions of propofol result from an inhibition of tonic sympathetic vasoconstrictor outflow.

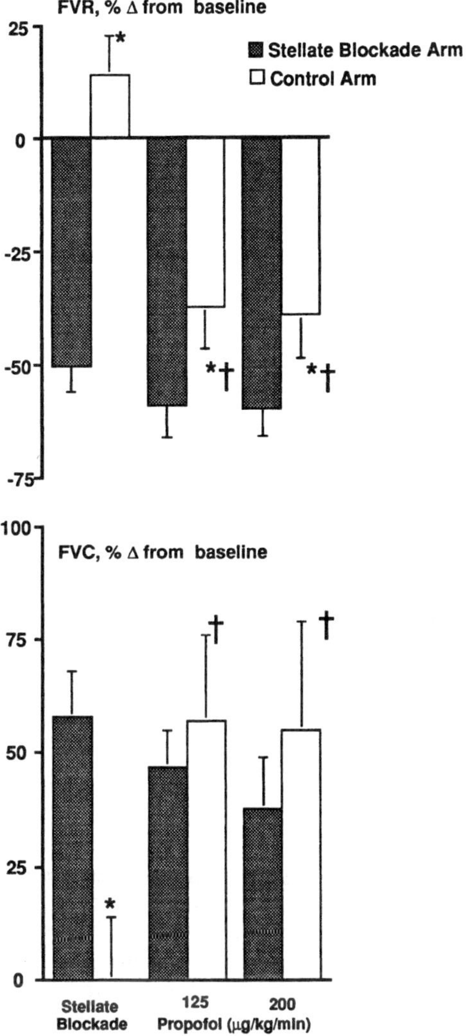

FIGURE 3.—Percentage changes from awake baseline in forearm vascular resistance (FVR) and forearm venous compliance (FVC) in the left arm after stellate blockade and in the control unblocked arm before and during propofol anesthesia. Stellate blockade decreased FVR and increased FVC on the side of the blockade. During propofol anesthesia, there was no further arterial or venous dilation in the sympathectomized arm, but significant dilation occurred in the unblocked control arm. Data are mean ± SEM. $*P < 0.05$ indicates significant difference between arms. $\dagger P < 0.05$ indicates significant change from prepropofol baseline. (Courtesy of Robinson BJ, Ebert TJ, O'Brien TJ, et al: Mechanisms whereby propofol mediates peripheral vasodilation in humans: Sympathoinhibition or direct vascular relaxation? *Anesthesiology* 86:64–72, 1997. Copyright American Society of Anesthesiologists, Inc. Used with permission of Lippincott-Raven Publishers.)

▶ This elegant clinical study comes from a group of investigators skilled in the use of techniques to evaluate sympathetic nervous function during anesthesia. The investigation extends previous work to explain why propofol causes a decrease in arterial blood pressure. The investigators demonstrated that the decreased peripheral resistance associated with propofol administration is mainly the result of an inhibition of sympathetic vasoconstrictor nerve activity and that in contrast to in vitro studies, propofol does not appear to have a direct effect on arterial or venous vascular smooth muscle. Thus there is a decreased sympathoinhibitory effect associated with propofol anesthesia. This effect may be particularly important for elderly patients with cardiac disease. In clinical practice, we might expect to see an exaggerated decrease in blood pressure with propofol in this group of patients because of their underlying disease and age-associated sympathetic nervous system dysfunction.

M. Wood, M.D.

Need for Basic Sciences in Anesthesiology

The Need for Basic Sciences in the Understanding and Practice of Anaesthesia

Burnstein RM, Jeevaratnam RD, Jones JG (Addenbrookes Hosp, Cambridge, England; Peterborough District Hosp, England)

Anaesthesia 52:935–944, 1997 9–23

Background.—How relevant are the basic sciences to the practice of anesthesia? This survey of British consultant and trainee anesthetists aimed to find out.

Methods.—Of 78 consultants, staff grades, and postfellowship trainees who were surveyed, 56 responded (72%). The survey, which was based on the topics covered in the Fellowship of the Royal College of Anaesthetists (FRCA) part I examination, had 2 parts. In the first part, respondents were asked to indicate 5 topics under 6 subject headings that were "essential to the understanding and practice of everyday anesthesia." The 6 topics were physiology, biochemistry and metabolism, pharmacology, statistics, physics and clinical measurements, and "other." In the second part, respondents were prompted by specific questions and topics (i.e., pulmonary circulation as regards the cardiovascular system) and were asked to determine their relevancy on a 10-point scale. Furthermore, they were asked to indicate whether they could deliver a tutorial on the subject to an FRCA candidate.

Findings.—In the first part, at least half of respondents indicated that knowledge of the following topics was essential: cardiovascular, respiratory, CNS, renal, and metabolic/endocrine physiology; metabolism; drug pharmacology, pharmacokinetics, and pharmacodynamics; principles of measurements; basic physical laws; and principles of monitors. Responses on the second part were generally in agreement with the items respondents listed as being important in part 1. In the second part, respondents said that about 65% of the basic science curriculum was relevant. Of those who thought a basic science concept was "essential," depending on the question, between 32% and over 90% were able to give tutorials on the topic.

Conclusion.—Many of the basic science concepts tested on the part I FRCA examination were considered to be unimportant to the everyday practice of anesthesia. In fact, only 12 items in the first part of the survey were rated as essential by more than 50% of respondents. And even though the respondent thought the topic essential, in some cases only one third could give a tutorial on the topic. These results indicate that the current part I FRCA examination tests basic science knowledge that appears to be irrelevant. Hopefully, these results will help define a better syllabus that tests the core basic science knowledge an anesthesiologist should have.

► I included this paper partly because it comes from Great Britain, a country in which nonphysicians do not practice anesthesia. The physician anesthesiologists involved in this survey were clearly in favor of basic science education, despite the fact that they only picked about 65% of the basic science curriculum to which they were exposed as being useful in understanding or practice of everyday anesthesia. Within that 65%, things got even worse. Although most people agreed that cardiovascular, CNS, and renal physiology were valuable, there was disagreement regarding some of the rest of the basic sciences. Worse, there were numerous areas in which anesthetists considered basic science knowledge to be "essential," yet they could not really give what the authors euphemistically call a "tutorial" on the subject.

In the United States, nonphysician anesthesia practitioners are unlikely to be as extensively grounded in the basic sciences as are physicians. Despite this, it has been exceedingly difficult, if not impossible, to show valid risk-adjusted provider-based differences in outcomes. I chose this study to opine that even though these British anesthetists *believed* in the importance of basic sciences, their "beliefs" are a bit unconvincing. In the abstract, the authors admitted the essentially subjective, emotional nature of this study when they substituted the word "believed" for the word "felt." They weren't even sure the anesthetists believed in what they said, but rather "felt" that way!

In truth, our drugs today are much better than in the past. Our monitors are even better, and our machines are also better. Perhaps the above facts serve to diminish the importance of basic science education in anesthesiology for those who practice it daily.

J.H. Tinker, M.D.

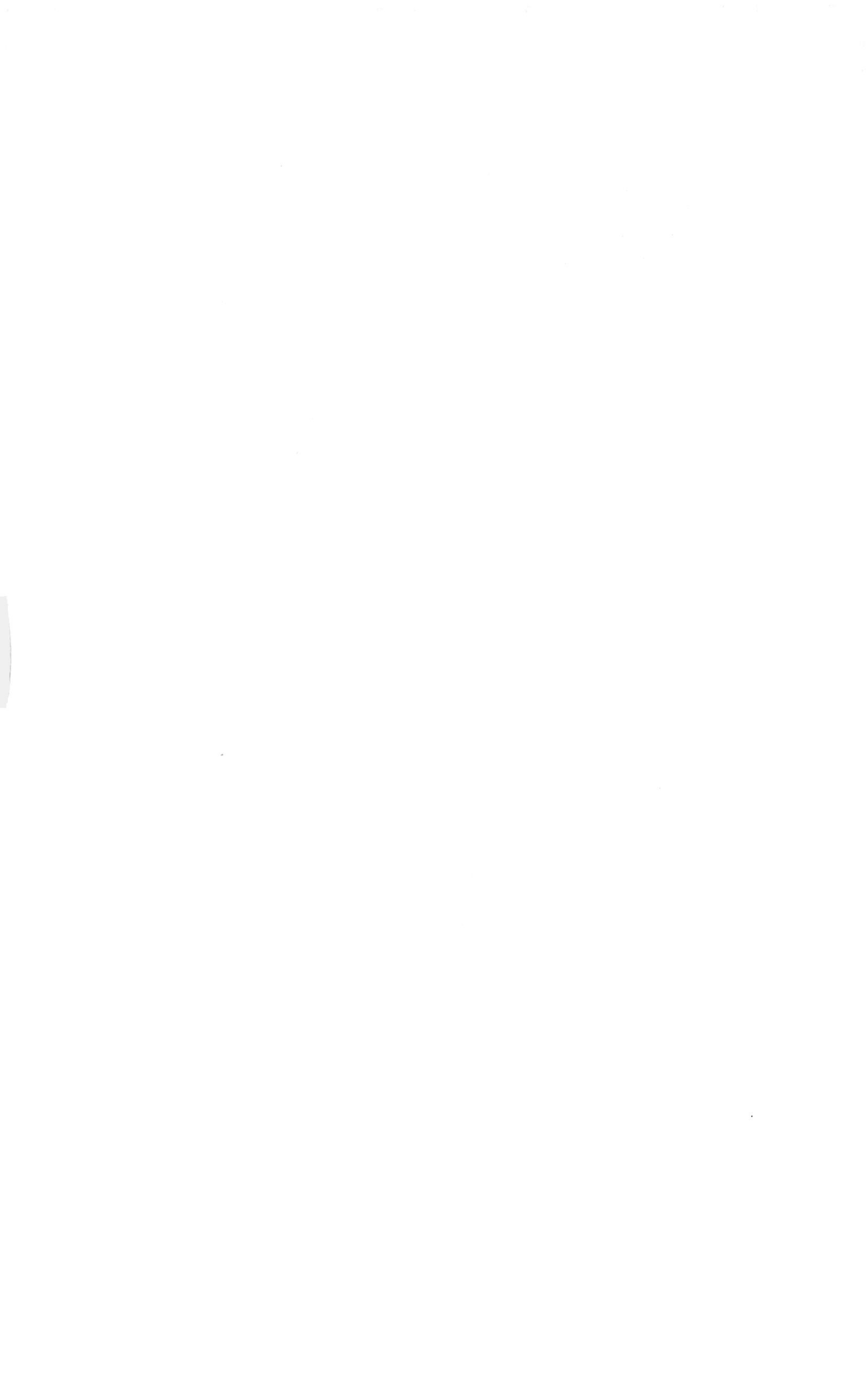

10 Medicolegal and Ethical Issues

Ethical Issues in Critical Care

The Supreme Court and Physician-assisted Suicide: The Ultimate Right
Angell M (Mem Sloan Kettering Cancer, New York)
N Engl J Med 336:50–53, 1997 10–1

Background.—The United States Ninth and Second Circuit Courts of Appeals recently decided that Washington and New York laws banning assistance in suicide were unconstitutional as applied to physicians and their terminally ill patients. If the United States Supreme Court allows this decision to stand, physicians in 12 states would be able to provide the means for terminally ill patients to kill themselves. About two thirds of the American public and more than half of the physicians currently support physician-assisted suicide. The medical and ethical aspects of this issue were discussed in an editorial in favor of physician-assisted suicide.

Editorial.—One of the most important ethical principles in medicine is respect for patient autonomy. When this principle conflicts with others, it should almost always take precedence. Another important point is that death is not fair and is often cruel. Although patients needing treatment, such as assisted ventilation or dialysis, to sustain life can hasten their deaths, if they wish, by having the life-sustaining treatment withheld, those not receiving such treatment may desperately need help that they cannot now get.

The Ninth Circuit Court made an analogy between suicide and abortion, stating that both were personal choices protected by the Constitution. Forbidding physicians to assist would, in effect, nullify these rights, according to that Court decision. States would be permitted to regulate assisted suicide as they do abortion, but they could not regulate it out of existence.

The argument that the physician's role in euthanasia is active—compared with the passive role in withdrawing life-sustaining treatment—is too physician-centered and not sufficiently patient-centered. Because assisted suicide, by definition, cannot occur without the patient's knowledge and participation, the patient's role in it is active. The voluntary nature of assisted suicide will, it is to be hoped, safeguard patients against the possibility of a "slippery slope," i.e., the potential for assisted suicide to lead to involuntary euthanasia. Many fear that economically and socially disadvantaged persons would be coerced into requesting assisted suicide. Although this is possible, there has been no evidence of widespread abuse. Another concern regarding legalized assisted suicide is that patients with depression may seek suicide rather than help for their depression. In such cases, physicians would be expected to use their judgment, just as they do in other life-and-death decision making.

Competent Care for the Dying Instead of Physician-assisted Suicide
Foley KM (Mem Sloan Kettering Cancer Ctr, New York)
N Engl J Med 336:54–58, 1997 10–2

Background.—The United States Supreme Court's review of the Second and Ninth Circuit Courts of Appeals decisions to reverse state bans on assisted suicide provides an opportunity to engage in a national discussion of how American medicine and society should address the needs of dying patients and their families. The author's essay argued for competent care for the dying instead of physician-assisted suicide.

Discussion.—On the issue of physician-assisted suicide, physicians generally fall into 1 of 3 groups. Supporters believe it is a compassionate response to a medical need and a way to re-establish patients' trust in physicians who have used technology excessively. Another group is opposed to the practice on moral grounds, stressing the need to preserve the professionalism of medicine and the commitment to do no harm. The last group is opposed because they believe the practice would be unregulatable. All 3 groups agree that a national effort is called for to improve care for the dying.

Physician-related barriers to appropriate, humane, and compassionate care for the dying range from attitudinal and behavioral barriers to educational and economic ones. Physicians do not know enough about their patients, themselves, or suffering to assist with dying as a medical treatment for relieving suffering. Legalized physician-assisted suicide would substitute for rational therapeutic, psychological, and social interventions that might enhance the quality of life for dying patients.

► These 2 editorials (Abstracts 10–1 and 10–2) offer conflicting viewpoints regarding the regulation of physician-assisted suicide (PAS) and are included to help educate anesthesiologists in formulating their own opinions regarding this contentious issue. Dr. Angell's argument in favor of PAS is based on the constitutional right of autonomy and on the belief that most discussions regarding end-of-life decisions are "too doctor-centered and not sufficiently patient-centered." She further states that good palliative care and PAS are not mutually exclusive and that the voluntary nature of PAS is "the best protection against sliding down a slippery slope." I disagree with her argument that data from the Netherlands (where PAS and euthanasia are practiced and condoned) fail to support a "slippery-slope" theory. Recently, a patient who suffered from depression only was granted physician-assisted death. Despite the presumed illegality of this case, no charges were filed.

Dr. Foley argues passionately that PAS undermines the moral framework of the practice of medicine and, in particular, palliative care. She believes that it would be inevitable for the courts to broaden PAS to include requests from proxies and, perhaps, active euthanasia. She expresses concern that the disadvantaged will be reluctant to seek health care for fear that they may be persuaded to pursue the economical and expedient pathway of PAS. In an era of capitated payments, this possibility does not seem to be too far-fetched.

Addendum: In June of 1997, the United States Supreme Court unanimously disagreed with the Circuit Courts' rulings that banning physician-assisted suicide was unconstitutional, thus supporting the beliefs extolled by Dr. Foley. However, the court left the door open for individual cases to be heard in the future and for individual states to enact their own laws. Finally, the Supreme Court emphasized the urgent need for palliative care, clearly delineating the "double effect" from euthanasia.

D.M. Rothenberg, M.D.

Physician-assisted Suicide and Patients With Human Immunodeficiency Virus Disease

Slome LR, Mitchell TF, Charlebois E, et al (San Francisco; Univ of California, San Francisco; San Francisco Gen Hosp)

N Engl J Med 336:417–421, 1997 10–3

Introduction.—Physician members of the Community Consortium, an association of health care providers for patients infected with HIV in the San Francisco Bay area, were surveyed about their views on physician-assisted suicide and the frequency with which they actually provided lethal doses of medications to patients with AIDS. The findings were compared with those of a similar survey conducted in 1990.

Methods.—The anonymous, self-administered questionnaire was given to all 228 physician members of the Community Consortium. Included in the survey were sections on demographic characteristics, professional and personal experience with AIDS, beliefs and attitudes regarding physician-assisted suicide, and actual participation in assisted suicide. The survey included a case vignette, in which a gay man, age 30, requested a prescription for a lethal dose of narcotics. The patient has severe wasting syndrome, is not responding to treatment, and appears to be mentally competent. Physicians were asked what course of action they would take if this patient were determined to obtain assistance in committing suicide.

Results.—Responses were received from 137 (60%) physicians, of which 19 were no longer in clinical practice. (Their returns were not analyzed.) Compared with respondents of the 1990 survey, physicians

TABLE 2.—Responses to the Case Vignette in 1990 and 1995

Question and Response	1990	1995
	no. (%)	
How likely would you be to prescribe a lethal dose of medication for Tom?*		
Very unlikely	20 (29)	18 (16)
Unlikely	20 (29)	19 (17)
Neither likely nor unlikely	9 (13)	22 (19)
Likely	13 (19)	47 (41)
Very likely	6 (9)	8 (7)
If Tom was adamant about getting assistance in committing suicide, what course of action would you take?†		
Refuse his request	10 (14)	18 (16)
Talk him out of it‡	16 (23)	12 (11)
Hospitalize him as danger to himself	2 (3)	1 (1)
Refer him to a mental health professional	41 (59)	50 (45)
Refer him to a suicide-prevention program	4 (6)	5 (5)
Refer him to clergy	11 (16)	17 (15)
Refer him to another physician	1 (1)	8 (7)
Refer him to the Hemlock Society	32 (46)	42 (38)
Grant his request§	24 (35)	56 (51)

Note: Only the physicians who responded to questions about the case vignette are included.

*There were 68 respondents in 1990 and 114 in 1995. $P = 0.005$ for the comparison of the distribution of responses between the 2 surveys.

†There were 69 respondents in 1990 and 110 in 1995. More than 1 response per physician was possible.

‡$P = 0.04$ for the comparison of the distribution of responses between the 2 surveys.

§$P = 0.05$ for the comparison of the distribution of responses between the 2 surveys.

(Reprinted by permission of *The New England Journal of Medicine,* from Slome LR, Mitchell TF, Charlebois E, et al: Physician-assisted suicide and patients with human immunodeficiency virus disease. *N Engl J Med* 336:417–421.)

completing the 1995 survey were more racially diverse, more likely to be heterosexual, and more likely to have treated a relatively high number of patients with AIDS. Respondents had received a mean of 7.9 direct and 13.7 indirect requests from patients for assistance; 53% said they had granted a request for assistance at least once (mean, 4.2 times). Responding to the case vignette, 48% of physicians said they would be likely or very likely to grant the patient's request for a prescription for a lethal dose of narcotics. Only 28% of respondents to the 1990 survey would have complied with such a request (Table 2).

Conclusions.—Physicians who regularly care for patients with HIV showed a greater acceptance of assisted suicide in 1995 than they did in 1990. The following 4 factors were positively associated with a physician's actual participation in a suicide: (1) having a higher intention-to-assist score (from responses to the case vignette); (2) having a higher number of patients with AIDS who had died; (3) having received a higher number of indirect requests from patients for assistance; and (4) gay, lesbian, or bisexual orientation on the part of the physician.

▶ Contrary to the positions of major medical and religious organizations, it appears that the majority of society (physicians included) favors legalizing physician-assisted suicide. This survey of physicians who care for HIV-infected patients merely reflects these societal beliefs. The majority (53%) of respondents stated they had, on at least 1 occasion, "granted an AIDS patient's request for assistance in committing suicide." It would be interesting to ascertain how these physicians determined what constituted lethality (i.e., type and dosage of drug) and how often their prescribed "therapy" failed to be "effective."

D.M. Rothenberg, M.D.

Practical Issues in Physician-assisted Suicide

Drickamer MA, Lee MA, Ganzini L (Veterans Affairs Connecticut Healthcare System, West Haven; Yale Univ, New Haven, Conn; Oregon Health Sciences Univ, Portland)

Ann Intern Med 126:146–151, 1997 10–4

Background.—The debate regarding physician-assisted suicide has centered on moral and legal considerations. The concrete effects that such legalization would have on practice have not been adequately explored.

Practical Issues in Physician-Assisted Suicide.—If physcian-assisted suicide becomes legal, physicians will have to gain expertise in understanding patients' motivations for requesting assistance with suicide. Physicians will also need expertise in assessing mental status, diagnosing and treating depression, maximizing palliative interventions, and evaluating external pressures on the patient. Physicians will be asked to give a prognosis on functional and cognitive decline along with life expectancy. Physicians will also need access to reliable information on effective medications and their dosages. A clinician's position on physician-assisted suicide will have to be open to discussion with the patient. Protecting a patient's right to confidentiality must be balanced against the need of health care professionals and institutions to be informed regarding a patient's choice. In addition, a patient's choice may affect insurance coverage and managed care options.

Conclusion.—These practical issues need further exploration. They have a role in the ongoing societal debate regarding physician-assisted suicide. Data are still lacking on the efficacy of palliative care and the treatment of depression in helping to remove the underlying reasons for requesting physician-assisted suicide; the differences in motivation between those who ask about physician-assisted suicide, those requesting it, and those who commit it; the ability of physicians to prognosticate in various situations; and appropriate methods for physician-assisted suicide.

► This article details the hurdles that will need to be overcome in implementing physician-assisted suicide. Of particular concern will be how to choose the optimal combination of drugs necessary to produce death. I could have only imagined the double-blinded, randomized studies that would have evolved had the United States Supreme Court legalized physician-assisted suicide. Outcome analysis, the focus of our current scholarly attention, would have taken on a whole new meaning.

D.M. Rothenberg, M.D.

Do Not Resuscitate Orders in the Perioperative Period: Patient Perspectives

Clemency MV, Thompson NJ (Emory Univ, Atlanta, Ga)

Anesth Analg 84:859–864, 1997 10–5

Background.—The American Society of Anesthiologists and the American College of Surgeons have published guidelines on the management of patients with do-not-resuscitate (DNR) orders in the perioperative period. However, there is no information on patients' views of this issue. The perspectives of terminally ill patients on the management of their DNR orders in the perioperative period, should they be offered surgery, were investigated qualitatively.

Methods and Findings.—Eighteen patients with DNR orders willing to discuss those orders and their intentions were interviewed. Patients' intentions for DNR orders centered on themes of "being ready to die" and concern about the financial and emotional cost to themselves and their families. Fifteen patients said they would agree to some kind of surgery, some of them would agree to palliative surgery and others to procedures unrelated to their primary illness. The different types of anesthesia and their risks were explained briefly to the patients, and they were asked how they wished their DNR orders to be respected during the perioperative period. Some patients said they would allow procedures in the operating room that would ordinarily not be allowed by a DNR order. In such situations, patients believed that their DNR orders should be suspended. Many patients said that their DNR orders should be discussed with them before surgery, and some wanted to be involved in decisions about specific procedures. Other patients were satisfied with discussing the intent of their orders.

Conclusion.—Many patients with DNR orders are willing to undergo anesthesia and surgery under certain circumstances. Anesthesiologists should be aware of their patients' opinions regarding their DNR orders to enhance preoperative discussion.

▶ This article is a nice attempt to qualify patients' understanding of perioperative DNR orders and reinforces the "required reconsideration" policy of both the American Society of Anesthesiologists and the American College of Surgeons. Although I agree with Drs. Clemency and Thompson in their conclusions regarding competent patients, the vast majority of patients with preoperative DNR orders who require surgery are, unfortunately, incompetent (personal observation). In this setting, the decision to rescind or maintain the DNR order during surgery is often overlooked by both surgeon and anesthesiologist, subjecting the patient to a procedure in which the preoperative advance directive is no longer protective.

D.M. Rothenberg, M.D.

Variable Expert Testimony

Variation in Expert Opinion in Medical Malpractice Review
Posner KL, Caplan RA, Cheney FW (Univ of Washington, Seattle; Virginia Mason Med Ctr, Seattle)
Anesthesiology 85:1049–1054, 1996 10–6

Objective.—Conflicting expert opinion in medical malpractice can result from bias arising from monetary compensation, from a personal affinity for individuals on one side, or from whether the expert review is based on implicit or explicit assessment. The level of agreement among objective medical expert reviewers of actual malpractice claims was measured when other sources of bias were eliminated or held constant.

Methods.—Fifteen pairs of anesthesiologists independently reviewed 103 closed claim files of 34 professional United States liability insurance companies for appropriateness of care. Agreement among pairs of reviewers was analyzed using the kappa statistic.

Results.—Each pair reviewed 2–15 claims. Reviewers agreed on 64 (62%) claims and disagreed on 39 (38%) claims ($\kappa = 0.37$). Care was deemed appropriate in 27% of claims, less than appropriate in 32%, and impossible to judge in 3%. Injuries were temporary or nondisabling in 42 claims (41%) and permanent and disabling in 50 claims (49%). Reviewers agreed on injury severity in 92 claims (89%) ($\kappa = 0.80$) and disagreed in 11 claims (11%). Reviewers agreed on appropriateness of care in 64% of claims for temporary or nondisabling injuries ($\kappa = 0.32$), but in only 60% of claims for permanently disabling injuries ($\kappa = 0.27$).

Conclusion.—Disagreement among medical experts in medical malpractice claims appears to be common.

► This is obviously an important subject for both our specialty and understanding the process of the advocacy system in areas where injury has been sustained after an operation. The fact that these anesthesiologists, who were taking special care to evaluate these cases objectively differed on the evidence of negligence on the anesthesia practitioners' part in over ⅓ of the claims, means that the divergent opinion is obviously common and that shopping by lawyers to find the right experts who will support their point of view could be a reasonable technique to promulgate their clients' interests. Those of us who believe that the system works should be rattled by this report, and further, if it weren't for the fact that trial lawyers populate Congress and state legislative bodies, this type of report should, in fact, push tort reform more towards a no-fault compensation process.

M.F. Roizen, M.D.

Informed Consent Issues

Physician–Patient Communication: The Relationship With Malpractice Claims Among Primary Care Physicians and Surgeons

Levinson W, Roter DL, Mullooly JP, et al (Oregon Health Sciences Univ, Portland; Johns Hopkins Univ, Baltimore, Md; Kaiser Found Hosps Ctrs for Health Research, Portland, Ore; et al)

JAMA 277:553–559, 1997 10–7

Background.—Malpractice litigation tends to occur at the conjunction of bad outcome and patient dissatisfaction. Patient dissatisfaction may occur as a result of communication problems. To evaluate the association between communication methods and malpractice litigation history, routine interactions between physicians and patients were taped and analyzed.

Study Design.—This study was designed to compare the normal communication style of physicians, with and without a history of malpractice litigation, and was stratified by years of practice and specialty. The study was conducted in 1993 in Oregon and Colorado and included primary care physicians and surgeons. Communication style was evaluated through audiotapes of 10 sequential office visits for each of the 124 physicians who participated in this study. The participating physicians were 94% male and 92% white. Patients were eligible if they were at least 18 years of age, spoke English, were not in acute distress, and were not on their initial visit to the physician. The participating patients were 85% white, 63% college-educated, and 45% male. The 1,265 audiotapes were coded for content by 3 trained, blinded coders using the Roter Interaction Analysis System.

Results.—Compared to primary care physicians with previous malpractice claims, those without claims spent more time on patient education and orientation, used more humor, and tended to use more facilitation. The physicians without prior claims spent more time with each patient than those with prior claims. Although these differences were relevant for primary care physicians, they could not be used to distinguish between surgeons who had prior malpractice claims and those who did not.

Conclusions.—This study of physician–patient interaction identified differences in the communication style between primary care physicians with no history of malpractice claims and those with a history of malpractice claims. Physicians and insurers can use these findings to improve communication and decrease the risk of malpractice litigation for primary care physicians. These communication behaviors did not explain the difference between surgeons with no history of malpractice claims and those with a history of claims. It cannot be assumed that these communication behaviors are equally appropriate or important for all specialty groups.

▶ This article offers an important yet simple lesson—friendly and compassionate doctors are rarely sued. In our quest to turn over cases in the name of efficiency, we have sacrificed establishing rapport, a characteristic that tends to separate doctors from technicians. In addition, I believe we have been circumspect in educating residents in the etiquette of proper bedside manner. Too often, an introductory conversation with the patient takes place *while* an IV is being inserted, without first gaining the patient's confidence by detailing the anticipated course of anesthesia care. Should the IV placement be unsuccessful, what type of message does this send to the patient? I for one would be thinking, "How will this doctor keep me alive if he cannot even insert an IV?" I realize we all work in a stressful and hectic environment, but when this is conveyed to a patient, it creates a situation ripe for litigation. It behooves all of us to spend the extra minute attempting to coax a patient to smile or laugh, not to prevent a malpractice claim, but to demonstrate that as anesthesiologists we are truly perioperative physicians.

D.M. Rothenberg, M.D.

Epidural Analgesia for Labour and Delivery: Informed Consent Issues

Pattee C, Ballantyne M, Milne B (Queen's Univ, Kingston, Ont)

Can J Anaesth 44:918–923, 1997 10–8

Introduction.—A 1985 survey of Canadian obstetric anesthetists indicated that anesthetists believed their patients were seldom or never adequately informed about epidural analgesia before labor. Eighty percent of respondents believed informed consent was their responsibility, but that it was not realistic to expect mothers to cope with informed consent information during labor. To further examine these findings, a patient survey was initiated to define complications for which patients wanted clear information; quantify the influence of pain, anxiety, opioid premedication, and the importance of level of education on a patient's level of satisfaction with the consent process; and determine how satisfactory epidural pain relief correlates with satisfaction with the consent process.

Methods.—Sixty patients were interviewed by survey in the hospital or by telephone call at home during the first 2 months after vaginal delivery. Patients were questioned regarding demographics, severity of labor pain, level of satisfaction with epidural anesthetic, risk of complications, and satisfaction with information they received. Questions were answered with yes or no or rated on a scale of 0–10.

Results.—Sixty-five percent of patients surveyed had their first epidural analgesia with this delivery. Pain relief was significant, with an average pain reduction of 70%. Patients considered it important to disclose epidural-related complications during the informed consent process (8.4/10), particularly complications with the highest morbidity and mortality for baby (9.3/10) and mother (7.0/10). The degree of satisfaction with the informed consent process was not affected by opioid premedication, anxiety, pain score, education group, or level of pain relief. Respondents indicated that the level of distress they experienced during labor was great, but that this discomfort did not compromise their ability to hear and comprehend information regarding the consent process (8.8/10).

Conclusion.—A survey performed during the postpartum period indicated that women wanted to be informed regarding all possible complications associated with epidural analgesia before delivery. Contrary to other reports, respondents reported nondisclosure of serious risks was unacceptable.

► This study confirms my long-standing opinion that the majority of obstetric patients want to receive adequate information regarding the risks and benefits of epidural analgesia, and that most would prefer to receive this information before the onset of labor.

D.H. Chestnut, M.D.

Postoperative Psychological Problems

The Influence of Psychological Variables on Postoperative Anxiety and Physical Complaints in Patients Undergoing Lumbar Surgery

de Groot KI, Boeke S, van den Berge HJ, et al (Erasmus Univ Rotterdam, The Netherlands; St Clara Hosp Rotterdam, The Netherlands)

Pain 69:19–25, 1997 10–9

Purpose.—Personality, coping behaviors, and anxiety can all affect postoperative distress. Although many studies have examined the effects of psychological factors on postoperative emotional and physical status, few have looked at the effects of state variables other than anxiety. Questions also remain about the effects of coping behavior. Patients undergoing lumbar surgery were studied to evaluate the influence of coping behavior, fatigue, and pain on postoperative anxiety and physical complaints.

Methods.—The study included 126 patients undergoing lumbar surgery. Each patient underwent a detailed preoperative assessment, including biographic and medical variables and measures of anxiety, fatigue, back and leg pain, and coping behavior. Postoperative indicators of distress were state anxiety and physical complaints.

Results.—Postoperative anxiety was significantly predicted by preoperative anxiety and leg pain, more so than by age, sex, or medical variables. Postoperative physical complaints were independently related to preoperative anxiety and fatigue. Preoperative coping behavior was not related to postoperative anxiety or physical complaints.

Conclusions.—In patients undergoing lumbar surgery, preoperative anxiety and leg pain are independent predictors of postoperative anxiety. Preoperative fatigue is an independent predictor of postoperative physical complaints, whereas coping is not related to postoperative anxiety or physical complaints. The risk of poor postoperative status may be elevated for patients with high levels of preoperative anxiety, fatigue, or leg pain. In addition to reassurance and education in reducing anxiety, patients facing lumbar surgery may benefit from measures to reduce fatigue and pain.

► An interesting point in this study is that preoperative anxiety predicted postoperative anxiety and preoperative fatigue predicted postoperative physical complaints. In addition, leg pain was an independent predictor of postoperative anxiety. This study points out the potential to help those patients with preoperative anxiety, leg pain preoperatively (whether it is a sign of anxiety or is related to the disease process itself), and preoperative fatigue, with more education, and other psychological means to help patients to cope with the postoperative period and speedy recoveries.

M.F. Roizen, M.D.

Routine Pregnancy Testing?

Should Pregnancy Testing Be Routine in Adolescent Patients Prior to Surgery?

Malviya S, D'Errico C, Reynolds P, et al (Univ of Michigan, Ann Arbor)
Anesth Analg 83:854–858, 1996 10–10

Background.—The need for routine preoperative pregnancy testing in adolescents is still debated. The reliability of adolescents' preoperative history for excluding pregnancy was determined..

Methods.—Four hundred forty-four girls aged 10–17 years undergoing 525 procedures were asked about the possibility of pregnancy before surgery. A urine pregnancy test was ordered for all patients, regardless of history.

Findings.—Patients having 508 of the procedures said there was no possibility of being pregnant. Eight said they might be pregnant. The parents of 6 girls responded for them, stating there was no possibility of pregnancy. Test data were not obtained for 17 girls because of patient or parent refusal or patient inability to void. One pregnancy test result was questionably negative, and the rest were negative. Follow-up in the questionable case showed that the patient was not pregnant.

Conclusions.—Preoperative histories obtained from this population of adolescents concurred with pregnancy test results. A detailed history, including data on last menstrual period, contraception, sexual activity, and the possibility of pregnancy, should be obtained for all postmenarchal patients before surgery.

► Because of present emphasis on cost containment, operating-room efficiency, and patient satisfaction, instead of subjecting every adolescent or adult woman of childbearing potential to the expense and inconvenience of a preoperative pregnancy test, it seems both practical and reasonable to rely on detailed history taking to ascertain pregnancy. Complete history and physical examination are fundamental to appropriate preoperative evaluation and subsequent surgical/anesthesia management. Routine pregnancy testing is another example of a screening test based on habit and medical-legal considerations rather than medical indications. This study shows that the same information may be obtained in a more cost-effective manner—by interviewing the patient!

C.P. Greenberg, M.D.

Aftermath of Anesthesia Disaster

Anaesthetic Disasters: Handling the Aftermath
Aitkenhead AR (Queen's Medical Centre, Nottingham, England)
Anaesthesia 52:477–482, 1997 10–11

Background.—Anesthesia occasionally results in death or serious injury. How to handle the aftermath of anesthestic disasters was discussed.

Discussion.—Close relatives should be informed of an anesthetic disaster in person by a health care team consisting of the anesthetist, the surgeon, a nurse from the operating room or surgical ward, a clergy member (when appropriate), and a social worker or interpreter. If trainee staff were involved in the incident, a member of the consultant staff of each specialty needs to be at the interview. Relatives must be informed as soon as possible, not at the convenience of the staff members. The interview should take place in a closed room that is not too small or too large and without interruptions. A leader should be designated to do most of the talking and should begin the interview by relaying the worst of the news. Suggesting that no one understands what went wrong is not appropriate. The facts should be explained, and the areas to be investigated should be indicated. However, particular staff members should not be incriminated, especially when the cause of the accident is not clear. Finally, staff members' spontaneous expressions of sorrow can be very comforting to the grieving family.

A number of formalities must be taken care of after an anesthetic disaster. The patient's general practitioner needs to be informed by phone and/or facsimile communication, and interest from the media must be addressed. The incident should also be reported at the departmental morbidity and mortality meeting. As soon as possible after the incident, the anesthetist should examine the patient's record and add as much detail as possible. All entries made after the event should be written in a different colored ink. These entries should include the date and time and should be initialed. Such formalities will help avoid any future suggestion that attempts were made to falsify the records. Also, a full factual account of the events should be written in the hospital notes.

Possible sequelae of anesthetic disasters include a coroner's inquest, criminal prosecution, disciplinary action, and civil litigation. The process of civil litigation is very stressful for the physicians involved and many cause psychological and physical problems as a result. Long-term support for the anesthetist involved in an anesthetic disaster is needed.

Conclusion.—Anesthetists receive little or no training in how to cope with the aftermath of a death or serious injury associated with anesthesia. Departments of anesthesia may wish to develop a plan for responding to anesthetic disasters to minimize the trauma and stress that inevitably result.

► I selected this article because I believe too little thought and attention are given to both supporting the patient's family and (just as important) the anesthesiologist's family when an anesthetic mishap occurs. I have been an anesthesiologist for over 25 years and this article struck an emotional cord.

M. Wood, M.D.

Subject Index

A

B

C

D

E

F

G

H

J

K

M

N

P

Q

R

S

T

U

V

W

X

Z

Author Index

A

B

C

D

E

F

G

M

N

O

P

W

Y

Z

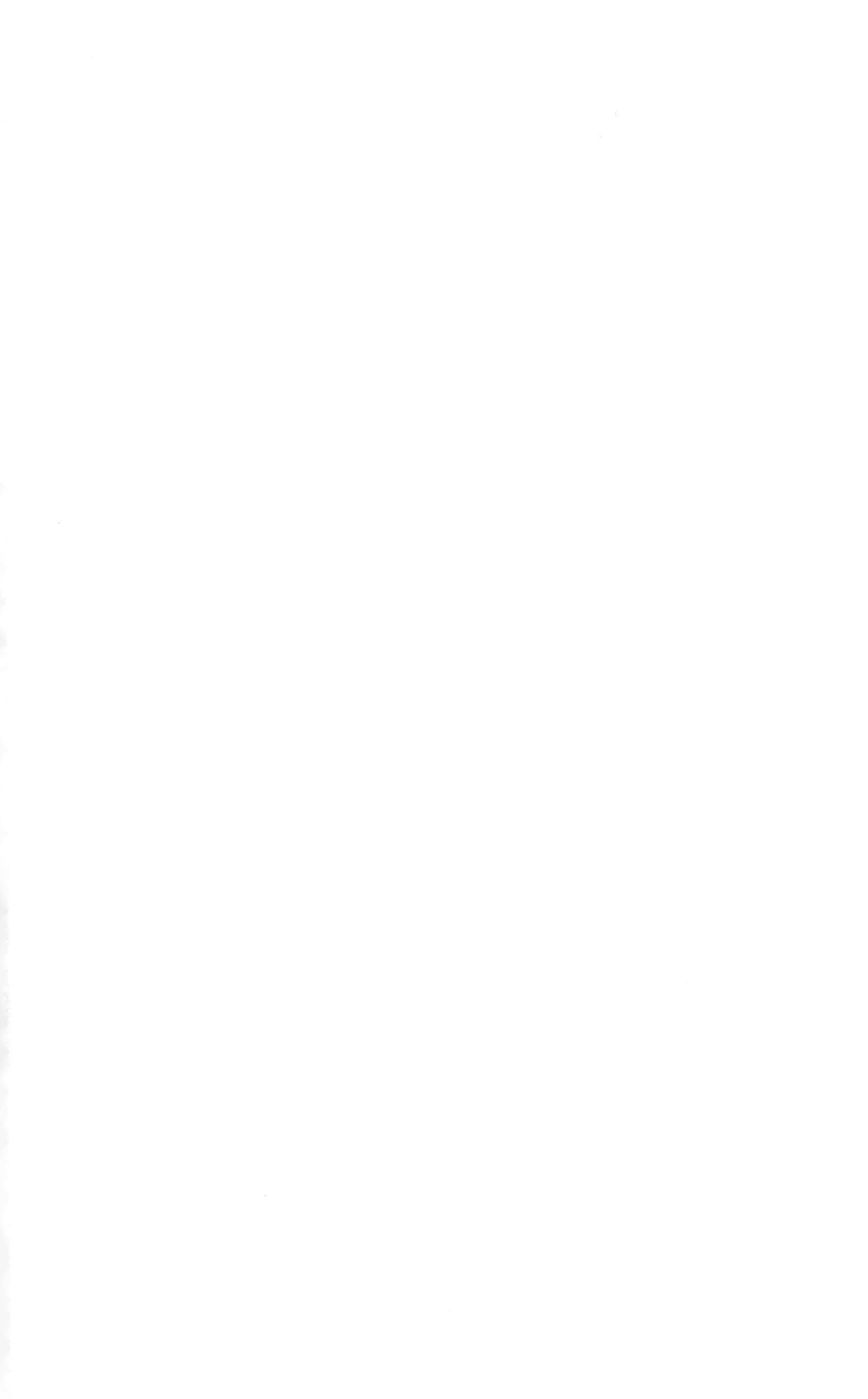